Pharmacology
for Dentistry

Pharmacology
for Dentistry

Dr. Surender Singh
All India Institute of Medical Sciences
New Delhi

PUBLISHING FOR ONE WORLD

NEW AGE INTERNATIONAL (P) LIMITED, PUBLISHERS
(formerly Wiley Eastern Limited)

New Delhi • Bangalore • Chennai • Cochin • Guwahati • Hyderabad
Jalandhar • Kolkata • Lucknow • Mumbai • Ranchi

Visit us at **www.newagepublishers.com**

Pharmacology is an ever-changing Science. The Author and Publisher of this book have checked with source believed to be reliable in their efforts to produce information that is complete and generally in accord with the standard accepted at the time of publication, but the author and publisher will not be held responsible for any inadvertent errors. Readers are advised to check the product information contained herein in the other sources i.e., product information sheet included in the package of each drug by respective pharmaceutical companies.

Published by New Age International (P) Ltd., Publishers
First Edition: 2007

ISBN : 81-224-2084-2

Rs. 295.00

C-07-03-1371

Printed in India at Chaman Offset, Delhi.
Typeset in-house

PUBLISHING FOR ONE WORLD

NEW AGE INTERNATIONAL (P) LIMITED, PUBLISHERS
(formerly Wiley Eastern Limited)
4835/24, Ansari Road, Daryaganj, New Delhi - 110002
Visit us at **www.newagepublishers.com**

In Loving memory of my dear sister

"BIMAL KANTA"

Preface

Pharmacology has undergone major intellectual changes in the recent years and has become increasingly important to all medical, dental and other health professionals. The graduate students of dentistry may have to handle medical emergency during various dental procedures on the dental chair. Besides this, dentists have to look into various drug associated interactions. The broad goal of teaching pharmacology to undergraduate students is to inculcate rational and scientific basis of therapeutics keeping in view the dental curriculum and profession. A sincere attempt has been made to present a complete text for undergraduate students of dentistry as per the new syllabus requirement (Dental Council of India, BDS course regulation, 2006).

The book is divided into thirteen sections, initial sections cover the general and autonomic pharmacology, followed by other sections of drug acting on different body systems. A detailed section is devoted only to dental pharmacology which covers all agents used in pharmacotherapy of dental conditions. The last section covers vaccine, sera and other immunological agents and drugs used in skin disorders. The chapters have been arranged in such a way that knowledge gained from initial chapters will be helpful to students for understanding subsequent chapters. The appendix contains the list of newly approved and banned drugs in India.

The classification adopted in the books provides pharmacological distinction among latest drugs with doses and routes of administration along with leading trade name(s) available in Indian market, but it should not be construed as the recommendation of those particular brands.

Thanks are due to New Age International (P) Ltd., N. Delhi for their keen interest and attention in bringing out this book in its present form. Further, I am indebted to all my friends and well wishers for their support and encouragement.

I would like to express my gratitude and indebtedness to all my family members for their sacrifice, affection and inspiration throughout the present work.

New Delhi **Surender Singh**

Contents

SECTION 3
Drugs Acting on ANS

SECTION 4
Drugs Acting on Cardiovascular & Urinary System

SECTION 5
Autacoids

SECTION 6
Drugs Acting on Blood

SECTION 7
Drugs Acting on GIT

SECTION 8
Drugs Acting on Endocrine System

SECTION 9
Chemotherapy

Section 10
Vitamins and Trace Elements

Section 11
Chelating Agents & Treatment of Poisoning

Section 12
Dental Pharmacology

Section 13
Miscellaneous

Appendices

Section 1

General Principles of Pharmacology

CHAPTER 1.1

Sources and Nature of Drug Dosage Form

INTRODUCTION

Pharmacology (derived from Greek words, *pharmacon*-drug; *logos*-discourse in) consists of detailed study of drugs – its source, physical and chemical properties, compounding, biochemical and physiological effects, pharmacodynamics (its mechanism of action), pharmacokinetics (absorption, distribution, biotransformation and excretion), therapeutic and other uses of drugs.

According to WHO definition 'Drug is any substance or product that is used or intended to be used to modify or explore physiological system or pathological states for the benefit of the recipient'.

Pharmacology has some major subdivisions:

Pharmacodynamics is the study of the biochemical and physiological effects of the drugs and their mechanism of action.

Pharmacotherapeutics deals with the use of drugs in the prevention and treatment of diseases and it utilizes or depends upon the information of drug obtained by pharmacodynamic studies.

Pharmacokinetics deals with the alterations of the drug by the body which includes absorption, distribution, binding/ storage, biotransformation and excretion of drugs.

Toxicology deals with the side/adverse effects and other poisonous effects of drugs, since the same drug can be a poison, depending on the dose.

Chemotherapy deals with the effects of drugs upon microorganisms and parasites without destroying the host cells.

Pharmacology also includes certain allied fields as:

Pharmacy is the science of preparation, compounding and dispensing of drugs. It is concerned with collection, identification, purification, isolation, synthesis and standardization of medicinal /pharmaceutical substances.

Pharmacognosy deals with the study of the sources of drugs derived from plants and animal origin.

Materia-medica: This is an older term and deals with the source, description (physical and chemical properties) and preparation of drugs.

Pharmacopoeia is an official reference containing a selected drugs/medicinal preparations with their description, tests for their identity, purity and potency and with their average doses. A few famous pharmacopoeia and other reference books are the Indian Pharmacopoeia (**IP**), the British Pharmacopoeia (**BP**); the United States Pharmacopoeia (**USP**); the British Pharmaceutical Codex (**BPC**); the National Formulary (**NF**) i.e. British National Formulary (**BNF**) and National Formulary (**NF**) of India. It is necessary for understanding the each aspects of pharmacology by dentists, as they have to prescribe the drug for the treatment of various dental conditions in general and other concurrently disease with many of the dental patients. The dentists should be aware of drug interactions and capable of handle any emergency during any dental procedure.

SOURCES OF DRUGS

'Drug' is derived from French word *'drogue'* means a dry herb. Drugs are obtained mainly from plants, animals, microbes and mineral sources, but a majority of them that are used therapeutically are from synthetic or semi-synthetic products.

PLANT ORIGIN

The pharmacologically active components in vegetable drugs are:

i. *Alkaloids* are basic substances containing cyclic nitrogen. The important alkaloids are obtained from:
   - Opium (*Papaver somniferum):* Morphine group.
   - Cinchona (*Cinchona officinalis*): Quinine etc.
   - Belladonna (*Atropa belladonna*): Atropine group.
   - *Pilocarpus* sp.: Pilocarpine.
   - Vinca (*Vinca rosea*): Vincristine, vinblastine.
   - *Rauwolfia serpentina* (root): Reserpine.
   - Coca (*Erythroxylum coca*): Cocaine.

ii. *Glycosides* are ether like organic structure combined with sugars, the non-sugar component called aglycone or genin. The important glycosides are:
   - Digitalis (*Digitalis purpurea, Digitalis lanata*): Digoxin etc.
   - Stropanthus (*Stropanthus kombe*): Stropanthin etc.
   - Senna (*Cassia acutifolia*): Sennoside etc.

iii. *Oils*
   a. *Fixed oils* are glycerides of oleic, palmitic and stearic acids. Mostly fixed oils are edible and used for cooking. The fixed oils used as drug are:
      - Castor (*Ricinus communis*): Castor oil.
      - Olive (*Olea europaea*): Olive oil.
      - Cocoa butter (*Theobroma cacao*): Theobroma oil used as emollient in skin cream and making suppositories.
      - Cod liver oil and shark liver oil: Rich source of vitamin A and D.
   b. *Volatile oil* or essential oil contains the hydrocarbon terpene. The important volatile oils are:
      - Turpentine oil, from species of pines, used as a counterirritant.
      - Lemon oil (*from Citrus limon*), used as flavouring agent.
      - Peppermint, cardamom and fennel used as carminative and flavouring agent.

- Oil of clove is mainly useful in relieving pain in toothache.

iv. *Resins* are produced by oxidation and polymerization of volatile oils. The different types of resins are:
- Oleoresins: Male fern extract used for tapeworm infestation.
- Gum resins: Asafoetida, used as carminative and antispasmodic.
- Oleo gum resin: Myrrh, it has a local stimulant and antiseptic properties and generally used in mouthwash.
- Balsams: Benzoin, used internally as expectorant and externally as astringent.
- Balsam Tolu, used as stimulating expectorant.

v. *Gums* are the secretory products of plants. On hydrolysis they yield simple sugar like polysaccharides. They are pharmacologically inert substances and mainly employed as suspending and emulsifying agent in various pharmaceutical products.

The widely used preparations are gum acacia and tragacanth.

vi. *Tannins* are nonnitrogenous constituents of plant. Chemically they are phenolic derivatives and are characterized by their astringent action. Tannins are generally employed in the treatment of diarrhoea and burns. The important plants which contains tannins are: Amla, Behera, Hirda (in combination form '*Triphala*'), Black catechu and Ashoka bark.

ANIMAL SOURCES

The different animal products after purification in a suitable dosage form for the treatment of disease are listed in table 1.1.1.

FROM HUMAN BEING

There are certain products which are obtained from human being e.g.

- Immunoglobulins: From blood.
- Placental extract: From placenta.
- Chorionic gonadotropin: From urine of pregnant women.
- Growth hormone: From pituitary gland.

FROM MICROORGANISMS

The different classes of drugs obtained/ isolated from microbes are:

- Penicillin: *Penicillium chrysogenum* and *notatum* (Fungus).
- Streptomycin: *Streptomyces griseus* (*Actino-mycetes*).
- Erythromycin: *Streptomyces erythreus* (*Actinomycetes*).
- Chloramphenicol: *Streptomyces venezuelae* (*Actinomycetes*).
- Tetracyclines: *Streptomyces aureofaciens* and *rimosus* (*Actinomycetes*).
- Polymyxin B: *Bacillus polymyxa*.
- Bacitracin: *Bacillus subtilis*.
- Nystatin: *Streptomyces nouresi*.
- Griseofulvin: *Penicillium griseofulvum*.

Apart from various other antibiotics obtained from microorganisms, there are other products that are also produced by microorganisms. They are:

- Streptokinase, an enzyme from gram positive cocci (*Streptococcus pyogenes*).
- Vitamin B_{12} (cyanocobalamin): *Streptomyces griseus*.

Table 1.1.1: *Classification of different animal products used as drug and surgicals.*

Drug	Category	Animal source
Insulin	Hormone	Pancreas of beef or pig
Thyroid extract/thyroxine	Hormone	Thyroid gland
Shark liver oil	Vitamin A	Livers of shark and allied species
Cod liver oil	Vitamin A and D	Livers of Gadus species
Antisnake venom	Immune serum	Blood of horse
Hyaluronidase	Enzyme	Testis of bull
Pepsin	Enzyme	Stomach of beef and pig
Surgical ligatures and sutures	Used in surgery	Intestinal tissues, tendons of animals.

Routes of Drug Administration

The drugs can be administered by a variety of routes, either locally or administered orally and by injection. To produce local effects, drugs are applied topically to the skin or mucous membranes. To produce systemic effects drugs are administered orally, rectally, parenterally or by inhalation route.

The choice of the route in a given situation depends upon the drug and the patient's condition (e.g. in unconscious and vomiting state), and urgency of treatment (whether the routine treatment or in emergency condition).

The important routes of administration are:

LOCAL ROUTES

The dosage forms applied locally to the skin are powders, paste, lotions, ointments, creams, plasters and jellies. They are used for their antiseptic, antipruritic, analgesic, local anaesthetic and other related effects.

The absorption of drug through the skin is proportional to the surface area covered and to their lipid solubility. The dermis layer is freely permeable to many fluids. Inflammatory and other related conditions which increase the cutaneous blood flow also enhance absorption of drugs. Absorption through the skin can be enhanced by induction (rubbing the oily vehicle preparation into the skin) also.

On the skin, drug is applied in the form of ointment, cream, lotion, paste, plaster, powder etc.

The topical application is also used on the mucous membranes i.e. nose, throat, eye, ear, bronchi, rectum, urethra, vagina and rectum.

In case of mouth and pharynx, the drug is used in the form of throat paints, lozenges, gargles or mouth washes.

In case of corneal application (in the form of ointments, drops), the drug may penetrate the anterior chamber and affect the ciliary muscle. The nasal mucosa is treated with drug solution in the form of spray or irrigation.

The bronchial mucosa and lungs are treated with inhalations, aerosols (in the form of fine powder with the help of nebulizer) e.g. salbutamol (ASTHALIN) inhaler.

Drugs may also be administered locally in the form of bougies, jellies for urethra, pessaries, vaginal tablets, creams and douches for vagina and suppositories for rectal administration.

Due to the rich blood and lymph supply to rectum the unionised and lipid soluble substances are readily absorbed from the rectum. The advantages of this route are that gastric irritation is avoided and easy administration by the patient himself.

Administration of drug in the form of liquid into the rectum is called enema, which may be soap water or glycerine-vegetable oil. It is used to remove the faecal matter and flatus and is used in constipation. Certain drugs are administered rectally for producing systemic effects also (e.g. aminophylline, indomethacin, paraldehyde etc.).

SYSTEMIC ROUTES

The drug administered through systemic routes (orally or parenterally), is absorbed into the blood, distributed along through the circulation and produce their desired effects.

Oral Route

This is the most commonly used route for drug administration. It is also the safest, most convenient and economical. But, there are some limitation of this route:

- Drug action is slow, thus not suitable for emergencies.
- Incapability to absorb some drugs, due to their physical characteristics i.e. polarity of the drug.
- Unpalatable and other irritant drugs can not be administered.
- Can not be used for unconscious and uncooperative patient.
- May not be useful in the presence of vomiting and diarrhoea.
- Drugs, which can be destroyed by digestive juices (i.e. insulin, penicillin G) or in liver (i.e. testosterone, nitroglycerine) can not be administered orally.
- The absorption of certain drugs is negligible e.g. streptomycin.

Enteric Coated Tablets

The drugs which are destroyed by the gastric juices in the stomach, are coated with keratin, shellac and cellulose acid phosphate. These substances are not dissolved by the acid juice of the stomach, but are dissolved in the intestinal juice (alkaline) only, which is useful in:

- Preventing gastric irritation and alteration of the drug in the stomach.
- To get the desired concentration of the drug in intestine.
- To delay the absorption of the drug.

Time Release/Sustained Release Capsules

It is a useful solid dosage form of drug, where the particles of the drug dissolve at different time intervals.

The *advantages* of time-release preparations are:

- Reduction in the frequency of administration of drug.

- Maintenance of therapeutic effect for longer time.
- To some extent decreased incidence of undesired effects.
- Appropriate for drugs with short half lives (less than 4 hours).

Sublingual Administration

The highly lipid soluble and nonirritating drugs (i.e. nitroglycerine, isoprenaline, methyltestosterone) in the form of tablets or pellet is placed under the tongue, where they rapidly dissolve and are absorbed quickly in the general circulation. The **advantages** of this routes are:

- Rapid onset of action.
- The degradation and metabolism of the drugs in the stomach and liver is avoided

PARENTERAL ROUTES

(par = beyond, enteral = intestinal)

The administration of drugs by injection directly into the tissue fluid or blood without having to cross the intestinal mucosa.

The advantages of parenteral routes are:

- Rapid action of drug.
- Can be employed in unconscious/ uncooperative patients.
- Drugs, which are modified by alimentary juices and liver can be given by this route.
- Drugs, which are not absorbed in small intestine or irritate the stomach can be administered by this route.

Disadvantages are:

- Less safe, more expensive.
- Inconvenient (painful) for the patient.
- Self medication is difficult.
- Chances of local injury at the site of injection.

The important parenteral routes are:

Subcutaneous

The non-irritant substances can be injected by this route. The rate of absorption of drug is constant and slow to provide a sustained effect. The site of injection is usually the outer surface of the arm, or front of the thigh. Self medication (e.g. insulin) is possible because deep penetration is not needed. Other drugs which are administered subcutaneously are adrenaline, morphine and certain hormonal preparations.

The other related subcutaneous routes are ***dermojet*** (by which, drug is projected from a microfine orifice using a high velocity jet) and ***pellet implantation*** (which provides sustained release of the drug over weeks and months e.g. testosterone).

Intramuscular

The soluble substances, mild irritants and suspensions can be injected by this route in the large skeletal muscles (deltoid, triceps, gluteus maximus, rectus femoris etc.). These muscles are less richly supplied with sensory nerves and are more vascular, so irritant solutions can be injected. Small volumes (up to 2 ml) are injected into the deltoid muscle, and small or large volumes (up to 10 ml) are injected into the gluteal mass.

The rate of absorption is reasonably uniform and the onset of action is rapid.

Intravenous

The drug is injected as a bolus or infused slowly directly into a vein to produce rapid action. It is also useful for certain irritant and hypertonic solutions, as they are rapidly diluted by the blood. Drugs in an oily vehicle or those which precipitate blood constituents or haemolyze erythrocytes should not be given by this route.

Intravenous route is the most rapidly effective and the desired blood concentration can be obtained with a definite dose but at the same time it is the most dangerous route of administration. For once the drug is injected there is no retreat. So, intravenous injection must usually be performed slowly and with constant monitoring of the patient. This route is usually reserved for emergencies when a rapid action is required and infusion of large amounts of fluids to overcome dehydration or to supply nutrition to patients who can not take food/fluids orally.

Intradermal

The drug is injected into the skin raising a bleb. This route is employed for vaccination e.g. BCG vaccine and for testing the sensitivity e.g. penicillin injection.

Intra-arterial

This route is useful in diagnostic studies, by which arterial blood sample may be withdrawn for blood gas studies. Certain cytotoxic compounds are administered by intra-arterial perfusion in localised malignancies.

Intrathecal or Intraspinal

For local and rapid effect of drugs on the meninges or cerebrospinal axis, drugs are injected directly into the spinal subarachnoid space. This is also used to produce spinal anaesthesia, or for introduction of a radio-opaque contrast-medium into the subarachnoid space for visualising the spinal cord.

Intramedullary

By this method, the drug is introduced into the bone marrow of the sternum or tibia. Blood is occasionally given by this route.

Intracardiac

In sudden cardiac arrest and other cardiac emergencies, the adrenaline is directly injected into the heart by a long needle in the left fourth intercostal space close to the sternum.

Intraperitoneal

This route is a common laboratory procedure, but it is seldom employed clinically in infants for giving fluids like glucose saline, as the peritoneum offers a large surface for absorption.

Intra-articular

Certain drugs (i.e. glucocorticoids) can be administered directly into a joint space for the treatment of local condition i.e. rheumatoid arthritis.

INHALATION ROUTE

The volatile liquids and gases are given by inhalation route. The drugs may be given as solid particles, as nebulized particles from solutions or in the form of vapours. The volatile substances include gaseous anaesthetics, amyl nitrite and vapours of liquid anaesthetics, gases like oxygen, carbon dioxide and helium.

Nonvolatile substances have to be broken down into small particles, and then inhaled as aerosols.

Drugs given by this route are quickly absorbed, which takes place from the vast surface of alveoli and produce rapid action. Various bronchodilators and mast cell stabilizers are used in the treatment and prophylaxis of bronchial asthma i.e. salbutamol (ASTHALIN) and sodium cromoglycate (FINTAL) inhaler.

DOSAGE FORMS AND ROUTES OF DRUG ADMINISTRATION

A dosage form is a medicated product specially designed for administration depending upon the routes to the patient for the diagnosis and treatment of disease.

The dosage form is broadly divided into solid dosage form, liquid dosage form and inhalations which are used both internally as well as externally.

Solid dosage form includes capsules, granules, effervescent granules, powders, tablets, insufflations, suppositories (pessaries, bougies and ear cone) etc.

Semisolid/liquid dosage form includes elixirs, emulsions, gels, linctus, mixtures, drops, solutions, syrups, tinctures, applicators, creams, enema, gargles, jellies, liniments, lotions, mouth washes, ointments, paints, paste, poultices etc.

Inhalation forms include aerosols, sprays etc.

SOLID DOSAGE FORM (INTERNAL USE)

Capsules: These are small gelatin contains shells. Capsules are of two types – hard & soft capsules.

Hard capsules are used for powdered drugs e.g. capsules ampicillin, tetracycline. In hard capsules, certain sustained released substance, which gradually release the drug in the respiratory tract (e.g. cap. theophylline).

Soft capsules are used for oils and solution of active drugs e.g. cap. vitamins A, A & D, E, garlic pearls, seven seas etc.

Soft capsules are also used for semisolid (ointment) e.g. eye applicaps of chloromycetin.

Granules: These are mixture of active medicament, sugar and some flavouring agent and then moistened to produce a coherent mass which is then passed through a sieve to form a granule. Granules are the unusual means of adminis tering drug that possess an unpleasant taste e.g. PAS (para-amino salicylic acid) granules.

Effervescent granules: It is a mixture of citric and tartaric acids with sodium bicarbonate and usually some sweetening agents (saccharin or glucose) may be added.

The powder granules should be dissolved with a prescribed amount of water and taken when it produce effervescence e.g. ENO powder used for indigestion, flatulence and heartburn etc.

Powder: Powder are medicaments in dried form. The powders are of different types:

- Simple or compound powder: The simple powder contain just one active ingredient (e.g. acetylsalicylic acid powder) and compound powder contain more than one active ingredient.
- Powders enclosed in cachets (e.g. ALCOPAR, ORS powder) and in capsules (e.g. ampicillin powder).
- Effervescent powder.
- Powder for external use e.g. NEBASULF, boric acid powder, zinc oxide powder, talc etc. Tooth powder may also be classified under this group.
- Powder with metal (e.g. mercury with chalk) used as purgative.
- Powder use after reconstitution e.g. syr. ampicillin for paediatric use.

Tablets: These are the most extensively used solid dosage form containing granulated or powdered drugs that are compressed or moulded into different shapes. These are different types of tablets according to their size, shape and uses:

- Simple tablets:
  - Are disintegrated readily e.g. tab aspirin.
- Soluble tablets:
  - Are dissolved in water to form solution for internal and external use (gargles) e.g. tab Disprin.
  - Also used for parenteral administration called hypodermic tablets e.g. atropine sulphate tablets.
- Scored tablets:
  - They may be easily divided if smaller doses are required (e.g. tab. Analgin).
- Lozenges:
  - Are solid preparation consisting mainly of sugar and gum and ensures slow release of medicaments and generally used for local action e.g. cough remedies – Strepcils, Vocacil.
- Pastilles:
  - Are solid medicated preparation intended to dissolve slowly in the mouth and softer than lozenges.
- Chewable tablets:
  - Are chewed in the mouth for systemic action e.g. tab. Digene, vitamin C (Suckcee), mebendazole (for paediatric use) etc.
- Buccal or sublingual tablets:
  - Are chewed and placed under the tongue. When it dissolved and exert their action e.g. tab. nitroglycerine.
- Implants:
  - Are tablets use for sustained action and implanted under the skin e.g. Deoxycortone acetone (for contraception).
- Depot tablets:
  - Are compressed tablets used for sustained systemic action e.g. tab. Asmapax Depot for asthmatic patients.

- Enteric-coated tablets:
  - Are coated with keratin, cellulose acetate phthalate, which do not dissolve in the stomach and only dissolve in alkaline juice of the intestine where the drug is liberated e.g. tab. erythromycin.

SOLID DOSAGE FORM (EXTERNALLY USED)

Collodions: These are the fluid preparation intended for external use. The vehicle of collodion are volatile (e.g. ethyl alcohol) in nature and when applied on the skin (with brush or rod) evaporates to the skin and leaving a flexible, protective film. The film producing agent is pyroxylin (nitrocellulose) and for flexibility colour oil is added.

It is generally used for small cuts and abrasions.

Dusting powder are free flowing and very fine in nature for external use.

Insufflations are dusting powder consisting medicaments that are blown by an insufflator (similar to atomiser) into various body cavities, nose, throat, ear etc., where it would be difficult to apply the powder directly.

Suppositories are conical or ovoid shape solid preparation made up of fat (cocoa butter oil or theobroma oil), a wax or a glycerine-gelatin jelly. They are used for insertion into the rectum, where they melt, dissolve and disperse and exert their action – local as well as systemic.

Pessaries are the same as suppositories for introduction into vagina. Pessaries are of two type:

- Moulded pessaries (as suppositories).
- Compressed pessaries – in different shapes.

Bougies used for nasal and urethral administration of drugs.

Ear cone for administration of drugs in ear.

Plasters are solid adhesive (with cloth) preparation applied to the skin to protect, soothe and lessen pain e.g. Mustard plaster, Capsicum plaster.

SEMISOLID/LIQUID DOSAGE FORM (INTERNAL USE)

Aqua are aqueous solution of volatile substance used as solvent in certain pharmaceutical preparation to mask the disagreeable taste of drug e.g. peppermint water.

Cachets are providing a means of administering nauseous or disagreeable powder in a tasteless form.

Elixir are liquid, oral preparation of potent or nauseous medicaments, which are pleasantly flavoured and coloured with suitable agents.

Emulsions are suspensions of fats or oils in water with the inclusion of an suitable emulsifying agent (e.g. gum acacia, gum tragacanth) e.g. Castor oil emulsion, Cod liver oil emulsion for internal use. One such emulsion is also used externally e.g. benzyl benzoate emulsion.

Gels are the aqueous colloidal suspension of insoluble medicaments (e.g. aluminium hydroxide as antacid in Digene gel).

Linctus are viscous, liquid oral preparation containing high proportions of syrup (sugar) and glycerin (for viscosity and its sweet nature) which produce a demulcent affect on the mucous membrane of the throat.

Mixture are liquid oral preparation, where the medicaments are in solution or suspension form. Mixture are generally not formulated for a long life and prepared freshly.

Paediatric drops are liquid oral preparation of small dose giving by a calibrated dropper intended for paediatric use.

Solution are aqueous solution containing one or more drugs. They are divided into different categories:

- Solution in dosage form for oral use/ external use e.g. strong iodine solution, hydrogen peroxide solution.
- **Parenteral solution** are sterile liquid or suspensions packaged in sterile containers, intended for parenteral administration.

There are other type of solutions that are used for peritoneal dialysis, anticoagulant solution, bladder irrigation and certain dermatological solution intended for application to broken surface.

Syrups are the liquid oral preparation made in concentrated sugar solution, mainly for paediatric use and for drugs which are unpleasant in taste.

Tinctures are the concentrated alcoholic preparation of vegetable drugs made by maceration process. (e.g. Tr. opium, Tr. lemon) used in different pharmaceutical preparation for oral use. Tr. Benzoin Co. is used externally.

SEMISOLID/LIQUID DOSAGE FORM (EXTERNAL USE)

Applications are liquid or semi-liquid preparation applied to the skin, and are usually emulsion or suspension in nature (e.g. antiparasitics application).

Creams are semisolid preparation (usually emulsion) for external use. They are oily and non-greasy in nature.

Ear/eye/nasal drops are solution of drugs that are instilled into a ear, eye and nose with a dropper. The eye drops are sterile solutions.

Enema are solution, suspension or emulsion (oil/water type) of medicament intended for rectal administration.

Gargles are aqueous solution used to prevent and for treatment of throat infections.

Irrigators are medicated solution used to treat urinary bladder, vagina and less often the nose infections. They are administered with a help of catheter (in bladder), vulcanite (for vagina) which are made up of thin, soft rubber or plastic tube. The nose irrigator is made up of glass.

Jellies are transparent or translucent, non-greasy medicated semi-solid preparation used externally, sometime containing local anaesthetic agent also e.g. Lignocaine jelly.

Liniments are liquid, semi-liquid and some-times semi-solid preparation used externally on the skin. Liniments are counter-irritant and stimulating type and are massaged or rubbed into the skin, and must not be applied to the broken skin e.g. liniment turpentine.

Lotions are liquid preparation applied to skin without friction. Lotions are used for soothing, astringent and antipruritic affects e.g. calamine lotion.

Mouth washes are liquid preparation similar to gargles but are use for oral hygiene.

Ointments are semi-solid greasy preparation for local application to the skin, rectum and mucous membrane also. The ointment base is usually anhydrous and contain the medicaments in solution or suspension. Ointments are used for its soothing, astringent, antiseptic and other selected actions e.g. chloromycetin eye ointment.

Paints are liquid preparation containing volatile solvent which quickly evaporate to leave a dry and resinous film of medicaments on the skin.

Throat paints are more viscous in nature (due to the high proportion of glycerine) which being sticky and adhere to the affected site and prolongs the action of the drug.

Pastes are semi-solid preparation for external application that differ from similar products (i.e. ointment) in containing a high proportion of finely powdered medicaments. They afford greater protection and are more absorptive. The base may be anhydrous or water soluble e.g. zinc oxide paste.

Poultices are paste like preparation for external application to reduce inflammation due to its heat retaining capacity. After heating, the preparation is spread thickly on a dressing gauze and applied as hot as patient can bear it, to the affected area.

INHALATION FORM

Aerosols are suspension of fine, solid or liquid particles in a medium like air or oxygen and administered with the help of nebulizers. They are used to apply drugs to the respiratory tract in asthmatic patients e.g. Asthalin (salbutamol) inhaler, Fintal (sodium cromoglycate) inhaler.

Sprays are preparation of drugs in oil or water, usually administered by atomizer or nebulizer. They are applied to the mucosae of nose or throat e.g. Tyrothricin spray.

Vitrellae are thin walled glass capsules containing volatile substance (drops) (e.g. amyl or octyl nitrite) and protected by absorbent cotton wool and an outer silk bag. This capsule is crushed and the vapours are inhaled in the treatment of angina.

❑❑❑

CHAPTER 1.2

Prescription Writing

Prescription is an order for medication written/issued by a physician, dentist or other registered medical practitioner and it is a part of the professional relationship among the physician, pharmacist and patient. It can also be defined as signed written order by a physician to pharmacist with certain directions for dispensing the prescribed drugs/formulations and their uses by the patient. It is the pharmacist's responsibility in this relationship to provide quality patient and pharmaceutical care that meets the medication needs of the patient. It is also the responsibility to advise the physician of drug sensitivities the patient may have, previous adverse drug reactions or allergy, or other medications that the patient may be taking which may alter the efficacy or safety of the newly or previously prescribed drugs.

Since pharmacist is the key person between physician and patient, he must establish and maintain the trust of the physician and patient. The important part in this relationship includes maintaining confidentiality. The medication being taken by a patient and the nature/severity of the illness is a private matter which must be respected.

There are two types of legal prescription according to Drugs and Cosmetics Act; those that can be obtained by prescription only and those that may be purchased without a prescription and one termed as non-prescription drugs or over-the-counter (OTC) drugs.

While a prescription can be written on any peice of paper (but it should contain all legal elements), it usually takes a specific printed form on pad that contains blank spaces for the required information. In certain emergency conditions it may be communicated telephonically or directly to the pharmacist by electronic means.

Elements of the Prescription

Prescription usually are written on printed pad of blanks, which consists of following parts.

(i) **Name and address of the prescriber:** Most prescription blanks are imprinted with the name, address, telephone numbers and other pertinent information (such as availability of the physician at particular time, if a physician is practicing in more than one hospitals) of the physician or his/her practice site. These printed information clarifies the physician's name when it is signed illegibly and address, telephone no. etc. which facilitates additional professional communication if required.

(ii) **Patient's name, age, sex, address and date:** The date of prescription should be written near the top of prescription form or at the beginning of the chart order. The patient's name, age, sex and address are necessary on the prescription and should be clearly spelled out.

(iii) **Superscription:** It consists of Latin symbol Rx meaning *take thau* or *you take* and it has been believed to be an innovation to Horus and Jupiter, the father of Gods whose help is wished to make the prescription effective.

(iv) **Inscription:** It is the principal part or body of the prescription which specify the medication, its strength, the dosage and direction for use by the patients. When writing the drug name, either the brand name (proprietary name) or generic name (non-proprietary name) may be used. Now a days, the majority of prescriptions are written for medications which are already prepared in various dosage forms by pharmaceutical manufacturers. Phamacists are required to dispense the trademarked products when prescribed, unless substitution of an equivalent product is permitted by the prescriber. Prescriptions requiring the pharmacist to mix ingredients are termed compound prescriptions, which containing the names and quantities of each ingredients, required and quantities of ingredients to be used may be indicated in the metric or apothecary system of weighs and measure.

(v) **Subscription:** This part of prescription consists of directions to the pharmacist for dispensing or preparing the prescription. With decreasing frequency of compounded prescriptions in a majority of prescriptions, the subscription only consists the name of dosage from (as tablet, capsule, syrup etc.) and the number of dosage units to be supplied.

(vi) **Signatura:** The word, usually abbreviated sigma or sig means *mark thou*. This part includes the direction for the patient. The instructions on how and when to take medications, the duration of therapy must be explained to each patient by the physician and by the pharmacist. To help patients remember to take their medication, physicians often give an instruction that particular medication be taken at or around meal times and at bed time. The direction for use must be clear and understandable to the patient and concise to avoid any toxicity and to obtain the maximum benefit from therapy. (table 1.2.1)

(vii) **Prescriber's signature and registration number:** This part consists of prescriber signature and registration number of respective medical or dental council which is also required as per law by every country.

Table 1.2.1 *Some commonly used Latin abbreviations in prescription writing:*

Abbreviation	Latin name	English meaning
ad	ad	up to
ad lib	ad libitum	as desired
aq.	aqua	water
q.s.	quantum sufficiat	as much as it sufficient
collut.	collutorium	a mouth wash
garg.	gargarisma	a gargle
liq.	liquor	a solution
past	pasta	a paste
pign	pigmentum	a paint
o.d	once in die	once daily
b.i.d	bis in die	twice a day
q.i.d	quarter in die	four times a day
s.o.s.	si opus sit	if needed
prim. luc	prima luce	early in the morning
o.m.	omni name	every morning
o.h.	omni hora	every hour
n.	nocte	at night
o.n.	omni nocte	every night
h.s.	hora somni	at bed time
a.c.	anti cibos	before meals
p.c.	post cibos	after meals
i.c.	inter cibos	between meals/food
pulv.	pulvis	powder
sol.	solutio	solution
stat.	statim	at once
tab.	tabella	teblet
caps.	capsula	capsule
tr.	tinctura	tincture
ung.	unguentum	ointment
ex.lact.	exlacte	with milk
ex. aq.	ex aqua	with water
p.r.n.	pro re nata	occassionally
dol. urg.	dolore urgente	when the pain is severe

CHAPTER 1.3

Rational Use of Drugs & Drugs Laws

RATIONAL USE OF DRUGS

Rational use of drugs means using drugs which are safe and effective. These drugs should be available at reasonable prices and could be stored conveniently. The drug should be the appropriate drug for the disease, should be administered at the right dose for the right period of time.

Following factors lead to irrational prescribing.

I. **A large number of commercial preparation:** There are large number of commercial preparations available in the market. It is difficult for the physicians to make a rational choice from the wide range of drugs available. However, by applying sound criteria for selection the most appropriate drug could be chosen.

II. **Physician's decision making process:** The knowledge about the pharmacological properties of the drugs, an ability to deal with demanding patient and aggressive drug promotion by pharmaceutical companies all influence the prescriber. An up-to-date knowledge about drugs and the ability to deal with the patient and the pharmaceutical companies will make it easier for the doctors to select the right formulation.

The rational use of drugs can be accomplished by applying the following approach:

1. **Patients' problem:** Try to find an explanation for the patients' problem. Take a detailed history of the illness and the drug history of the patient.
2. **Diagnosis:** An accurate diagnosis is a prerequisite for rational therapy.
3. **Therapeutic objectives:** This should be arrived at from the prognosis of the disease or relieving a symptom or preventing a disease or a combination of these.
4. **Selection of drug treatment (drug):** The approach towards selection of a drug treatment is divided into two phases:
   a. Determine the options available to treat a health problem. Sometime simple advice may be all that is necessary and drug therapy may not be needed.

b. Evaluate the drugs on the basis of the following criteria: Efficacy, safety, suitability, cost, ease of administration and storage requirements.

5. **Start the treatment:** Describe the drug and start drug administration. Inform the patient about the beneficial effects as well as side effects of the drugs and how to deal with.
6. **Result of treatment:** The results of the drug therapy should be assessed periodically.

Rational Prescribing

Rational prescribing is to prescribe drugs to treat a particular health problem effectively and safely at an affordable cost. Therefore selection of a drug to treat a particular disorder should be based on a systematic approach towards its rational use.

I. **Selection of a drug:** If a drug is really needed to treat a health problem, then its selection involves the following steps:
   i. Accurate diagnosis is the prerequisite for rational therapy. However, if a tentative diagnosis is made due to the limited local resources, then it should be reviewed in the light of response to the therapy.
   ii. Select group of drugs effective to treat the particular health ailment.
   iii. Compare the effective groups of drugs and then select a drug on the basis of following criteria:

- **Efficacy:** Efficacy of a drug is not only based on pharmacodynamic but also on pharmacokinetic parameters, which have special importance in certain situations where onset and duration of drug effect is to be considered.
- **Safety:** Drug with fewer serious side effects in normal doses should be preferred.
- **Suitability:** Dosage forms should be such that it does not only guarantee the desired effect but can also be handled easily by the patient and due consideration should be given for contraindications and interactions.
- **Cost:** More expensive dosage forms may be an important factor for non-compliance. So, the cost factor should be considered while selecting a drug. The less expensive drug treatment may be preferred.
- **Storage conditions:** If all other things are equal then the drug which can be stored more easily should be selected.

II. **Monitoring of treatment:** The treatment can be monitored by the following methods:
   i. Passive monitoring: Information is given to the patient regarding the possible side effects with the necessary cautions. The patient is therefore well informed and able to do his monitoring.
   ii. Active monitoring: Make an another appointment for active determination of relief or side effects due to drug therapy.

Knowledge about the drugs are constantly changing. New drugs are introduced in the market and more information about existing drugs appear constantly. Therefore the doctor has to keep themselves updated.

SELECTION OF ESSENTIAL DRUGS

Essential drugs are those drugs that satisfy the health needs to the majority of the population. These should always to available in adequate quantities and in appropriate dosage forms.

The selection of the essential drugs should be based on the established health need for the drugs. The list should be reviewed periodically. Changes in the essential drugs list are made according to changes in the health needs, epidemiology of the diseases for which the drugs are prescribed and on therapeutic advances.

The WHO list of Essential Drugs published at regular intervals is a model list which could be used at the national, regional, hospital and primary health centre levels (given in appendix III).

DRUGS LAWS

The Drugs and Cosmetics Act, 1940 and rules 1945 have been passed with the objectives of regulating the import, manufacture, distribution and sale of drugs & cosmetics. The Act and rules have been amended from time to time and the latest and major amendment was made in 1982. Schedules G & H have been revised and new schedule X have been added and schedules E, I & L have been deleted. According to the Act, now there are four categories of drugs:

i. Drugs specified in schedule C, C_1 & X.
ii. Drugs not specified in schedule C, C_1 & X.
iii. Drugs specified in schedule C & C_1 (excluding those specified in schedule X).
iv. Drugs specified in schedule X.

Schedule M (Good Manufacturing Practice – GMP) and schedule Y (clinical trials etc.) were introduced in 1988.

Drugs and Cosmetics Rules have been divided into 18 parts each dealing with a particular subject. There are 2 schedules to the Act and 26 schedules to the Rules, which are as follows:

SCHEDULES TO THE ACT

First Schedule – Names of Books under Ayurvedic, Siddha and Unani Tibb systems.

Prior to independence, a Health Survey and Development Committee was appointed in the Year 1943. The committee underscored the future role to be played by the indigenous systems of medicine of India. In 1946, the conference of Health Ministers resolved that adequate provisions should be made at the Centre and provinces for research in indigenous systems of medicine, Ayurveda and Unani. The conference also recommended for starting educational and training institutions of these systems. In pursuance of the recommendations of the Health Ministers's conference, a number of committees were appointed by the Government of India, famous of them being Colonel R.N. Chopra (1946) and C.G. Pandit (1949) Committees. These committees recommended detailed outline for the development of Indian systems of medicine.

The Government of India established in 1969 a Central Council for Research in Indian Medicine and Homeopathy (CCRIMH) to develop scientific research in different branches of Indian systems of medicine – Unani Medicine, Ayurveda, Siddha, Yoga, Naturopathy and Homeopa-

Table 1.3.1: *Schedules to the rules*

- **A:** Proforma for application for the licences, issue and renewal of licences, for sending memoranda under the Act.
- **B:** Rates of fee for test or analysis by the Central Drugs Laboratory or the Government Analyst.
- **C:** List of biological and special products whose import, sale, distribution and manufacture are governed by special provisions.
- **C_1:** List of other special products whose import, sale, distribution and manufacture are governed by special provisions.
- **D:** List of drugs exempted from the provisions of import of drugs.
- **E_1:** List of poisonous substances under the Ayurvedic (including Siddha) and Unani systems of medicine.
- **F*(i)*:** Space, equipment and supplies required for a blood bank.
  ***(ii)*:** Minimum requirement for grant of licence to procure blood components from whole human blood.
- **F_1 Part I:** Provisions applicable to the production of bacterial and viral vaccines.
  Part II: Provisions applicable to the production of all sera from living animals.
  Part III: Provisions applicable to the manufacture and standardization of diagnostic agents (bacterial origin).
- **F_2:** Standards for surgical dressings.
- **F_3:** Standards for sterilized umbilical tapes.
- **FF:** Standards for ophthalmic preparations.
- **G:** List of substances that are required to be used only under medical supervision and which are to be labelled accordingly.
- **H:** List of prescription drugs.
- **J:** Diseases or ailments which a drug may not purport to prevent or cure.
- **K:** Drugs exempted from certain provisions relating to the manufacture of drugs.
- **M:** Good Manufacturing Practices (GMP) requirements of factory premises, plants and equipments.
- **M_1:** Requirements of factory premises etc. for manufacture of homeopathic preparations.
- **M_2:** Requirements of factory premises for the manufacture of cosmetics.
- **M_3:** Requirements of factory premises for manufacture of medical devices.
- **N:** List of minimum equipment for efficient running of a pharmacy.
- **O:** Standards for disinfectant fluids.
- **P:** Life periods of drugs.
- **P_1:** Pack sizes of drugs.
- **Q Part I:** List of dyes, colours and pigments permitted in cosmetics and soaps.
  Part II: List of colours permitted in soaps.
- **R:** Standards for condoms made of rubber latex intended for single use and other mechanical contraceptives.
- **R_1:** Standards for medical devices.
- **S:** Standards for cosmetics.
- **T:** Requirements of factory premises and hygienic conditions for Ayurvedic (including Siddha) and Unani drugs.
- **U:** Particulars to be show in manufacturing, raw material and analytical records of drugs.
- **U_1:** Particulars to be shown in manufacturing, raw material and analytical records of cosmetics.
- **V:** Standards for patent or proprietary medicines.
- **W:** List of drugs which are to be marketed under generic names only.
- **X:** List of drugs whose import, manufacture and sale, labelling and packaging are governed by special provisions.
- **Y:** Requirements and guidelines on clinical trials for import and manufacture of new drugs.

thy. Research activities in these systems continued under the aegis of the CCRIMH until 1978, when it was split into four separate research councils, one each for Unani Medicine, Ayurveda and Siddha, Yoga and Naturopathy, and Homeopathy, so as to further develop these systems in consonance with the basic philosophies of the respective systems. Also, with a view to streamlining education and regulating practice in Indian systems of medicine – Ayurveda, Unani Medicine and Siddha, the Government of India set up by an Act of Parliament, Indian Medicine Central Council Act 1970, the Central Council of Indian Medicine (CCIM).

In 1995, the Government also set up a full-fledged Department of India Systems of Medicine & Homeopathy (ISM & H) in the Union Ministry of Health & Family Welfare to further boost the development of Unani Medicine and other Indian systems of medicine. The Department of ISM & H has been renamed as Department of Ayurveda, Yoga & Naturopathy, Unani, Siddha and Homeopathy (AYUSH).

Second Schedule – Standard to be complied with by imported drugs and by drugs manufactured for sale, sold, stocked or exhibited for sale or distributed.

In addition the following appendices are also prescribed:

Appendix

I. Data required to be submitted with application for permission to market a new drug.

II. Format for submission of clinical trial reports.

III. Animal toxicity requirements for clinical trials and marketing of a new drug.

IV. Number of animals for long term toxicity studies.

V. Patient consent form for participation in a phase I clinical trial.

VI. Four groups of fixed dose combinations and their data requirements.

NARCOTIC DRUGS & PSYCHOTROPIC SUBSTANCES ACT & RULES

Opium was brought under legislature control as far back as in 1857. The primary aim of the Opium Act was the protection of the public welfare by preserving health & eliminating undesirable social and moral effects which are associated with indiscriminate use of opium. Govt. of India passed the Dangerous Drug Act in 1930 with a view to control certain operations in the dangerous drugs and to centralise and vest the same in the central government.

Further to "consolidate and amend the law relating to narcotic drugs, to make stringent provisions for the control and regulation of operations relating to narcotic drugs & psychotropic substances, and concerned matters", the "Narcotic Drugs & Psychotropic Substances Act & Rules was passed in September 1985.

THE MEDICINAL & TOILET PREPARATIONS (EXCISE DUTIES) ACT & RULES

The Medicinal and Toilet Preparation Act was passed in 1955 and Rules were passed in 1956 and came into force in April,

1957 to provide for the collection of levy and collection of duties of excise on medicinal and toilet preparations containing alcohol, narcotic drugs or narcotics.

THE DRUGS & MAGIC REMEDIES (OBJECTIONABLE ADVERTISEMENTS) ACT

The Drugs & Magic Remedies Act, 1954 was passed with the objective of controlling the advertisement of drugs in certain cases, to prohibit the advertisements for certain purposes for remedies alleged to possess magic qualities and to provide for related matters. The Act as well as Rules came into force in April, 1955 and was amended in 1963.

NEW DRUG POLICY

The drug policy was announced for the first time in 1978 on the basis of the recommendations of Hathi Committee report 1975. To provide the new thrust and direction in the policy frame, some new modifications were announced vide Drug policy, 1986. In 1994, new Drug policy guided the better & effective implementation of policy through newer provisions, rationalization, liberalization, minimizing control on drug & pharmaceutical industry sector and encouraging the indigenous research & development.

THE DRUGS (PRICE CONTROL) ORDER

Under section 3 of Essential Commodities Act, 1955, the central government is empowered to control the production, supply, distribution etc. of essential commodities including drugs. The Drugs (Price Control) Order, 1955 has been promulgated to ensure equitable distribution of essential bulk drugs and to fix the maximum retail prices of drug formulations.

THE PREVENTION OF FOOD ADULTERATION ACT & RULES

Food & drugs are generally controlled through a common administration i.e. FDA (Food & Drugs Administration in various states/country). The main objective of the Prevention of Food Adulteration Act is to make provision for the prevention of adulteration of food. The Act was passed in 1954 & Rules under the Act were passed in 1955.

THE MEDICAL TERMINATION OF PREGNANCY (MTP) ACT & RULES

The MTP Act, 1971, Rules 1971 and Regulation, 1975 provide for the termination of certain pregnancies by registered medical practitioners and related matters.

THE POISONS ACT

The Poisons Act was passed in 1919 with the objective of consolidating and amending the laws regulating the import, possession for sale & sale of poisons.

According to the provisions of the Act, the Central Government has been empowered to regulate the importation of poisons into India whereas the various state governments have been empowered to make rules regarding the possession and sale of poison within their respective territories.

❑❑❑

CHAPTER 1.4

Pharmacokinetics (Absorption, Distribution, Metabolism and Excretion of Drugs)

Pharmacokinetics is the study, which determines the rapidity and concentration of the drug in the body and its duration of appearance at the target organ, i.e. onset, time of peak action and duration of action and by these also determine the route(s) and frequency of administration of drug.

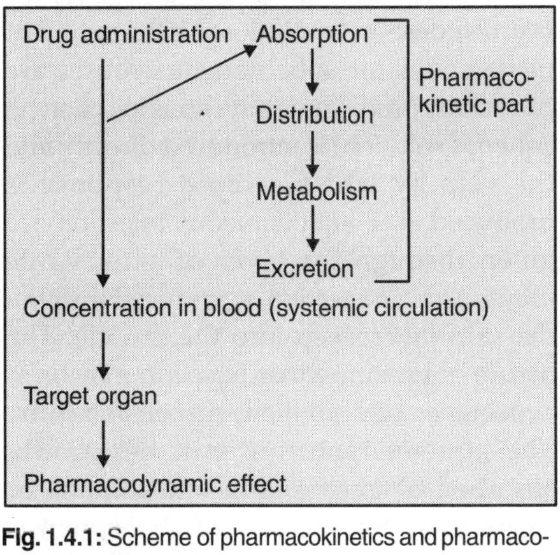

Fig. 1.4.1: Scheme of pharmacokinetics and pharmacodynamic processes.

ABSORPTION

Absorption is the entry of drug with blood via the biological membrane from the site/route of administration.

It is the movement of drug with the circulation from its site and route of administration.

Biopharmaceutics is the study of factors influencing the extent and rate of absorption and release of a drug from its various physicochemical properties and dosage forms and the therapeutic response obtained after its administration.

The rate and total amount of drug absorbed is dependent upon many factors, which are:

BIOLOGICAL FACTORS

The biological factors which affect the drug absorption are:

Passage or Drug Through Body Membranes

After a drug is administered in any form/route, it must reach the site of action and remain there for a particular period, so as to yield the desired effect. During their way to site of action, drug molecules have to cross one or more membranous barrier, which are lipoidal in nature, and having different sizes of pores.

The substance with higher water partition coefficient values can penetrate through natural membranes easily as compared to those having lower value. The natural substances like amino acids, bile salts, glucose readily pass through body membranes even if their molecules are too large.

Site of Absorption

The site of absorption is mainly localised in mouth (for buccal administration), stomach, intestines or colon.

Certain vasodilators (like nitroglycerine) and hormones which can penetrate the buccal mucosal wall will only be kept in buccal cavity or under the tongue. It provides rapid onset of action and prevention of gastrointestinal interactions.

The absorption in stomach depends upon the gastric emptying, gastrointestinal motility and its pH.

- Codeine, which is absorbed in the intestine fails to give quick relief if its emptying from the stomach is delayed.
- Benzylpenicillin if allowed to stay longer in the stomach, much of its activity is lost.

The other important factors controlling the rate of gastric emptying by influencing the gastric motility are the volume of the meal, its temperature, its viscosity and physical position.

The gastrointestinal pH has its own effect on the drug absorption. The range of pH in stomach is 1 to 3.6, in duodenum is 5 to 7 and 7 to 8 in ileum and colon.

Presence of Food and Other Salts

Normally, the presence of food in the GIT reduces the rate of absorption of drugs. Tetracycline, when given in full stomach, the blood level are reduced by 55 to 80% as compared with fasting individuals. The griseofulvin absorption is enhanced by giving it with fatty meals.

Bile salts have favourable effect on the absorption of drugs mainly due to their surface activity.

Routes of Administration

The drugs are mostly given by mouth, which is considered already in previous sections, the other routes of administration of drugs in relation to absorption are being discussed here.

Parenteral administration: This route is applicable for drugs which are inactivated by gastrointestinal tract or absorption is poor when given orally or there is a urgency for fast response in small dose. Intramuscular, intravenous, or subcutaneous routes are commonly used. The intravenous injection (in aqueous solution) is introduced directly into the vein by which a rapid response is produced. The subcutaneous injection are given through the layer of skin, while intramuscular injection, introduced through the skin layer deep into the muscle. The nature of intramuscular injection may be in aqueous or oily solution/suspension form. The aqueous solution will be rapidly absorbed as compared to oily solution or suspension. So, the rate of absorption is dependent on the nature of the preparation.

Inhalational administration: The absorption of drug takes places through lungs and the absorbing membrane is very thin and surface area is quite large. The lipid soluble drugs are readily absorbed from the nasal mucosa, as these drugs diffuse more rapidly.

Topical administration: It is employed for local action in the form of ointments, creams, jellies etc. for its antiseptic and local anaesthetic action. The lipid soluble drugs penetrate the skin easily and rapidly.

Rectal administration: The drug is also administered rectally in the form of suppositories and enema preparations which are absorbed from the colon.

PHYSICO-CHEMICAL FACTORS

The physicochemical factors affecting the absorption are lipid solubility, dissolution rate, salt from complexation, viscosity and drug stability in the GIT.

Lipid Solubility Dissociation Constant and pH

The drug solution of weak acid in the stomach (pH = 1.0; acidic) will be in more unionized form, which is more lipid soluble and gets more easily absorbed in the stomach.

A solution of weak base in stomach, less unionized is most unabsorbable e.g. quinine.

The high pH in intestine favours the absorption of weak bases.

Dissolution Rate

All the drugs in any solid dosage form or suspension when administered will first change into drug solution in body fluids. So, dissolution rate is important factor affecting the rate of absorption.

When a drug is more rapidly or completely absorbed from solution, it is very likely that its absorption will be dissolution rate limited.

Salt Form

The sodium or potassium salts of weak acids have higher absorption rate than those of acids themselves. For example, the biological activity of sodium salt of novobiocin (weak acid) is twice as compared to its calcium salt, and about 50 times larger in comparison to its free acid.

The dissolution rate of tolbutamide sodium is much greater than the rate of its free acid.

Crystal Form

The metastable forms are preferred in pharmaceutical preparations due to their higher solubility and dissolution rate e.g. the amorphous form of novobiocin is absorbed readily as compared to its crystalline form.

Complexation

The complexation of calcium of the mucosal cells reduces the absorption of certain drugs e.g. the barbiturates and sulfonamides. Presence of EDTA increases the absorption of mannitol.

Viscosity

Viscosity limits the dissolution rate and thereby affect the rapid absorption e.g. aqueous solution of sodium salicylate showed its rapid appearance in plasma while the same drug in suspension form failed to reach the target as quickly as with aqueous solution.

PHARMACEUTICAL FACTORS

These factors are mainly related to the various dosage form of pharmaceuticals. Their absorption depends upon their physical nature like aqueous solution, suspension, powder, tablets, capsules etc.

Aqueous Solutions

The aqueous solution are most quickly absorbed. But due to their poor stability, solubility limitation and packaging problems, most of the drugs are not designed in aqueous solution unless unavoidably needed in some specific preparations.

In aqueous suspensions, the particle size is the important factor for their stability, dissolution and absorption of drug e.g. sulphadimethoxine when given in suspension form is absorbed much quickly as compared when given in tablet form. Penicillin V, when given in aqueous suspension gives much higher initial blood level as compared to the tablets or capsules.

Solid Forms – Powders, Capsules, Tablets

Powder: When drug is given in the form of powder its absorption is largely dependent upon particle size, interaction with other diluents and dissolution rate.

The micronized powder gives much higher concentration in blood as compared to ordinary powder and tablets.

Capsule: The absorption of capsule is also dependent on their type e.g. hard capsule and soft capsule. The hard capsule dissolves much more readily in gastrointestinal tract as compared to soft capsules.

Tablets: After swallowing, the tablet first disintegrates into granules and primary solid particles and then into solution by dissolution for absorption. There is a specific disintegration and dissolution time for each tablet specified in the various pharmacopoeias. The absorption of any tablets is dependent on their disintegration and dissolution time, which may be affected by adding certain pharmaceutical additive e.g. dissolution can be increased by increasing the starch content, binders can retard the dissolution as they delay disintegration.

BIOAVAILABILITY

The bioavailability of any drug is defined as its rate and extent of absorption. This is mainly used to describe the biological availability of a drug from a preparation and is calculated/determined in terms of amount or rate of presence of drug in various body fluids like blood, urine etc.

It is also used to indicate a measurement of rate and relative amount of an administered drug in general circulation.

Bioavailability, after determining the rate and amount of drug absorbed, and the duration of drug's presence in the body fluid gives an idea about the therapeutic efficiency and toxicity.

The extent of absorption of a drug can be estimated by comparing the total area under the drug concentration in the blood versus time curve or the total amount of unchanged drug excreted in the urine after administration of drug and compared to the administration of standard (standard may be an intravenous injection, where the bioavailability of a drug reaches 100%).

For bioequivalence studies, the two formulations of same drug is administered orally as single dose. Figure 1.4.2 shows that in the study the different parameters are obtained. Firstly the peak height which represents the highest concentration of the drug reached in the blood at a particular time i.e. time of peak concentration. The area under the curve (AUC) represents the total amount of drug absorbed into the circulation.

The percent availability can also be calculated from *urine data:*

$$\text{Percent availability} = \frac{\text{Total amount of drug excreted in urine after oral administration}}{\text{Total amount of drug excreted in urine after intravenous administration}} \times 100$$

From *blood data:*

$$\text{Percentage availability} = \frac{\text{AUC (Oral)}}{\text{AUC (IV)}} \times 100$$

AUC = Area under the curve (Total amount of drug absorbed into the circulation).

Distribution of Drug

After absorption, the drug may be distributed into various body fluids like intestinal fluid, transcellular fluids e.g. fluids in the gastrointestinal tract, CSF etc.

The drug is distributed in such a pattern which reflects physiological factors and physicochemical nature of drug. These patterns of distribution depend on various factors.

PLASMA PROTEIN BINDING

Most of the drugs are transported bound to nonspecific sites on plasma proteins, mostly to albumin (for acidic drugs) and to α_1-acid glycoprotein (for basic drugs). Binding to other proteins like ceruloplasmin and transcortin generally occurs to a much smaller extent. The binding is usually reversible and depends on the individual compound.

The binding of drugs to plasma proteins limit its concentration in tissue and glomerular filtration of the drug. Since only unbound drug is in equilibrium across membranes and this process does not immediately change the concentration of free drug in the plasma. The free drug is cleared from the plasma by the liver and kidneys, which is rapidly replaced by

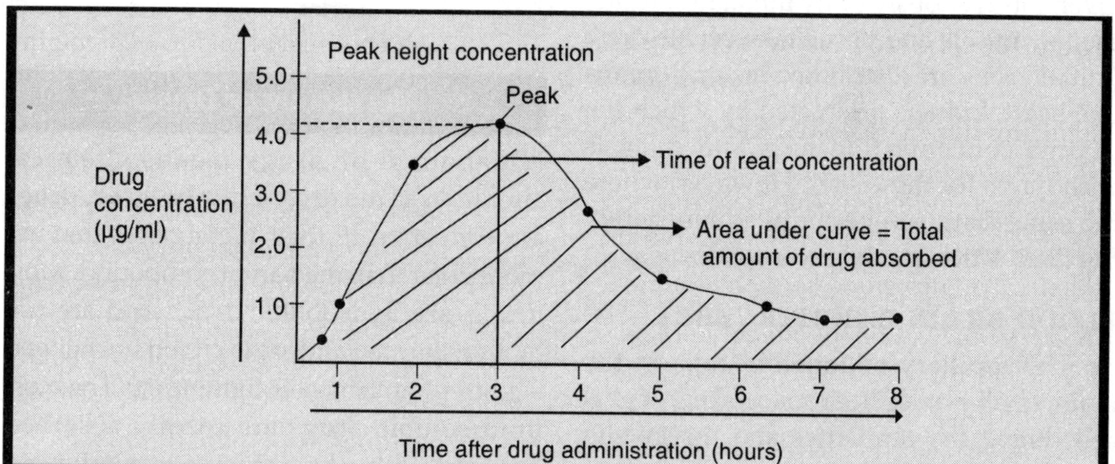

Fig. 1.4.2: Drug concentration in the plasma after oral administration (area under the curve versus time plot).

dissociation from plasma proteins and redistribution from the tissue.

Since, only unbound drug in the plasma is available for distribution. Therefore, higher the degree of protein binding, greater is the proportion which remains in the blood which makes the drug long acting, as bound fraction is not available for metabolism or conversion unless it is actively excreted by the liver or kidney.

Other drug reservoirs are cellular and fat reservoir. The accumulation of drug in the cells may be the result of active transport or binding. Many drugs are accumulated in muscle and other cells in higher concentration than in the extracellular fluids. Many lipid soluble drugs are stored in the neutral fat, and act as the important reservoir.

REDISTRIBUTION

In general, the termination of drug effect is usually by metabolism and excretion, but it can also be due to the redistribution of drugs. The highly lipid soluble drugs when given intravenously or by inhalation route, the fat, muscle and tissue take up the drug (initially they are distributed in other organs like heart, kidney, brain etc.) by which the plasma concentration falls and drug is withdrawn for these sites. However, where the same drug is repeatedly administered, the drug action can be prolonged.

BLOOD BRAIN BARRIER (BBB)

The capillary endothelial cells in the brain, small extracellular space, sheet of glial cells lining the capillaries and the myelin sheath together constitute the barrier, so called blood-brain barrier. There is another barrier, called blood-CSF (cerebrospinal fluid) barrier, which is located in the choroid plexus. The penetration of any drug through these barriers is dependent on their lipid solubility and ionization. Both barriers are lipoidal in nature and restrict the entry of non-lipid soluble drugs. Only lipid soluble drugs are able to penetrate and produce their action on central nervous system. The best example is levodopa in the treatment of parkinsonism, the dopamine (which is ultimately required in the brain) does not enter the brain but its precursor levodopa crosses the blood-brain barrier, changes into dopamine and produce their action.

PLACENTAL BARRIER

The placental membranes are also lipoidal in nature and lipophilic drugs (also nonlipid soluble drugs to some extent) can easily cross the placental barrier. It is a contact between the foetal blood and the maternal blood. Drugs are transferred through this barrier by simple diffusion method, once across this, drug molecules circulate in the foetal blood before diffusing back.

METABOLISM OF DRUGS

Metabolism of drugs means chemical alteration of the drug in the body i.e. drugs are converted to their metabolites that are more polar than the parent compound. Most drugs, are hydrophilic drugs and are not biotransformed and are excreted unchanged e.g. streptomycin, neostigmine etc. The most lipid soluble drugs are readily absorbed from the filtrate by diffusion through renal tubular cells. Thus, the enzymatic biotransformation of drugs to more polar and less lipid soluble metabolites enhances their excretion and reduce their volume of distribution. The primary site of drug metabolism is liver. The other organs like kidney, intestine, lungs and plasma are also involved in drug metabolism.

Many active drugs, during metabolism are converted into one or more active metabolites and produce effect due to the collective effect of parent drug and their metabolites e.g. phenacetin is converted into paracetamol, phenylbutazone into oxyphenbutazone, primidone into phenobarbitone, amitriptyline into noriptyline, imipramine into desimipramine and codeine into morphine. Certain drugs (parent drug) are inactive as such and has little or no biological activity called '**prodrug**,' but it is metabolized to a pharmacologically active compound. For example, levodopa is converted into dopamine which is effective in the treatment of parkinsonism, the anticancer drug cyclophosphamide is biologically inert but is converted into a active cytotoxic compound aldophosphamide, and another anticancer drug fluorouracil is changed into fluorouridine monophosphate, etc.

The drug metabolism in liver usually undergoes three general types of enzymatic reactions:

1. Oxidation-reduction and hydrolysis or stage I reaction.
2. Conjugation or stage II reaction.

The first stage I reaction i.e. oxidation-reduction are generated by a common hydroxy-lating enzyme system (cytochrome P450 system; CYP), which is located in endoplasmic reticulum of the liver cells. The CYP important isoenzymes in human being are CYP3A4/5, CYP2C19, 2CYP2D6, CYP2C8/9, CYP2E1 and CYP1A1/2 which are responsible for metabolism of large number of drugs. Hydrolytic enzymes are mostly located in the cell cytoplasm or in plasma and conjugation enzymes are associated with cytoplasm and endoplasmic reticulum.

OXIDATION

Oxidative reactions involve addition of oxygen/negatively charged radical or removal of hydrogen/positively charged radical.

The different oxidative reaction are:

Hydroxylation

It may be followed by oxidation to form a ketone or in the case of oxidative dealkylation to form an unstable intermediate, examples are:

Ring hydroxylation	:	Phenobarbital in to p-hydroxyphenobarbital.
		Cortisol into 7-β-hydroxycortisol.
Epoxidation	:	Benzene into benzene 1,2-epoxide.
N-oxidation	:	Drug containing amino groups can undergo N-oxidation i.e. imipramine into imipramine N-oxide.
O-dealkylation	:	This reaction probably involves formation of an unstable hydroxy methyl intermediate i.e. codeine into morphine.
Oxidative deamination	:	Amphetamine into phenylpropanone-2.

REDUCTION

The different type of reduction reactions are azo, nitro and keto group reductions. The important one is azoreduction, and example includes conversion of prontosil into sulfonamide, which was the first antimicrobial agent in treating the systemic bacterial infections.

HYDROLYSIS

It is a cleavage of drug molecule by taking up a molecule of water. The most hydrolytic enzymes are found outside the endoplasmic reticulum, and in higher concentrations in liver, kidney and plasma. The metabolism of an ester by an enzyme esterase results in the formation of an acid and alcohol. The examples are meperidine, procaina-mide, pethidine and lidocaine etc. Meperidine is catalyzed by esterases to be changed into meperidinic acid and procainamide is catalyzed by amidases.

CONJUGATION REACTION (STAGE II OR SYNTHETIC REACTIONS)

The conjugation reaction involves the chemical combination of the reactive group with a molecule provided by the body e.g. glucuronic acid, sulfate, glycine. This conjugation reaction decreases the drug activity to give a pharmacologically inactive compound, which is highly water soluble, that increases the rate of drug excretion.

Glucuronide Conjugation

This is the most common single metabolic reaction undergone by drugs, which occurs in the liver. These reactions are catalyzed by a family of enzymes known as uridine diphosphate (UDP) glucuronyl transferases. These enzymes are present in liver, kidney, intestine and lungs.

The compounds with a hydroxyl or carboxylic acid groups are easily conjugated with glucuronic acid which is derived from glucose.

The examples are aspirin, phenacetin, morphine, chloramphenicol, metronidazole, steroidal hormones etc.

Sulfate Conjugation

Sulfate conjugation is catalyzed by a family of enzymes known as 'sulfotransferases', which are present in the cell cytoplasm of liver and other organs. Example are chloramphenicol and sex steroids etc.

Acetylation

This reaction is catalyzed by enzymes 'N-acetyltransferases' that utilize acetyl-CoA as a cofactor, and are present in the cell cytoplasm of the liver, intestine, kidney and lung.

Examples:

$$\text{Isoniazid} \xrightarrow[\text{Acetyl CoA}]{\text{N-acetyl-transferase}} \text{N-acetylisoniazid}$$

Other examples are sulfonamides, PAS etc.

Methylation

This reaction is catalysed by enzyme 'methyl-transferases' (catechol-o-methyl-transferase) and generally uses S-adenosylmethionine as a methyl donor. Examples are conversion of norepi-nephrine into normetanephrine, which has less than one percent of the vasoconstrictor activity of the parent compound.

Glutathione Conjugation

It is an important pathway in the detoxification of a large variety of chemical toxic substances. Forming a mercapturate is normally a minor pathway like naphthalene (an aromatic compound) is excreted in the urine as N-acetylcysteine derivatives called as mercapturic acid.

Glycine Conjugation

Certain drugs having carboxylic acid groups are often inactivated by conjugation with glycine for example, salicylic acid.

FACTORS AFFECTING DRUG METABOLISM

AGE

In general, infants and older (human or animals) tend to be more sensitive to the action of the drugs. The impairment of drug metabolism in the new born infants usually results from a diminished capacity to deactivate drugs and consequently to more prolonged pharmacological action and to increased toxic reactions.

NUTRITION

Protein or calcium deficiency impairs drug metabolism in animals, due to decreased activity of the microsomal enzymes of the liver. The sleeping time by hexobarbitone is increased as a result of prolonged protein malnutrition. Acetylsalicylic acid has been shown to be more toxic to animals on a diet deficient in protein and magnesium.

The rates of metabolism are also impaired in vitamin deficiency states (especially vitamin A, vitamin B_2, C and E). Starvation in mice leads to decrease in the rates of metabolism of certain drugs like pethidine, acetanilide, hexobarbitone etc. Ethanol increases the hepatic content of monooxygenase enzymes and cytochrome P450 on chronic ingestion.

DISEASE CONDITIONS

Patients with liver disease may exhibit an increased sensitivity of many drugs. Patients with obstructive jaundice, hepatitis, cirrhosis shows reduce ability to synthesize glucuronide and sulfate conjugates.

Experimentally induced obstructive jaundice in animals (by ligation of bile ducts) decreases rate of metabolism of certain drugs like hexobarbitone, chlorpromazine, codeine etc.

SEX

The sex difference in the metabolism of drugs has not been observed in human beings. However, in rats, the pharmacological activity of a drug is more prolonged and the toxicity more marked in females than males, a difference which has been attributed to the more rapid metabolism of the drugs by the hepatic microsomal enzymes of the male rat.

PREGNANCY

During late pregnancy in rats, the conjugation of drugs with glucuronic acid (a major pathway for the deactivation of drugs) is reduced to about 50%. Certain oxidative metabolic transformations of drugs are also inhibited in pregnancy.

HORMONAL EFFECTS

The hormones of adrenal glands, thyroid and pancreas exert various effects on the metabolism of drugs. Adrenalectomy of certain species e.g. rat impairs the metabolism of certain drugs, which can be reversed by administration of cortisone or prednisolone. Administration of ACTH, adrenaline or thyroxine impairs the hepatic microsomal metabolism of drugs. Thyroidectomy reduces the metabolism of a number of drugs like barbiturate induced sleeping time is prolonged in thyroidectomized animals. Alloxan or streptozotocin induced diabetes in rats also reduced the metabolism of hexobarbitone thus prolonging the sleeping time.

EFFECTS OF THE INTESTINAL MICROFLORA

The metabolic transformation of many drugs is catalysed by various enzyme of the intestinal microflora. The anaerobic microflora and colon are rich in reductases which may be responsible for a significant proportion of the azoreductase and nitroreductase activity. The enzymes and other factors that may produce change in the nature of intestinal microflora might also produce changes in the metabolism pattern of the drugs.

GENETIC FACTOR – SPECIES DIFFERENCES

Species differences in the metabolism of drug may be due to the difference in the rate of metabolism or in their metabolites difference. Certain drugs have been found safe and non-toxic in animals, but when they were tested in human beings severe toxic effects were observed. For example, when sulfanilamide was tested in dog it was found safe and non-toxic, but when it was administered to human being, certain toxic effects like the hematuria, renal failure were observed.

Likewise, in certain case it was opposite. In human beings, phenacetin is generally free from toxic side effects, but in dogs it undergoes deacetylation.

PHARMACODYNAMIC FACTORS

Effects of Protein Binding

Acetylation of sulfonamides is reduced by protein binding, but the formation of glucuronide conjugates is unaffected.

EXCRETION OF DRUGS

The excretion of drugs has been known to take place through different routes mainly kidneys, skin, lungs and alimentary tract. Only few drugs are eliminated through skin and via lungs (only for volatile drugs like chloroform, ethyl alcohol, ether etc.). Drugs which are poorly absorbed are excreted in faeces. So kidneys serve as the primary and major organ for removal of most drugs, which is constituted by the microunits called 'nephron'. Three major processes that are involved in the excretion of drugs through kidneys are:

i. Glomerular filtration,
ii. Tubular secretion, and
iii. Passive diffusion.

Glomerular filtration: The rate of drug filtration is determined by the glomerular filtration rate (GFR) by using a substance like 'inulin', which when injected is filtered by the glomeruli and does not undergo either reabsorption or secretion by the renal tubules. The highly protein bound drugs like phenylbutazone, digoxin etc. are excreted slowly. Factors affecting the GFR of drug also can influence the rate of drug clearance. For example inflammation of the glomerular capillaries may increase GFR. Molecular configuration of drugs may also influence the GFR.

Tubular secretion: The active secretory systems can rapidly remove the protein-bound drugs from the blood and transport them into tubular fluid as the drugs that are bound to proteins are not readily available for excretion by filtration. The drugs known to be secreted by organic anion secretory system (i.e. strong acids) are salicylates, chlorothiazide, probenecid, penicillin etc. and cation (i.e. bases) includes catecholamines, choline, histamine, hexamethonium, morphine etc.

Passive diffusion: Passive diffusion can occur in both the ways in proximal and distal convoluted tubules. The lipophilic drug molecules are reabsorbed from the glomerular filtrate into the blood stream.

The pH of the urine can affect the rate of passive diffusion and hence drug excretion. The changes in urinary pH affect tubular reabsorption of partially ionized drugs. The effect of change in urinary pH on excretion of drugs is more with the drugs having pH values between 5 to 8. The excretion of basic drugs can be increased by making the urine more acidic by using the acidifying salt i.e. ammonium chloride.

PULMONARY EXCRETION

Volatile lipophilic substances like volatile general anaesthetics, ethyl alcohol, paraldehyde are excreted by the lungs. These volatile substances and certain gases that enter the body through the respiratory tract in the form of aerosol are excreted by this route.

Ethanol, having high blood gas solubility is excreted very slowly by the lungs and nitrogen oxide, which are not very soluble in blood, will be excreted rapidly. The excretion of these drugs may be affected in the presence of lung disease conditions, which may precipitate the drug toxicity.

BILIARY EXCRETION

Certain drugs are excreted in urine only in small amounts but appear in high concentrations in the bile for example, erythromycin, novobiocin, tetracycline, phenolphthalein etc. The abnormality or any disease related to liver may impair bile secretion which can lead to the accumulation of certain drugs like probenecid, digoxin etc. This can also lead to decreased drug metabolism and decreased rates of secretion of drugs into bile.

Certain drugs that are secreted by the liver into the bile and then to small intestine are not eliminated out through the faeces, so that the drugs will re-enter the blood that perfuses the intestine and again carried to the liver (repeatedly reabsorbed from the intestine and re-excreted in the bile) and thereby prolongs the action by the so called '***enterohepatic circulation***'.

EXCRETION IN OTHER BODY FLUIDS

Sweat and Saliva

The excretion of drugs through sweat and saliva is primarily dependent upon the diffusion of the non-ionized, lipophilic form of the drug across the epithelial cells of the glands. The compounds like lithium, potassium iodide and heavy metals are present in these secretions.

Milk

The excretion of drugs into the mother's milk will depend upon the amount of drug in blood, its lipid solubility and the extent of its active excretion. A highly lipid soluble drug should tend to accumulate in milk fat. As milk has a lower pH (6.5), the basic drugs are more concentrated in it. The drugs which are excreted in milk include sulfonamides, penicillin, tetracycline and other antibiotics, morphine, lithium, antithyroid drugs, antineoplastic agents, radioactive iodine etc.

So these drugs should be avoided or breast feeding should be suspended in lactating mothers as these drugs have effect on the infants.

CLEARANCE

Clearance may be defined as the rate of urinary excretion divided by the average concentration of excreted substance in the plasma.

Clearance can be calculated as:

$$Cl = \frac{\text{Rate of elimination}}{C},$$

where C is plasma concentration.

Drugs are eliminated by (i) **first order kinetics** or (ii) **zero order kinetics**. Majority of drugs obey first order kinetics i.e. a constant fraction of the drug is eliminated in each equal interval of time. The rate of drug elimination is directly proportional to plasma concentration. They are eliminated exponentially i.e. first order kinetics.

BIOLOGICAL HALF-LIFE ($t^{1/2}$)

It is the time it takes for the blood concentration of the drug in the body to be reduced by 50 percent.

When a drug of single compartment distribution is given intravenously, a semi-log plasma concentration time plot is obtained (Fig. 1.3.4), which has two slopes, one is due to distribution and another which is due to the drug elimination.

The elimination half life (t½) from elimination phase is

$$t½ = \frac{\text{Log } 2}{k}$$

k = Elimination rate constant (total amount of drug in the body removed per unit time).

$$k = \frac{CL}{V}$$

Clearance is the measure of the body's ability to eliminate a drug.

$$\text{Therefore } t½ = 0.693 \times \frac{V}{CL}$$

And, having known the biological half-life (t½), the elimination rate constant (kE) can be calculated

$$kE = 0.693/t½$$

VOLUME OF DISTRIBUTION (Vd)

It relates the amount of drug in the body to the concentration of drug in the blood or plasma.

$$Vd = \frac{\text{Amount of drug (in body)}}{\text{Concentration of drug (in blood/plasma)}}$$

REPEATED DRUG ADMINISTRATION

When the drug is repeated at short intervals, it accumulates in the body until elimination balances input and steady state plasma concentration is attained. When the doses are widely spaced, there is enough time for each dose to be cleared before the next dose in given.

The common pattern of drug administration is to attain the steady-state concentration, which correlates with the steady effective concentration of the drug at the site of action.

The figure shows the different types of drugs with different plasma half life, but the steady state concentration is maintained on repetitive dosing in all the three type of drug.

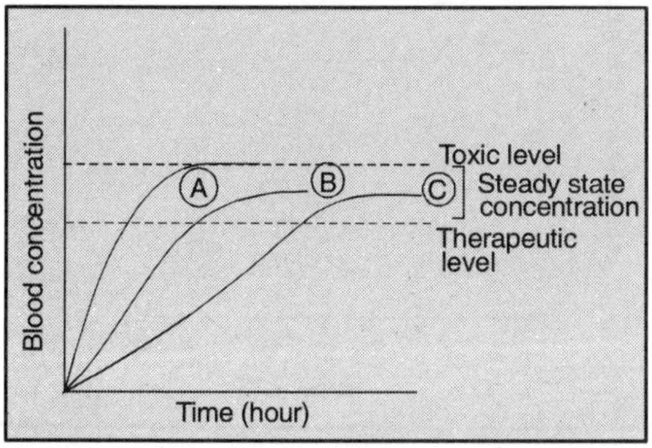

Fig. 1.4.3: Drug concentration vs time curve of repeated dosing.

Drug : A = Drug with long plasma half life given in initial loading dose followed by constant maintenance dose.

B = Drug with short plasma half life given in constant repetitive dose.

C = Drug with long plasma half life given in constant repetitive dose.

LOADING DOSE

It is a single or many quickly repeated doses given in the beginning of treatment to achieve target concentration rapidly.

DOSAGE INTERNAL

Most of the drugs are given in divided dose daily, the dosing interval is determined by the plasma half life. The drugs with long half lives may be given once or twice daily while drugs with shorter plasma half lives may require constant dosing or with short dosing interval.

When any drug is administered, it produces its desired effect in a particular time at receptor site and remain there at therapeutic level for particular time and after that its therapeutic efficacy declines. So the next dose should be given in between this period so that the steady state concentration is maintained and no toxic effects are produced due to high dose.

The graph shows that the drug reaches at the therapeutic level in 3½ hours after oral administration and achieve its peak concentration in 4½ hours and decreases below the mini-mum effective concentration (MEC) in 10 hours.

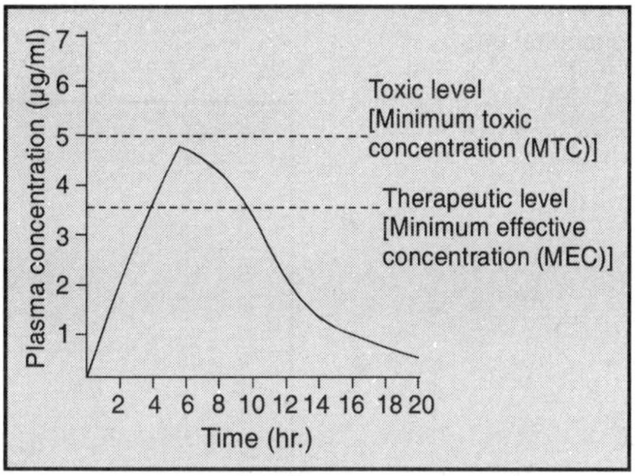

Fig. 1.4.4: Drug concentration in plasma vs time curve of drug administered orally.

Now for maintaining the serum concentration above the MEC for longer duration, the second dose of drug should be given about 7 to 8 hours after the first dose, otherwise when it is given after 7 to 8 hours it will take extra time to reach the MEC or if it is given prior to 7 to 8 hours the second dose in combination with the first dose effect crosses the minimum toxic concentration (MTC).

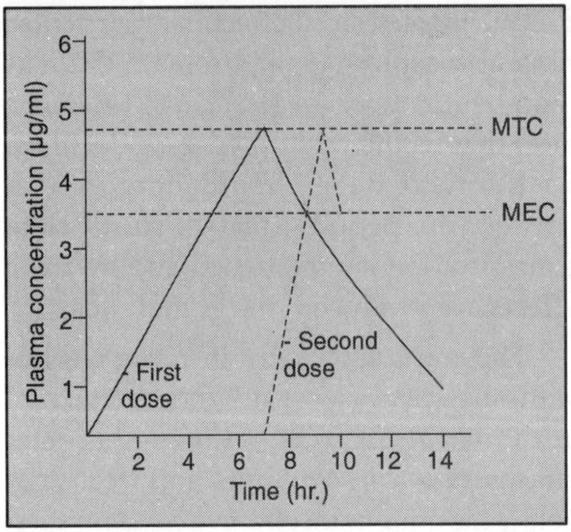

Fig. 1.4.5: Shows the administration of 2nd dose between the 7-8 hours interval which maintains the drug plasma levels above minimum effective concentration.

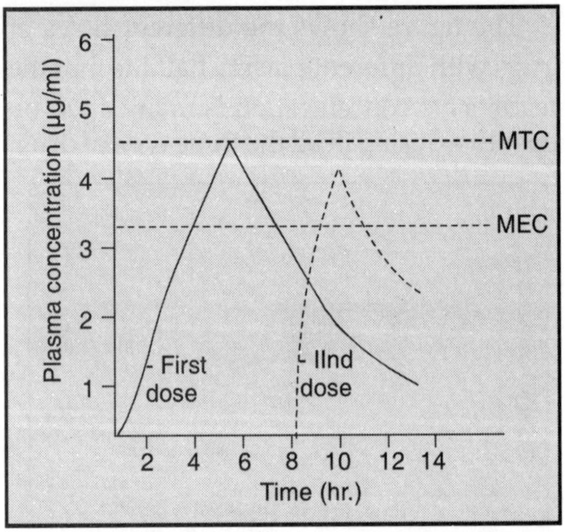

Fig. 1.4.6: Shows the administration of 2nd dose after 7-8 hours interval which does not maintain the drug plasma concentration at MEC level.

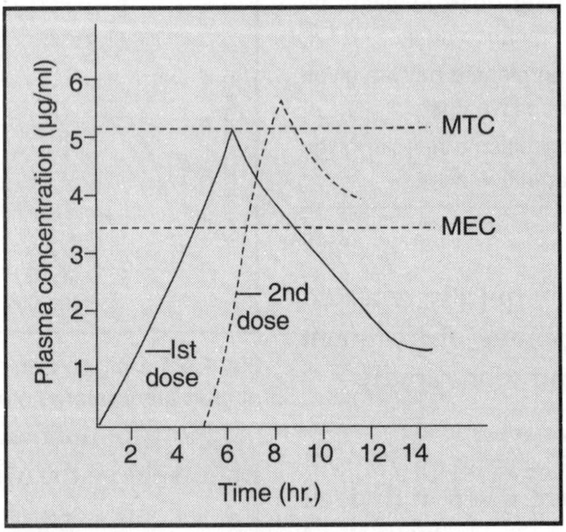

Fig. 1.4.7: Shows the administration of 2nd dose before 7-8 hours interval which crosses the MTC which may produce toxic effects of drugs.

CHAPTER 1.5

Pharmacodynamics

(Mode of Action of Drugs)

Pharmacodynamics is the study of drug effects (biochemical and physiological) and their mechanism of action. When the drug reaches its site of action it has a pharmacological effect which may be responsible for an eventual therapeutic effect and also responsible for the adverse effects as well as some other effects which may be of no clinical importance.

Site and Mechanism of Drug Action

The site of drug action means where a drug acts and mechanism means how the drug acts. Drug which act only at the site of application (i.e. localized region) are termed as **local** or **topical action** for example, ointments, paste, creams and certain other local preparations used externally produce only local effect. The local anaesthetics like lignocaine, procaine produce anaesthesia (local) in a localized region only.

The second type of action is **systemic** or **general action** which produce their action after absorption, for example, general anaesthetics act centrally after absorption, and often drugs like antibiotics, antacids, and so many other drugs acts systemically.

The proper localization of the site of drug action can be determined pharmacologically. When a new drug is introduced its screening gives an idea about the site and mechanism of drug action, for example, if any drug is said to be antihypertensive in nature and by blocking this action by prior administration of an antihistaminic, it will gives an idea that the drug may act in the same place and same mechanism as histamine. The use of certain blocking agents also help in suggesting the probable site of action of drugs.

Types of Drug Action

The drug may produce their effects by:

i. Stimulation.
ii. Depression.
iii. Irritation.
iv. Replacement.
v. Bactericidal and cytotoxic action. Stimulation

STIMULATION

Stimulation is an increase in the selective activity of specialized cells, which increases the secretion from a gland, for example, morphine stimulates vagus, acetylcholine stimulates exocrine glandular secretions, high dose of CNS stimulant picrotoxin produces convulsions.

DEPRESSION

It is a reduction/decrease in the activity of specialized cells. For example barbiturates depress central nervous system, quinidine depresses myocardium. Certain drugs stimulate one type of cells but depress others e.g. morphine stimulates the vagus and chemoreceptor trigger zone but depresses the vomiting and cough centres. Similarly acetylcholine stimulates intestinal smooth muscle but depresses SA node in the heart.

IRRITATION

It is the effect of drugs on the growth, nutrition and morphology of living tissues which induce a gross change in cellular function. Such drugs produce a nonselective, often noxious effects and is particularly applied to less specialized cells and causing a mild inflammation or irritation, corrosion and necrosis of cells. The other cellular changes produced by irritation are precipitation of protein (astringent effect) and when these agents as applied locally to the skin to relieve deep seated pain by increasing the blood flow to the site (counter irritant action) e.g. liniments to relieve muscular pain (turpentine oil liniment).

REPLACEMENT

It includes certain drugs, which are used to replace some missing endogenous component of the body or when the production of endogenous components is reduced e.g. thyroxine is used to replace natural thyroid hormone secretion in hypothyroidism, insulin in diabetes mellitus, levodopa in parkinsonism, hydroxycobalamin (vitamin B_{12}) and ferrous salts in the treatment of conditions associated with their deficiency.

BACTERICIDAL AND CYTOTOXIC ACTION

The *bacteriostatic* activity which is inhibition of growth and multiplication of bacteria and *bactericidal* activity, which is bacterial death, is induced by certain types of antibiotics. Cytotoxic action is selective for invading cancer cells and altering them without affecting the host cells.

FACTORS MODIFYING DRUG ACTION

The drug action can be modified either quantitatively (in which the action of drug is increased or decreased) or qualitatively (in which the type of response is altered).

The factors are:

1. **Age:** In newborn infants, the glomerular filtration rate and tubular transport is immature, which takes 5 to 7 months to mature. Also, the hepatic drug metabolism capacity is also inadequate (that is why chloramphenicol can produce '*grey baby syndrome*'), and due to the higher permeability of blood brain barrier, certain drugs attain high concentration in the CNS.

The dose of a drug for children is often calculated from adult dose.

$$\text{Child dose} = \frac{\text{Age}}{\text{Age} + 12} \times \text{Adult dose}$$

Children are more susceptible to special adverse effects of drugs and in the elderly, the renal function is on decline and doses of drugs have to be reduced.

2. **Body size/weight:** The average adult dose refers to individuals of medium body build. For obese or lean individuals, doses of drug may be calculated by the formula:

$$\text{Adult dose} \times \frac{\text{Weight (kg)}}{70}$$

Dose can be calculated more accurately by body surface area (BSA).

$$\text{Individual dose} = \frac{\text{BSA } (m^2)}{1.7} \times \text{Average adult dose}$$

3. **Sex:** Females require lower dose than males. Drugs given during pregnancy can affect the foetus. There are certain physiological changes that take place during pregnancy, which can alter the drug disposal.
4. **Species and racial difference:** In animal species, rabbits are resistant to atropine and rat and mice are resistant to digitalis.

Among human beings, blacks require higher and Mongols require lower concentration of atropine and ephedrine to dilate their pupils.

5. **Genetics:** In certain individuals, the same dose may produce their effect 5-6 times more among others, which is due to their differing rate of drug metabolism, e.g. haemolysis occurs with primaquine in a person with glucose-6-phosphate dehydrogenase (G-6-PD) deficiency.
6. **Routes and time of administration:** The different routes of administration may affect the intensity of drug effect e.g. magnesium sulphate, when used orally acts as a purgative, in local application it relieves inflammation of wound or boil and when it is used intravenously it causes depression of CNS and reduce convulsions.

The time of administration can also affect drug response e.g. INH and rifampicin (anti-tubercular drugs) are taken in early morning empty stomach. The corticosteroids when taken in morning as single dose cause less adrenal-pituitary suppression.

7. **Pathological conditions:** Several disease conditions influence the drug disposal and action of drug. For example:

In liver disease:

- Bioavailability of drug (having first pass metabolism) is increased, which is due to diminished hepatocellular function.
- Protein binding of drugs (acidic) is reduced.
- Metabolism and elimination of some drugs is reduced.

In kidney disease:

- The kidney disease affects the pharmaco-kinetics of certain drugs.
- Clearance of drugs (e.g. digoxin, glycosides) is reduced.
- Plasma albumin is altered in structure in patients with renal disease.
- In renal failure, the permeability of blood-brain barrier is increased so that the

drugs like morphine, barbiturates, phenothiazines, benzodiazepine can produce more CNS depression.

In gastrointestinal disease:

- The absorption of orally administered drug is altered e.g. achlorhydria reduces aspirin absorption.
- Absorption of amoxycillin is reduced in coeliac disease.

Other important diseases in which the drug action is altered are:

- The hyperthyroid patients are relatively resistant to inotropic action but more prone to arrhythmic action of digoxin.
- In congestive heart failure the drug elimination is retarded due to decreased perfusion and congestion of liver, also reduced glomerular filtration and increased tubular reabsorption.
- In head injury, morphine (in normal dose) can cause respiratory failure. In severe pain, hypnotics may cause mental confusion.

8. **Tolerance:** Tolerance is a condition when there is a requirement of higher dose of a drug to produce a given response.
9. **Drug resistance:** It is tolerance of micro-organisms to inhibitory action of antimicrobials e.g. staphylococci to penicillin.
10. **Other drugs:** Drugs may modify the response to each other by pharmacokinetic or pharmaco-dynamic interaction between them.

Tachyphylaxis is the rapid development of tolerance in which there is a marked reduction in response even after repeated doses of a drug. It is not necessary that tolerance develop equally to all the action of the drug, e.g. tolerance of morphine occurs to its analgesic and euphoric action and not to its constipating and miotic actions. Likewise in phenobarbitone, tolerance occurs to its sedative action and not to its anti-epileptic action.

Cross tolerance is development of tolerance to pharmacologically related drugs e.g. morphine and barbiturates.

Chemical Character of Drugs

STRUCTURE ACTIVITY RELATIONSHIP (SAR)

The effect of certain structural compounds in relation to its activity, duration of action and mechanism can be altered by changing the structure of drugs of known activity. A new product can show different reactions, different relation between the drugs and cell constituents and perhaps even new mechanism of action.

The structure activity relationship is useful in synthesis of new active compounds with more specific actions with lesser unwanted effect, and to know about their mechanism of action.

Drug Receptors

The drug receptors are macromolecular sites which are situated on the surface or inside the effector cells with which specific agonist combines to produce its response. Antagonist prevents the action of an agonist on a receptor, but does not have any effect of its own (Fig. 1.5.1).

Receptors are mostly protein macromolecules. The cholinergic, adrenergic, histaminergic and other receptors are 'physiological receptors' on which certain drugs act which mediate the responses to transmitters, autacoids etc. Another type of receptor is 'drug receptors', which do not have any known physiological ligands, for example thiazide receptor, benzodiazepine receptor etc.

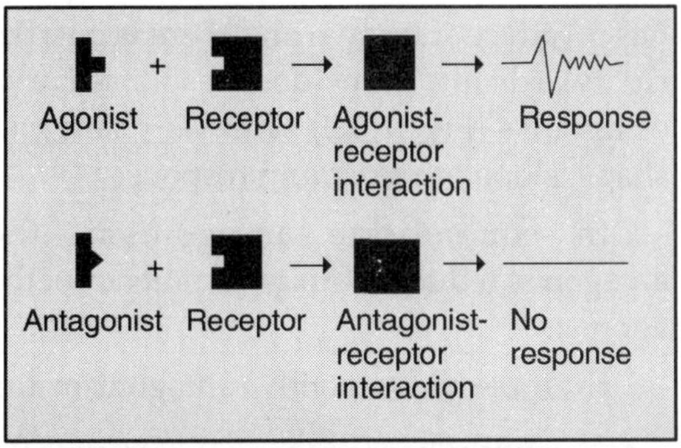

Fig. 1.5.1: Drug-receptor interaction: The agonist completely fits (interact) with the receptor site to produce a pharmacological response and antagonist only partially fit with the receptor site and is unable to produce any pharmacological response, and also prevents the agonist from combining with the receptors.

The ability of a drug to get bound to a receptor is termed as the **'affinity of the drug'** for the receptor. The ability of the drug to produce a pharmacological response after its interaction with the receptor is known as **'intrinsic activity of the drug'**, it also determines the degree of receptor response. The agonists produce a maximal receptor response (high intrinsic activity), partial agonists have intermediate intrinsic activity and antagonists have low intrinsic activity and high affinity for the receptors.

On the basis of affinity and efficacy, the drugs can be classified as **agonists**, which have both affinity as well as high intrinsic activity and can mimic the effects of the endogenous substance after combining with the receptor (e.g. methacholine produces the effect of acetylcholine at cholinergic receptors). **Antagonists** have only the affinity but no intrinsic activity. These drugs bind to the receptor, but do not mimic (rather block) or interfere with the binding of an endogenous agonist (e.g. atropine block the effect of acetylcholine on cholinergic-muscarinic receptors). **Partial agonists** have full affinity to the receptor but with lower intrinsic activity [e.g. pentazocine is a partial agonist at μ receptor (subtype of opioid receptor)]. **Inverse agonist** or **negative antagonists** have full affinity towards the receptor but their intrinsic activity is absolutely negligible and may be zero or in minus.

RECEPTOR TYPE

On the basis of molecular structure and nature of transduction mechanism, receptor can be classified into following categories:

i. G-protein and second messengers.
ii. Ligand-gated channels.
iii. Cytokine receptors.
iv. Tyrosine kinases.
v. Intracellular receptors.

COMBINED EFFECT OF DRUGS

SYNERGISM

When two drugs are given simultaneously, and the action of one drug is increased by the other, they are treated as

synergistic. In the synergism, the drugs can have action in the same direction or when given alone, one may be inactive. Synergism can be additive or supradditive in nature.

ADDITIVE

When the effect of two drugs are in the same direction. For example when aspirin is combined with paracetamol the combined effect is analgesic/antipyretic.

Another important example is combination of theophylline and ephedrine as bronchodilator, combination of sulfonamides as antibacterial etc.

SUPRADDITIVE

In this the effect of combined therapy is greater than the individual effect of the one drug. Examples are:

- Levodopa and peripheral dopa-decarboxylase inhibitor, carbidopa or benserazide in the treatment of parkinsonism.
- Sulfonamide and trimethoprim (well known preparation 'Septran') as antibacterial.

DRUG ANTAGONISM

Antagonism describes the situation, when one drug decreases or inhibits the action of another. The antagonism may be ***physical*** in which the physical property of the drug can affect the absorption of another drug, ***chemical*** in which two drugs react chemically and form a biologically inactive compound. This type of reaction may be used in the treatment of drug poisoning. For example in cyanide poisoning nitrites form methaemoglobin which has high affinity for cyanide radical and forms cyanomethaemoglobin and after sodium thiosulphate injection forms sodium thiocyanate which is easily excreted in urine.

On receptor basis, drug antagonism will be of two types competitive and noncompetitive antagonism.

COMPETITIVE ANTAGONISM

In competitive antagonism, the antagonist binds with the same receptor as agonist. If the log dose response curve with agonist is obtained in the presence of antagonist, it will be found that antagonist has no effect of its own and there is parallel rightward shift in the dose response curve of agonist (Fig. 1.5.2) with no change in shape, slope or maximum response.

In competitive antagonism, the antagonist reduces affinity i.e. potency of the agonist.

Example of competitive antagonism are:

- Acetylcholine (as agonist) – atropine (as antagonist).
- Acetylcholine – d-tubocurarine.
- Isoprenaline – propranolol.

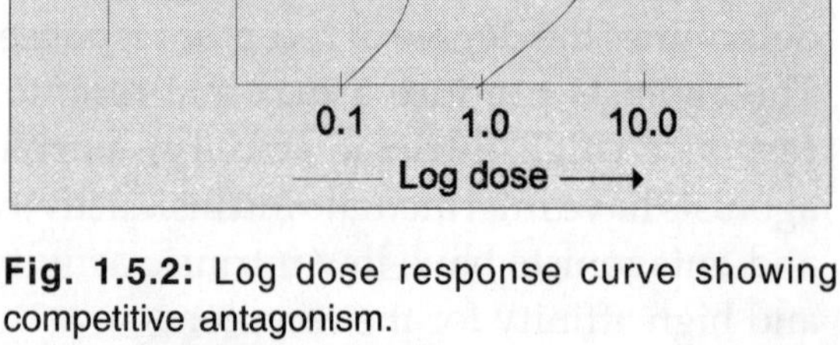

Fig. 1.5.2: Log dose response curve showing competitive antagonism.

NONCOMPETITIVE ANTAGONISM

In this type of antagonism, antagonist binds to another site or receptor. The antagonist is not displaced by a high concentration of the agonist on the same receptor and the log dose response curve is flattened and its slope and maximum response will be decreased.

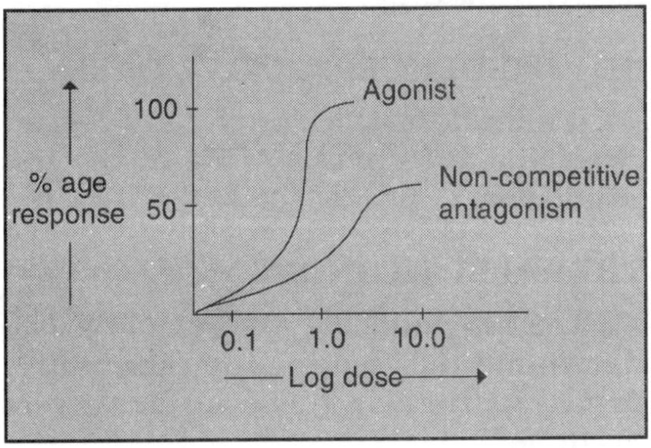

Fig. 1.5.3: Log dose response curve showing non-competitive antagonism.

In noncompetitive antagonism, the antagonist apparently reduces intrinsic activity i.e. efficacy of the agonist and the response depends only on the concentration of the antagonist. Examples are noradrenaline – phenoxybenzamine.

Dose – Response Relationship

The relationship between the dose and the response depends on the object, percent response measured and drug employed. By increasing the dose of a drug there is increase in the pharmacological response. The response to a drug is related to its molar concentration presented to the cells.

There are two types of dose-response curve:

HYPERBOLIC OR EXPONENTIAL TYPE OF DOSE-RESPONSE CURVE

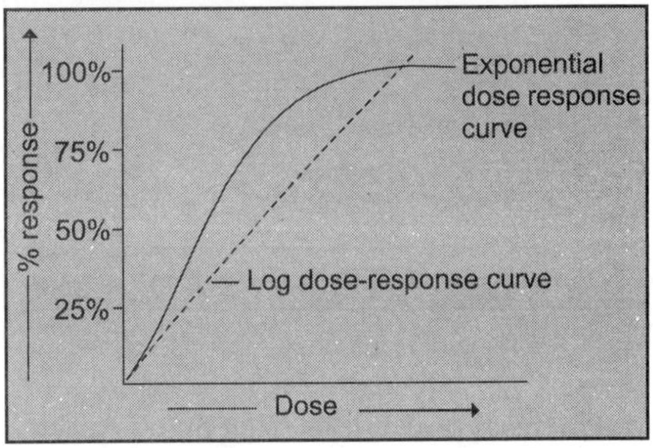

Fig. 1.5.4: Hyperbolic or exponential dose-response curve.

In this the magnitude of response is proportional to the concentration of the drug present.

If the log dose of a drug is plotted against the percentage response, the relationship becomes linear, which is termed as **log-dose response curve**.

SIGMOID TYPE DOSE-RESPONSE CURVE

In this type, the response is quantal or 'all or none' type. If dose-response curve is plotted, no significant response is observed till a certain steady or threshold level is attained. The dose with which it is obtained is called **'ceiling dose'**. Beyond this point, there is no further increase in the therapeutic effect which remains unchanged even after increasing the dose of the drug. This type of response gives a sigmoid type dose-response curve.

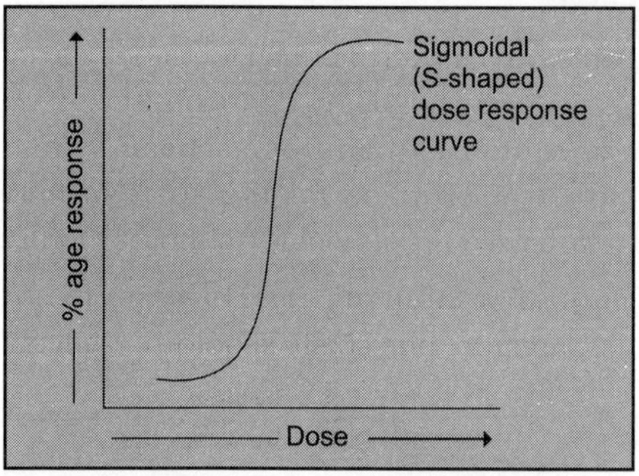

Fig. 1.5.5: Sigmoid type dose-response curve.

In this type of curve, if log dose is plotted against the percentage response, the shape of the curve remains unchanged. This log dose-response curve is useful in bioassays.

LD_{50} (MEDIAN LETHAL DOSE)

It is the dose which kills 50% of the experimental animals (i.e. 50% mortality) receiving the drug.

ED_{50} (MEDIAN EFFECTIVE DOSE)

It is the dose which produced a desired effect (i.e. effective) in 50% of the test population.

THERAPEUTIC INDEX

The LD_{50} and ED_{50} are employed to determine the therapeutic index for a particular drug, which assesses the safety of the drug.

$$\text{Therapeutic index (TI)} = \frac{Ld_{50}}{Ed_{50}}$$

❑❑❑

CHAPTER 1.6 Adverse Drug Reactions

Adverse Drug Reactions

Adverse drug reaction is an undesired or unintended effect of the drug, occurs at dose normally used by human being. The adverse drug reaction requires treatment or decrease in dose if it is due to poisoning or overdose.

Adverse drug reaction may be defined as 'any response to a drug which is noxious (injurious) and unintended, and which occurs at doses of an appropriately given drug used in man for prophylaxis, diagnosis or therapy excluding therapeutic failures.'

Adverse drugs reactions are not rare and have increased in number, which may be due to irrational use of multiple drug therapy, availability of most of the drugs as OTC (over the counter) i.e. without prescription and self medication by the patients.

Adverse effects can be based on the pharmacodynamics of the drug i.e. ***side effects*** (occur at therapeutic dose of the drug), ***toxic effects*** (occurs at overdose or poisoning) and ***drug withdrawal symptoms*** (i.e. withdrawal of narcotic drugs) and secondly, the effects which are individual to individual like drug allergy (hypersensitivity to drugs), idiosyncracy.

Other types are ***teratogenicity*** (drug causing foetal abnormalities), ***carcinogenicity*** (drug causing cancer), ***iatrogenicity*** (drug induced diseases).

Side Effects

There are undesirable and unavoidable pharmacological effect of the drug, which occur at therapeutic dose. These unwanted effects of many drugs are based on their pharmacological actions. Some important examples are:

- Atropine causes dryness of mouth as side effect which is due to its antisecretory effect, and due to this action atropine is used in peptic ulcer.
- Acetazolamide (a carbonic anhydrase inhibitor) used as diuretic by increasing bicarbonate excretion and thus acidosis occur as side effect which is related to its pharmacological action.

Side effects are also based on different facet of action (or side effects unrelated to its pharmacological or therapeutic effect). All antihistaminics except few newer compounds e.g. astemizole, terfenadine etc. cause sedation which is unrelated to its therapeutic action i.e. antiallergic action.

The history of pharmacology revealed that certain drugs have been developed from the observation of their side effects for example sulfonamide produce hypoglycemia and acidosis as side effect, which further gave an idea for developing a new compound related to sulfona-mide – sulfonylurea as hypoglycemic agent and acetazolamide as diuretic.

Toxic Effects

Toxic effects develop due to excessive pharmacological action of drug, which may be due to overdose or continuous use of drug for prolonged period.

The overdose toxicity occurs when the high dose of drug is required for the specific treatment or the drug is taken accidentally or with the intention of suicide. The effects are predictable and dose related. For example delirium by the use of atropine and respiratory failure by morphine occur due to their overdoses. The well known antitubercular drug, streptomycin causes vestibular damage and deafness on prolonged use.

Drug Allergy and Idiosyncrasy

HYPERSENSITIVITY (DRUG ALLERGY)

Drug allergy is a cell-mediated immune reaction producing symptoms, which are unrelated to the pharmacological effects of the drug. It results from previous sensitization to the drug itself or a particular chemical with similar structure.

The B-lymphocytes, when exposed to antigens mature into immunoglobulin secreting cells after proliferation, which often have the appearance of plasma cells.

The immunoglobulins (Ig) are secreted by B-lymphocytes in the later stage of their development into plasma cells. IgG, IgA, IgM, IgE and IgD are immunoglobulins, out of these IgG is the major one.

Based on the mechanism of immunological reactions, the allergic responses have been divided into four categories:

TYPE-I (ANAPHYLACTIC REACTION)

They are mediated by IgE antibodies. On exposure to the drug, antigen and antibody reaction takes place on mast cells and basophils releasing various mediators e.g. histamine, leukotrienes, 5 hydroxytryptamine (5-HT), prostaglandins etc., which are responsible for immediate immune reactions like skin reaction, anaphylactic shock, asthma etc. These reactions occur immediately after challenge and are termed as immediate hypersensitivity.

TYPE-II (CYTOLYTIC REACTION; DELAYED IGG/IGE MEDIATED)

These reactions are mediated by IgG and IgE antibodies, which bind to the target cells (cells in the circulating system). On reexposure antigen-antibody reaction takes place on the surface of these target cells and cytolysis occur. Example are penicillin-induced hemolytic anaemia, sulfonamide-induced granulocytopenia and quinidine-induced cytopenic purpura.

TYPE-III (ARTHUS REACTION IGG MEDIATED)

These reactions are predominantly mediated by IgG. The antigen-antibody complexes are deposited in the vascular endothelium, where a destructive inflammatory response occurs. *Serum sickness*, clinical symptoms include fever, skin eruptions, arthralgia and lymphadenopathy. The reaction usually subsides in 6-12 days.

The drugs inducing serum sickness are sulfonamides, penicillin etc. Sulfonamides also cause ***Stevens-Johnson syndrome***, a form of immune vasculitis, which is characterized by the reactions including arthritis, nephritis, myocarditis and certain mental symptoms.

TYPE-IV (DELAYED HYPERSENSITIVITY)

These reactions are mediated by production of sensitized T-lymphocytes. On contact with antigen, an inflammatory reaction is generated which includes contact dermatitis, fever and photosensitization.

Drugs which cause these types of reactions are penicillin, sulfonamides, tetracycline, phenylbutazone, salicylates etc.

TERATOGENICITY

Teratogenicity is derived from the word 'teratos' mean 'monster.' Teratogens may act directly on the foetus, e.g., thalidomide and anticancer drugs act directly on the foetus, or act indirectly on placenta e.g., vitamin A, 5-HT.

It is clear that the major foetal damage occur by drug when it is taken in early pregnancy (i.e. first 2-9 weeks when organogenesis takes place.)

The teratogenic drugs can affect different stages of pregnancy i.e.

- At fertilization and implantation stage (i.e. conception to 3 weeks).
- Organogenesis period (3 to 9 weeks), and
- In growth and development period (i.e., after 9 weeks).

The drugs, which are proven to be teratogenic are thalidomide, anticancer drugs (specially methotrexate), sex hormones (androgens, progestins, stilboesterol) corticosteroids, warfarin, antithyroid drugs (which can cause foetal goitre and hypothyroidism), oral antidiabetic drugs, and social drugs including tobacco, alcohol etc.

CARCINOGENICITY

Certain drugs affect the genes and structural changes in the chromosomes. The drugs that cause cancer are called as carcinogenic drugs, for example, oral contraceptives increase the incidence of benign liver tumors, vaginal adenocarcinoma in the female offsprings of women who have taken stilboesterol during her pregnancy for abortion purpose.

Drugs producing carcinogenic effects are anticancer/antineoplastic drugs, radioisotopes like P^{32}, I^{131} and hormonal therapy etc.

Idiosyncrasy

It is genetically determined abnormal reactivity to a drug. The abnormal reaction to the drug are precipitated sometime because of genetically determined total absence or reduced activity of some enzyme in the body of the recipient, e.g., primaquine produce haemolysis in individuals with glucose-6-phosphate dehydrogenase (G-6-PD) deficiency. Blacks require higher concentration of atropine to dilate their pupil. Certain individuals feel excitement and mental confusion after taking barbiturates. The short acting skeletal muscle relaxant succinylcholine may produce respiratory paralysis and prolonged apnea in individuals whose plasma contain an atypical pseudocholinesterase enzyme.

Poisoning

Poison is a substance which endangers life due to its toxic reaction/poisoning on certain vital functions in the body. The poisonous substances may be the toxins, very high doses of drug, industrial chemicals/gases, household chemical like insecticides-DDT, BHC, etc.

For the treatment of poisoning, a selective antidote (which antagonises the action) may be given e.g., nalorphine and naloxone in case of morphine poisoning, atropine in case of anticholinergic drugs, dimercaprol in mercury and penicillamine in lead poisoning, etc.

MANAGEMENT OF POISONING

- Maintain a clear airway/adequate ventilation (for inhaled poisons).
- Washing the eyes and other surface of the body (for local poison entering from the surface).
- Gastric lavage (with hypertonic saline solution, apomorphine injection for ingested poison).
- Activated charcoal (to bind the unabsorbed drug) 10-30 g in suspension in 200 ml water.
- Identify the poison and specific antidotes should be given.
- Maintenance of blood pressure and other related body function by fluid infusion, pressor agents, depending upon the condition of the patient.
- The nonspecific antidotes are also given, for example anticonvulsants in convulsions.
- Forced diuresis by furosemide, mannitol etc. and altering the urinary pH– ***increasing the pH*** of urine favours ionisation of acidic drugs like salicylates, phenobarbital etc. whereas ***reducing the pH*** favours ionisation of basic drugs like pethidine, amphetamine etc.
- Haemodialysis and haemoperfusion which is a passage of blood through a charcoal or adsorbent resin column may be instituted, depending upon the patient's condition.

(Detailed treatment of poisoning is discussed in chapter 11.1)

❑❑❑

CHAPTER 1.7

Drug Interactions

Drug interactions may be defined as an alteration in duration and/or onset of action of the pharmacokinetic and/or pharmacodynamic of one drug produced by another drug. The multiple drug therapy produced a combined effect, which may be antagonistic or synergistic in nature. In antagonism the effects of one drug are reduced or abolished by the second drug, and in synergism the effects may be additive or potentiative in nature, which may be harmful or useful to the patient in a particular disease.

The clinically established drug interactions can be minimized to some extent by the avoidance of combined drug therapy, which are proven to be incompatible.

But, in certain cases, the single drug is effective only to a certain degree or stage of disease condition. The multiple/combined drug therapy is required in many medical and dental conditions.

- To produce a desired pharmacodynamic/ therapeutic effect which is not obtained by single drug, e.g. in the treatment of hypertension, a single drug is effective only in very low percentage of patients. Likewise, in the treatment of heart failure, a combined therapy of diuretic with vasodilator and/or cardiac glycoside has to be given to achieve a adequate cardiac output and control over edema. Multiple drug therapy also required in chemotherapy of cancer, tuberculosis and certain infectious diseases.
- To minimize the side effects of drugs e.g. to supplement potassium by giving potassium sparing diuretic with digitalis.

The use of combined drug therapy can not be avoided in certain cases to attain a desired therapeutic level, but the risk of incompatibility/interactions involved in the treatment increases.

The drug interactions may be divided into:

i. *Pharmacokinetic,* which occur at the level of absorption, distribution, metabolism and excretion of one drug by another.
ii. *Pharmacodynamic,* which occur at the site of drug action involving the receptors.

Table 1.7.1: *Drug interactions at the sites of absorption.*

i.	**Interaction due to the formation of chelate complex**		
	Antacids	Tetracycline, isoniazid, atenolol, chlorpromazine penicillamine, digoxin, ranitidine	Decreased absorption
	Antacids	Bishydroxycoumarin	Increased absorption
	Cholestyramine	Warfarin, phenylbutazone, digitoxin, cephalexin and chlorothiazide	Decreased absorption
	Activated charcoal	Tolbutamide, theophylline, phenytoin, digoxin, carbamazepine, valproate	Decreased absorption
	Activated charcoal	Piroxicam, theophylline & phenobarbital	Increased absorption
	Mineral oils	Fat soluble vitamins	Decreased absorption
	Iron preparation	Methyldopa	Decreased absorption
ii.	**Interaction due to the alteration in gastric pH**		
	Antacids	Cimetidine	Decreased absorption
	Cimetidine	Tetracycline	Decreased absorption
iii.	**Interaction due to increase in gastric motility**		
	Metoclopramide	Digoxin, cimetidine	Decreased absorption
	Metoclopramide	Chlorothiazide, acetaminophen	Increased rate of absorption
iv.	**Interaction due to decrease in gastric motility**		
	Antacids	Isoniazid, phenytoin, propranolol and benzodiazepines	Decreased rate of absorption
	Amitriptyline	Bishydroxycoumarin	Increased absorption
v.	**Interaction due to alteration of gut**		
	Cimetidine	Lidocaine, propranolol, verapamil, imipramine	Increased absorption

PHARMACOKINETIC INTERACTIONS

The drug may interact with the another drug at any point during their absorption, distribution, metabolism and excretion.

Drug Interactions Involving Absorption

Important drug interactions include antacids which contain calcium, magnesium or aluminium that interfere with absorption of tetracycline by forming a 'chelate' with the metals; carbonates prevent absorption of iron; cholestyramine interferes with the absorption of certain drugs like warfarin, thyroxine and digitalis glycosides.

Some important drug interactions at the site of absorption are shown in table 1.7.1.

Drug Interactions Involving Distribution

After absorbed into blood many drugs are bound to plasma proteins, the portion of the drug which is being transported in the bound form is inactive (pharmacologically) and only the free part or molecule that diffuse into the tissues produce their effect.

The most important drug interaction caused by displacement from plasma proteins occur with coumarin anticoagulants. Phenylbutazone displaces warfarin from its binding site thereby causing bleeding. Tolbutamide is displaced by dicumarol resulting in severe hypoglycemia (See table 1.7.2).

Drug Interactions During Metabolism

This type of interaction occurs when the metabolism of a drug is inhibited or decreased by another drug.

Certain drugs induce the hepatic microsomal enzyme system i.e. enzyme induction, which decreases the effectiveness of other drugs, for example, if phenobarbital is suddenly discontinued without lowering the dosage of coumarin, severe hemorrhage can occur.

Some important drug interactions during metabolism are shown in table 1.7.3 & 1.7.4.

Drug Interaction During Excretion

The renal drug clearance is influenced by alterations in glomerular filtration rate and tubular reabsorption or secretion rate.

The tubular secretion of penicillin is inhibited by probenecid, so that the blood concentration and its half life (therapeutic effects) is prolonged with the simultaneous use of these two drugs. Phenylbutazone can block the renal tubular reabsorption of uric acid, leading to uricosuria.

Quinidine inhibits the tubular secretion of digoxin which consequently raises the plasma digoxin concentration, which may be associated with toxicity. Certain other drugs also increase the digoxin concentration like verapamil, amiodarone, spironolactone etc.

Table 1.7.2: *Interactions caused by displacement of drugs from plasma protein binding sites.*

Drug displaced	Displacing agent
Coumarin	Diazoxide, ethacrynic acid, phenylbutazone, NSAIDs
Tolbutamide	Dicumarol, phenylbutazone
Phenytoin	Tolbutamide, NSAIDs
Diazepam	Heparin

NSAIDs = Nonsteroidal antiinflammatory drugs.

Table 1.7.3: *Drugs that induce the metabolism.*

Drug (inducing part)	Drug induced
Chloral hydrate	Bishydroxycoumarin
Phenobarbital	Bishydroxycoumarin, digitoxin, phenylbutazone, phenytoin
Phenytoin	Carbamazepine, cimetidine, theophylline, oral

Table 1.7.4: *Drugs inhibit the metabolism of other drugs.*

Drug causing inhibition	Drug inhibited
Bishydroxycoumarin	Tolbutamide
Disulfiram	Phenytoin, theophylline, warfarin
Isoniazid	Phenytoin
Phenylbutazone	Tolbutamide, phenytoin

Ammonium chloride increases urinary volume with acidification of urine. The excretion of amphetamine is decreased in relatively alkaline urine and has proved useful in 'the treatment of amphetamine intoxication'.

PHARMACODYNAMIC INTERACTIONS

Pharmacodynamic interactions take place at the site of drug action. When two or more drugs with similar pharmacological effects are administered together, an additive or synergistic effect is usually seen.

These type of interactions are of two types:

The ***direct pharmacodynamic interactions*** occur when two drugs either act on the same site or on two different sites with a similar effect.

When two drugs act on same site, they are either antagonist or synergist. For example:

Antagonism: Reversal of the effect of opiates with naloxone.

Reversal of anticholinergic effects with tricyclic antidepressants and physostigmine.

Synergism: Increased anticoagulation of warfarin with clofibrate, corticosteroids, tetracycline, vitamin K and naloxone.

Arrhythmias with the use of b-adrenoreceptor antagonists and verapamil together.

The ***indirect pharmacodynamic interactions*** are unrelated to the effects of the object drug, for example:

- Drugs which alter potassium content may have effect on the therapeutic effect of cardiac glycosides, which are enhanced by potassium depletion e.g., potassium-sparing diuretics, corticosteroids and purgatives.
- Diuretics like frusemide may attenuate the effects of oral hypoglycemic drugs.
- Drugs like salicylates, dipyridamole, phenylbutazone decrease the ability of platelets to aggregate, and thus impairing the haemostasis if warfarin induced bleeding occurs.
- The nonsteroidal antiinflammatory drugs like aspirin, indomethacin and phenylbutazone causes ulceration in gastro-intestinal tract which provides a site for bleeding in patients on anticoagulants.

The pharmacodynamic interactions are relatively common in practice, but they can be minimized if the interactions are anticipated and appropriate precautions are taken by avoiding irrational and unnecessary drugs combination.

Table 1.7.5: *Some clinically important drug interactions.*

Drug affected	Drug interacting	Effect
Gastrointestinal system		
Carbenoxolone	Amiloride, spironolactone	Inhibition of ulcer healing.
Cimetidine	Antacids	Reduced absorption if taken simultaneously.
Metoclopramide	Anticholinergic drugs such as atropine, benzhexol, propantheline, narcotic analgesics	Antagonism – they have opposing effects on gastrointestinal activity.
Cardiovascular system		
Antiarrhythmic drugs	Any combination of two or more	Increased myocardial depression.
Disopyramide	Potassium salts, amiodarone	Hyperkalaemia, increased risk of ventricular arrhythmias due to prolongation of QT interval.

Contd.....

Drug affected	Drug interacting	Effect
Lignocaine, mexiletine, tocainide.	Diuretics: Bumetanide, ethacrynic acid, frusemide, thiazides	Antagonised by hypokalaemia.
Lignocaine	Cimetidine, propranolol	Increased risk of lignocaine toxicity.
Verapamil	Beta-adrenoceptor blocking drugs	Asystole, hypotension.
Digoxin & other cardiac glycosides	Diuretics: Bumetanide, ethacrynic acid, furosemide, thiazides	Increased toxicity.
	Cholestyramine, colestipol	Reduced absorption.
	Phenobarbitone, rifampicin	Inhibition (Digitoxin only)
Digoxin	Amiodarone, quinidine, quinine	Potentiation may occur.
	Nifedipine, verapamil	Potentiation may occur.
Diuretics	Indomethacin	Antagonism.
	Carbenoxolone, corticosteroids, corticotrophin, estrogens	Hypokalaemia.
Aldosterone antagonists: Amiloride, triamterene	Captopril, potassium supplements, trilostane	Hyperkalaemia.
Heparin	Aspirin, dipyridamole.	Potentiation.
Adrenaline, noradrenaline	Beta-adrenoceptor blocking drugs	Potentiation of hypertensive effect.
Respiratory system		
Theophylline	Cimetidine, erythromycin, influenza vaccine, oral contraceptives	Potentiation.
	Carbamazepine, phenytoin, rifampicin, sulphinpyrazone	Plasma concentration of theophylline may be reduced.
Antihypertensive drugs		
Captopril	Antiinflammatory analgesics such as indomethacin, phenylbutazone, corticotrophin, estrogens, oral contraceptives	Reduced effects.
	Alcohol, antidepressants, hypnotics, sedatives, tranquillizers, fenfluramine, levodopa, vasodilators such as nitrates, nifedipine, verapamil	Potentiation.
	Potassium supplements, potassium sparing diuretics.	Hyperkalaemia.
Clonidine	Beta-adrenoceptor blocking drugs	Increased risk of clonidine withdrawal hypertension.
	Tricyclic antidepressant	Antagonism.
Beta-adrenoceptor blocking drugs	Indomethacin	Antagonism of antihypertensive effect.
	Nifedipine	Severe hypotension and heart failure occasionally.
	Sympathomimetic amines such as adrenaline, amphetamines, phenylephrine	Severe hypertension reported.
Labetalol	Cimetidine	Potentiation possible because of reduced metabolism.

Contd.....

Drug affected	Drug interacting	Effect
Infections		
Aminoglycosides e.g. gentamycin etc.	Ethacrynic acid, furosemide, skeletal muscle relaxants	Increased ototoxicity, increased neuromuscular blockade.
Cephalosporins	Ethacrynic acid, furosemide, gentamycin	Increased nephrotoxicity.
Chloramphenicol	Phenobarbitone	Reduced plasma concentration of chloramphenicol & increased levels of phenobarbitone.
Dapsone	Probenecid	Reduced excretion: Increased side effects.
Griseofulvin	Phenobarbitone	Impairs absorption.
Ketoconazole	Antacids, anticholinergic drugs, cimetidine, ranitidine	Decreased absorption.
Metronidazole	Alcohol	'Antabuse' reaction.
Tetracycline	Antacids, dairy products, oral iron, sucralfate, zinc sulphate	Reduced absorption.
Malignant disease & immunosuppression		
Azathioprine mercaptopurine	Allopurinol	Potentiation: Increased toxicity.
Cyclosporin	Ketoconazole	Increased plasma concentration of cyclosporin.
Methotrexate	Aspirin, phenylbutazone, probenecid	Delayed excretion: Increased toxicity.
	Antiepileptics, cotrimoxazole, pyrimethamine	Increased anti-folate effect.
Central nervous system		
A. *Analgesics*		
Aspirin	Metoclopramide	Potentiation.
Ketoprofen, naproxen	Probenecid	Increased plasma concentration.
Paracetamol	Cholestyramine, metoclopramide	Reduced absorption.
B. *Antiepileptics*		
General	Tricyclic antidepressants, oral contraceptives	Increased seizure activity.
Carbamazepine	Cimetidine, dextropropoxyphene, erythromycin, isoniazid	Potentiation.
Ethosuximide	Carbamazepine	Reduced plasma concentration of ethosuximide.
Phenobarbitone, primidone	Phenytoin, sodium valproate	Increased sedation, increased blood levels of phenobarbitone.

Contd.....

Drug affected	Drug interacting	Effect
C. *Psychotropic drugs*		
Hypnotics & sedatives	Alcohol, antidepressants, antihistaminics, narcotic analgesics	Potentiation.
Tricyclic anti-depressants	Alcohol	Potentiation of sedative effect.
	Oral contraceptives	Reduced effect.
	Phenothiazine derivatives	Increased side effects.
Imipramine	Cimetidine	Potentiation.
Lithium	Diuretics, diclofenac, indomethacin, phenylbutazone	Potentiation.
	Acetazolamide, aminophylline, sodium bicarbonate	Increased lithium excretion.
	Haloperidol	Increased risk of extra pyramidal effects.
Endocrine system		
Antidiabetic drugs	Alcohol	Antabuse like reaction.
	Beta-adrenoceptor blocking drugs, MAO inhibitors	Potentiation.
	Corticosteroids, corticotrophin, diazoxide, diuretics (bumetanide, furosemide, thiazides), oral contraceptives	Antagonism.
Metformin	Alcohol	Increased risk of lactic acidosis.
Corticosteroids, corticotrophin	Diuretics (bumetanide, ethacrynic acid, furosemide, thiazides)	Increased potassium loss.
Cortisone, dexamethasone, hydrocortisone, prednisolone, prednisone.	Barbiturates, carbamazepine, phenytoin, primidone, rifampicin	Reduced effect.
Gynaecology		
Oral contraceptives	Barbiturates, carbamazepine, dichloralphenazone, phenytoin, primidone, rifampicin.	Reduced effect.
	Oral antibiotics such as ampicillin, tetracycline	Reduced effect.

❑❑❑

Section 2

Drugs Acting on CNS

CHAPTER 2.1 General Anaesthetics

General anaesthetics are the group of drugs which bring about a reversible loss of pain sensation and consciousness. The depth of anaesthesia appropriate for the conduct of surgical procedures can be achieved by a wide variety of drugs, either alone or by a combination of drugs, each drug for a specific purpose. General anaesthetics can be administered by a variety of routes, but intra-venous or inhalation administration is preferred, because the effective dose and the time course of action are more predictable when these techniques are used.

The general anaesthetics are divided into two main groups (table 2.1.1).

Inhalational Anaesthetics

NITROUS OXIDE (N_2O)

It is a colourless, odourless, noninflammable gas which is approx. 1½ times heavier than air. It is non-irritating with a sweet taste.

Nitrous oxide is used for induction and maintenance of anaesthesia. It is widely used as carrier gas for other volatile agents in general anaesthesia. The usual concentration used is 70 percent N_2O + 30 percent O_2 along with some muscle relaxants or other potent anaesthetics. Nitrous oxide, if administered along with air, it produces a stage of excitement and delirium and also produce amnesia. Hence, the name 'laughing gas.'

It is eliminated unchanged from the body, via the lungs. Despite its high fat solubility, it is rapidly eliminated through lungs within 2 to 5 minutes after its withdrawal.

Nitrous oxide, due to its analgesic action in subanaesthetic concentration, is **employed for** minor operation like tooth extraction, for obstetrical analysis, painful procedures such as changing dressing of burns. It is cheap and very commonly used.

Prolonged administration of nitrous oxide as in cases of tetanus, **may cause** bone marrow depression and agranulocytosis.

CYCLOPROPANE

It is a colourless gas with sweet odour and taste, available as liquid under pressure. It produces analgesia without loss of consciousness in 1 to 2 percent concentration, in 6 to 8 percent it produces loss of consciousness while

Table 2.1.1: *Classification of general anaesthetics.*

I.	**Inhalational anaesthetics**	
i.	***Gases***	
	Nitrous oxide	70-80% with other agents
	Cyclopropane	5-25%
ii.	***Volatile liquids***	
	Ether (Diethyl ether)	3-10%
	Trichloroethylene (TRILENE)	0.25-0.75%
	Halothane (FLUOTHANE)	0.5-2.0%
	Methoxyflurane (PENTHRANE)	0.1-0.3%
	Enflurane (ETHRANE)	1-3.0%
	Isoflurane (FORANE)	0.8-2.0%
II.	**Intravenous anaesthetics**	
i.	***Ultra short acting barbiturates***	
	Hexobarbitone (sodium salt)	
	Thiopentone sodium	3-5 mg/kg as 2.5% solution
	Methohexitone sodium (BREVITAL)	1-3 mg/kg as 1% solution
ii.	***Non-barbiturate intravenous anaesthetics***	
	Propanidid (EPONTOL)	5-10 mg/kg as 5% solution
	Ketamine (KETMIN)	2 mg/kg IV, 6.5-13 mg/kg IM
	Droperidol (INNOVER) + Fentanyl	Droperidol 2.5 mg + fentanyl 0.05 mg/ml; 4-6 ml is diluted in glucose solution and infused over 10 min
	Diazepam (CALMPOSE)	0.2-0.4 mg/kg slow IV
	Lorazepam (ATIVAN)	0.05-0.1 mg/kg slow IV
	Midazolam	0.05-0.1 mg/kg slow IV

20 to 25 percent is required to produce surgical anaesthesia. It has a low blood solubility. The induction and recovery are rapid and smooth. Blood pressure and cardiac contractility are well maintained with cyclopropane even on prolonged administration. Muscle relaxant activity is fairly good. Because of its highly inflammable and explosive nature, the close circuit has to be used to conserve the drug and to keep its concentration in the operating room low.

Because of its smooth induction and non-irritant to the respiratory passage, **the danger of overdosage must be watched for**. Cyclopropane also sensitizes the myocardium to adrenaline and may produce a variety of cardiac irregularities such as tachycardia and fibrillation. That is the reason for avoiding cyclopropane anaesthesia in pheochromocytoma and thyrotoxicosis. Cyclopropane shock (in patients with sepsis) is another drawback, which produces a sudden fall of blood pressure with collapse.

VOLATILE LIQUIDS

ETHER (DIETHYL ETHER)

It is a colourless, volatile liquid with a pungent odour and produces irritating vapours which are inflammable and explosive. It is one of the first substances to be employed for general anaesthesia. It is a potent agent and produces full anaesthesia when inhaled in low concentration. A concentration of 10 to 15% in the inspired air is usually required for induction. It produces prolonged and unpleasant induction with salivation and marked respiratory secretions. For this atropine must be given prior to anaesthesia for inhibition of these secretions.

Respiration and blood pressure are generally well maintained because of reflex stimulation and high sympathetic tone.

Because of its slow induction and recovery, irritant property and other disadvantages ether is rarely used these days and may be occasionally used as a supplement to nitrous oxide-oxygen mixture in children.

TRICHLOROETHYLENE

It is a clear, colourless liquid with a characteristic odour but a blue dye is added for distinction from chloroform. It is a potent analgesic with a rapid onset of action but muscular relaxation with this agent is inadequate. Induction and recovery are slow.

It may **produce** tachypnoea and bradycardia and sensitizes the myocardium to adrenaline and cardiac arrhythmias can occur probably due to hypoxic release of adrenaline.

Now-a-days, it is occasionally used in obstetrics, burns dressings etc. as a self medication analgesic.

HALOTHANE

It is a volatile liquid, non-irritant and non-inflammable. It is most widely used volatile anaesthetic due to its smooth and rapid induction. It inhibits laryngeal and pharyngeal reflexes in upper planes of surgical anaesthesia.

Halothane **causes relatively greater depression of respiration**. It inhibits intestinal and uterine contractions. Cardiac output is also reduced by 20 to 50 percent when anaesthesia is induced by inspiration of halothane at 0.8 to 1.2 percent concentration, which is necessary for surgical anaesthesia. Heart rate is slowed during anaesthesia, tachyarrhythmias may also occur in the presence of halothane.

Halothane causes dose-dependent reductions of renal blood flow and glomerular filtration rate as a result of fall in blood pressure.

Hepatitis occurs in susceptible individuals with repeated use.

It causes decrease in uterine muscle tone.

Elimination of halothane may continue for 24 to 48 hours after prolonged administration. Recovery is smooth and reasonably quick. It is currently one of the most popular anaesthetic used due to its non-irritant, non-inflammable, pleasant and rapid action.

ENFLURANE

It is a clear, colourless, noninflammable liquid with a mild, sweet odour and considered to be a useful alternative to halothane. Induction of anaesthesia, appropriate for surgery may be achieved within 10 minutes after approximately 4 percent enflurane in inhaled. Arterial blood pressure decreases progressively as the depth of anaesthesia is increased with enflurane, about the same degree as it does with halothane inhalation. The anaesthesia produces rapid induction with quick recovery.

Enflurane can be used for prolonged operations such as cholecystectomy and other abdominal surgery which requires profound muscular relaxation. It stimulates salivary and respiratory secretions. Uterine relaxation is similar to halothane.

No unusual effect on the gastrointestinal tract has been reported with enflurane anaesthesia, however, certain evidence of hepatic impairment has been obtained during and after surgical anaesthesia. Hepatic necrosis probably occurs with enflurane in rare instances.

Heart rate decreases little and reduction of cardiac output is less marked. Fall in blood pressure is similar to that caused by halothane, arrhythmias are rare.

ISOFLURANE

It is a isomer of enflurane and its chemical and physical properties are similar to enflurane, but it is approximately 1½ times more potent, more volatile. It has a lower blood: gas solubility coefficient than enflurane. It produces rapid induction and recovery.

Systemic arterial blood pressure decreases progressively with increasing depth of anaesthesia with isoflurane. It also increases heart rate but arrhythmias are not precipitated. Isoflurane depresses respiration as concentration is increased. Uterine and skeletal muscle relaxation is similar to enflurane.

During anaesthesia, depression of renal blood flow, decrease in rate of glomerular filtration and urinary flow are reported but these changes are rapidly reversed during recovery.

METHOXYFLURANE

It is a clear, colourless liquid with a sweet and fruity odour. It is noninflammable and non-explosive in air or oxygen in anaesthetic concentrations. It is the **most potent inhalational anaesthetic** which has a good analgesic and muscle relaxant properties. Renal blood flow, glomerular filtration rate and urine flow are reduced as with the halothane.

It also **produces the respiratory** and **cardiovascular depression** as with halothane but bradycardia is more prominent.

Methoxyflurane damages renal tubules leading to inability to concentrate urine and uraemia. Because of its renal toxicity, it should not be used to achieve profound anaesthesia nor for prolonged periods of time.

This agent is **used** due to certain advantages i.e. it provides profound analgesia and good relaxation of skeletal muscles, uterine contractions are not inhibited and postoperative nausea and vomiting are not troublesome. But, due to its renal toxicity, its use as a general anaesthetic is limited.

DESFLURANE

It is a noninflammable, non-irritant agent and chemically related to ether. Induction with this agent is smooth and rapid. The respiratory, hemodynamic and other changes caused by desflurane are similar to those of isoflurane. This agent is undergoing clinical trial.

SEVOFLURANE

This is also a new compound and undergoing clinical trial. It is noninflammable, non-irritant agent. It produces more rapid induction and termination of anaesthesia than observed with other inhalational agents. The respiratory and circulatory effects of sevoflurane resemble those of isoflurane.

INTRAVENOUS ANAESTHETICS

Intravenous anaesthetics are mainly used for rapid induction of anaesthesia, which is then maintained by an inhalational agent. They also serve to reduce the amount of maintenance anaesthetics.

In this section the agents having anaesthetic properties will be discussed. More details of each class of drug and their uses in other circumstances are presented elsewhere.

BARBITURATES

THIOPENTONE SODIUM

It is an ultra short acting thiobarbiturate. The sodium salts are highly soluble in water yielding a very alkaline solution (pH 10.5 to 11), which must be prepared freshly before injection. Induction is generally smooth and takes approximately 10 to 30 seconds.

Thiopentone sodium is usually given as 92.5 percent solution, initially 100 to 150 mg over 10-15 seconds and repeated if necessary depending upon the patient's response after 20-30 seconds. On repeated administration the extracerebral sites are gradually filled up and lower doses produces anaesthesia which lasts longer.

Because of its poor analgesic property, the painful procedures should not be carried out under its influence unless an opioid or nitrous oxide has been given.

Thiopentone **depresses respiration transiently**. Blood pressure falls immediately after injection but recovers rapidly. It does not sensitize the myocardium to adrenaline.

Thiopentone also has been sometimes used for rapid control of convulsions.

Adverse effects include laryngospasm, which occurs generally when respiratory secretions or other irritants are present. Shivering and delirium may occur during recovery. Postoperative pain induces restlessness. Nausea and vomiting are uncommon. It can precipitate acute intermittent porphyria in susceptible individuals.

METHOHEXITONE SODIUM

It is preferred to thiopentone sodium for short procedures and out patients due to its rapid recovery. It is approximately three times more potent than thiopentone sodium with quicker and briefer action.

The only **disadvantages** associated with its use are that induction is less smooth, restlessness is more common, as is coughing and hiccup.

NON-BARBITURATE INTRAVENOUS ANAESTHETICS

PROPANIDID

It is an oily liquid eugenol derivative and less potent than thiopentone. It is a very short acting intravenous anaesthetic and specially used for very short outpatient operations and dental procedures.

Adverse effects include laryngospasm, high incidence of hypersensitivity reactions, tachycardia, respiratory depression and sometimes hypotension. Local irritation and thrombophlebitis occur due to the alkalinity of the solution. It is occasionally used as an alternative to thiopentone.

KETAMINE

It is a new non-barbiturate anaesthetic agent and pharmacologically related to phencyclidine, a hallucinogen. Intravenous ketamine produces unconsciousness and analgesia within 30 seconds. It can be given by intramuscular route also. It acts on the cerebral cortex and subcortical areas.

The drug increases the heart rate, cardiac output and blood pressure which is due to sympathetic stimulation. Respiration is not depressed, muscle tone increases and reflexes are not abolished during anaesthesia. Ketamine has been recommended for short operations, unpleasant therapeutic and diagnostic procedures in children, operation in shocked patients and in obstetrics.

Adverse reactions include delirium, hallucinations and unpleasant dreams. It should not be used in hypertensives and in patient with ischaemic heart disease.

FENTANYL-DROPERIDOL COMBINATION

Fentanyl is a potent short acting analgesic related to pethidine and belongs to group of 4-acyl-anilinopiperdines. Droperidol is a rapidly acting potent neuroleptic butyrophenone derivative related to haloperidol. In combination, these agents produce a state of 'neuroleptanalgesia.'

The fixed dose combination of fentanyl (0.05 mg) and droperidol (2.5 mg/ml), 4 to 6 ml is diluted in glucose solution and infused IV over 10 minutes.

Patient remains drowsy but conscious. Respiratory depression is marked and predictable. There is slight fall in blood pressure. Heart rate often decreases but myocardium is not sensitized to adrenaline.

It is **recommended** for endoscopies, angiographies, burn dressings etc.

DIAZEPAM

It may be **used** to produce light sedation and amnesia for unpleasant procedures by intravenous injection. It has also been used for induction and to supplement nitrous oxide anaesthesia. The benzodiazepines are further discussed in chapter 'Sedative and hypnotics' in detail.

ETOMIDATE

It is a new intravenous anaesthetic agent with poor analgesic property. It has a briefer duration of action than thiopentone. It produces little cardiovascular and respiratory depression. A single intravenous dose produces loss of consciousness within 10 seconds and a state of anaesthesia.

ALPHADONE

It is a slower acting steroid anaesthetic which is a combination of two preganedione derivatives, alphaxolone and alphadolone acetate. It produces analgesia and sleep lasting 20-30 minutes. It is less irritant, blood pressure and respiration are not much affected. It has been **used** as an inducing agent in place of thiopentone but due to hypersensitivity reactions its use is very limited.

Preanaesthetic Medication

Preanaesthetic medication refers to the use of drugs before the administration of an anaesthetic agent, which makes it more pleasant and safe to the patient

The **aims** of preanaesthetic medication are:

1. Reduce the anxiety and apprehension without producing much drowsiness.
2. To facilitate a smooth and rapid induction.
3. To relieve preoperative and postoperative pain or to supplement the analgesic action of anaesthetics.
4. To provide amnesia for preoperative and postoperative period.
5. To suppress respiratory and other secretions and vagal stimulation caused by anaesthetics.
6. To minimize certain undesirable effects produced by anaesthetic agents like bradycardia and vomiting.

To achieve all the objectives, a combination of 2 or 3 drugs is used depending on the need. The commonly employed drugs are opioids, sedative-hypnotics, antianxiety agents, anti-cholinergics, neuroleptics and antiemetics.

OPIOIDS

These are the most commonly used drugs. Morphine (10-15 mg IM), pethidine (50-100 mg IM) are frequently used drugs for their sedative and analgesic property. They reduce the anxiety and apprehension, produce pre- and postoperative analgesia, help in smooth induction. They also reduce the amount of anaesthetic required. However, they have certain **disadvantages**:

- They depress respiration.
- May cause fall in blood pressure during anaesthesia.
- Can precipitate asthma, as these drugs are histamine liberators.
- Pethidine may produce tachycardia by its vagolytic action.
- Morphine can interfere with pupillary signs of anaesthesia.

SEDATIVE-HYPNOTICS

The barbiturates like pentobarbitone, secobarbitone or butobarbitone (100 mg oral) have been used to provide sedation and to relieve apprehension before operation.

Non-barbiturate sedatives like chloral hydrate, paraldehyde and glutethimide may be used.

Promethazine (50 mg IM), an antihistaminic with sedative, antiemetic and anticholinergic properties is generally used in children as it causes little respiratory depression.

ANTIANXIETY DRUGS

The tranquillizers like benzodiazepines (diazepam 5-10 mg oral, or lorazepam 2 to 4 mg IM, IV are now preferred for preanaesthetic medication because they produce tranquillity, have better muscle relaxant property and smoothen induction. Other tranquillizer compounds include phenothiazines which possess sedative, antiemetic and antihistaminic properties. They can be given orally as well as parenterally.

ANTICHOLINERGICS

Atropine (0.06 mg IM, IV) or scopolamine is generally given in combination with morphine to block the vagal action so as to reduce the salivary and bronchial secretions.

They also prevent vagal bradycardia and hypotension during operation. Hyoscine produces amnesia and antiemetic effect also.

NEUROLEPTICS

Chlorpromazine (25 mg), triflupromazine (10 mg) or haloperidol (2-4 mg) IM are used as preanaesthetic medication. They reduce anxiety, emesis and help in smooth induction.

However, these compounds potentiate respiratory depression.

ANTIEMETICS

Droperidol and hydroxyzine (25-50 mg IM) is sometime used for their antiemetic activity. Hydroxyzine has antianxiety, antihistaminic and anticholinergic properties also.

❑❑❑

CHAPTER 2.2

Sedative & Hypnotics

Sedative (anxiolytic) are the agents which reduce anxiety and exert a calming effect with little or no effect on motor or mental functions.

Hypnotics are the drugs which produce drowsiness and encourage the onset and maintenance of sleep. They are classified into different categories (Table 2.2.1.)

BARBITURATES

Barbiturates are the derivatives of barbituric acid. They are general CNS depressants. They can cause sedation, hypnosis and general anaesthesia depending upon the particular barbiturates used and its dose.

Pharmacological Actions

CNS: Barbiturates produce depression of central nervous system in dose dependent manner. In small dose, barbiturates relieve anxiety and are generally used as sedative. In hypnotic dose, it produces sleep resembling normal physiological sleep. Hypnotic dose of barbiturates produce motor incoordination.

Pain: Barbiturates do not have any analgesic effect.

Anaesthesia: The ultra short acting barbiturates produce general anaesthesia (details are given in chapter 'General anaesthetics').

Anticonvulsant action: In anaesthetic dose all barbiturates e.g. phenobarbitone, mephobarbitone possess anticonvulsant action. Phenobarbitone is drug of choice for the treatment of grandmal epilepsy (details are given in chapter 'Antiepileptic drugs').

CVS: In hypnotic dose, hypotension and decrease in heart rate occurs. In toxic dose, there is a severe decrease in blood pressure due to ganglionic blockade.

Respiration: In higher dose, barbiturates depress the respiration. It depresses the sensitivity of respiratory centre to CO_2.

GIT: They depress the tone and motility of GIT, but thiobarbiturates may stimulate the intestinal smooth muscles.

Kidney: They directly depress the tubular reabsorption of sodium, reduce urine flow and increase ADH release.

Table 2.2.1: *Classification of sedative and hypnotics.*

I. **Barbiturates**	
Phenobarbitone (LUMINAL)	15-30 mg TDS (as sedative) 60-100 mg HS (as hypnotics)
Butobarbitone (SONERYL)	15-30 mg TDS, 100-200 mg HS
Pentobarbitone (NEMBUTAL)	30 mg TDS, 100 mg HS
Secobarbitone (LIPATON)	30 mg TDS, 100 mg HS
II. **Benzodiazepines**	
i. **Used as hypnotics**	
Diazepam (CALMPOSE)	5-10 mg HS
Nitrazepam (NITROSUN)	5-10 mg HS
Midazolam (FULSED)	0.02-0.1 mg/kg/hr IV infusion
ii. **Used as antianxiety agents**	
Diazepam (CALMPOSE)	2-10 mg BD-TDS
Chlordiazepoxide (LIBRIUM)	10-25 mg BD-TDS
Lorazepam (TRAPEX)	1-2 mg BD-TDS (oral/IM)
Alprazolam (ALPRAX)	0.5-4 mg/day
Oxazepam (SEREPAX)	15-30 mg OD-TDS
iii. **Used as antiepileptic agents**	
Diazepam	10-25 mg/day IM/IV
Clonazepam (CLONOTRIL)	0.5-4 mg TDS
III. **Newer nonbenzodiazepine compounds**	
Zopiclone (ZOPICON)	7.5 mg HS
Zolpidem (SOBRIUM)	10 mg HS
Zaleplon (ZAPLON)	10 mg HS

Liver: They induce microsomal drug metabolising enzyme thus they increase the rate of metabolism of number of drugs.

Pharmacokinetics

They are well absorbed from the GIT. They are widely distributed in body. Rate of entry into CNS is dependent on lipid solubility. Ultra short acting barbiturates are highly lipid soluble and quickly enter the brain. Redistribution to various tissues terminate their action and they are slowly released from the tissues and gradually metabolised in the liver. They are partly metabolised and partly excreted unchanged in urine.

Adverse Effects

Intolerance effects include headache, vomiting, diarrhoea, nausea.

Hangover especially with long acting barbiturates. Excitement and restlessness, neuralgic pain, allergic reactions include swelling and erythematous dermatitis. They produce physical dependent and have abuse potential.

Therapeutic Uses

- To produce hypnosis.
- To produce sedation.
- Anticonvulsant action: Phenobarbital is drug of choice.

- For general anaesthesia: Ultra short acting barbiturates are used.
- As preanaesthetic medication.
- As obstetrical analgesia.

Barbiturate Poisoning

It produces severe toxic manifestations. Either suicidal or accidental intake of toxic doses of barbiturates is characterized by depressed respiration, circulatory shock, pupils are initially constricted & then dilated due to asphyxia, hypothermia, renal failure and pulmonary complications such as acute pulmonary edema.

Treatment of Acute Barbiturate Poisoning

- Gastric lavage to remove unabsorbed drug. Emesis can be produced by apomorphine and activated charcoal is administered to adsorb the unabsorbed drug.
- Maintenance of respiration:
  - Oxygen inhalation.
  - Endotracheal intubation or tracheostomy.
  - Mechanical ventilation.
- Intravenous fluids.
- Forced diuresis: Diuretics like mannitol and furosemide can be used.
- Alkalinization.
- Prophylactic antimicrobial therapy to avoid any secondary infection e.g. pneumonia and infection due to tracheostomy or urinary catheterization.
- Dialysis (peritoneal or haemodialysis).

BENZODIAZEPINES

Benzodiazepines are commonly used anxiolytics in clinical practice because these agents exhibit good efficacy, are relatively safe and have minimum toxicity. They are indicated for short term relief of anxiety. Benzodiazepines have no action on respiration and cardiovascular system. They have no action on other body systems. They have a muscle relaxant action, probably due to CNS depressant action and have anticonvulsant action. They have lower abuse liability. Benzodiazepines when administered cause sedation, hypnosis, muscle relaxation, relieve anxiety and some have anticonvulsant action.

Benzodiazepines exert their pharmacological **effect mainly by potentiation of neural inhibition in CNS which is mediated by GABA**.

Pharmacokinetics

The pharmacokinetic profile is different with different compounds. Diazepam after oral administration is completely and rapidly absorbed from the proximal small intestine. Oxazepam is least rapidly absorbed while lorazepam is an intermediately absorbed between these two. They are metabolised in liver by dealkylation and hydroxylation and excreted in urine as glucuronide conjugates. They cross the placental barrier and are secreted in milk.

Adverse Reactions

The common side effects are drowsiness, lethargy, ataxia. They also cause behavioural changes and dose dependent impairment of visual motor coordination. Other side effects which occur rarely are vertigo, headache, allergy, photosensitization, leucopenia, impaired sexual function and menstrual irregularities.

Therapeutic Uses

- As antianxiety agent.
- As hypnotic.
- As anticonvulsant.
- As preanaesthetic medication.

DIAZEPAM

Being highly lipophilic it is quickly absorbed from the gastrointestinal tract. The kinetics of redistribution of diazepam is complicated by enterohepatic circulation. Initially there is high concentration in CNS after intravenous injection, then due to redistribution of drug the concentration starts falling in brain. It has a plasma half life of more than 20 hours. Diazepam is metabolised in liver to pharmacologically active metabolite, desmethyldiazepam which has a long plasma half life (80 hrs). It crosses the placental barrier and when given before labour may cause hypotonia and mild respiratory depression in neonates.

It is **indicated** as hypnotic, in anxiety, tension, muscle spasm, psychosomatic and behaviour disorders, dysmenorrhoea, cerebral palsy, upper motor neuron spasticity, sedative for surgical procedures, labour, tetanus, eclampsia and epilepsy.

LORAZEPAM

It provides prompt relief from a variety of symptoms associated with anxiety and in anxiety associated with depression.

It is readily absorbed when given orally. Peak concentrations in plasma occur approximately 2 hours following administration. The halflife of unconjugated lorazepam in human plasma is approximately 12 to 16 hours. At clinically relevant concentration, lorazepam is approximately 90 percent bound to plasma proteins. It is conjugated to inactive glucuronide metabolite and is excreted in urine.

The most frequent **adverse reactions** reported are sedation, followed by dizziness, weakness and unsteadiness. Less frequent adverse reactions include disorientation, depression, nausea, change in appetite, headache, sleep disturbance, agitation, dermatological symptoms including very serious reactions, eye-function disturbance, together with various gastrointestinal symptoms and autonomic manifestations. The incidence of sedation and unsteadiness increases with age.

It is **used** in anxiety disorders or anxiety associated with depressive symptoms, as pre-surgical medication.

OXAZEPAM

It is **used** in tension, anxiety disorders, anxiety associated with alcohol withdrawal, agitation and irritability in older patients and psychoneurosis.

Adverse effects include sedation, vertigo, dizziness, disorientation, blurred vision and dependence.

MIDAZOLAM

Midazolam is a new, short acting benzodiazepine with sedative properties, twice as potent as diazepam. It is also used as an anaesthetic inducing agent.

The mechanism of action of midazolam though not clearly understood is probably similar to other benzodiazepines i.e. **through interference with GABA reuptake**. It has a relatively high affinity for benzodiazepine receptors.

It is rapidly absorbed following intramuscular administration with more than 90 percent bioavailability.

Adverse effects include local effects like redness and phlebitis, apnoea (usually seen on IV administration). Rarely nausea, vomiting, headache, drowsiness, hiccups and retrograde amnesia may occur.

It is **indicated** for preoperative sedation, conscious sedation prior to short diagnostic or endoscopic procedures, induction of general anaesthesia prior to administration of other anaesthetic agents.

ALPRAZOLAM

CNS agents of the 1,4 benzodiazepine class presumably exert their effects by binding at stereo specific receptors at several sites within the central nervous system (CNS). Alprazolam like other benzodiazepines **exerts its anxiolytic action by potentiating GABA activity**. GABA is a neurotransmitter which inhibits the CNS activity. Alprazolam acts preferentially in midbrain, ascending reticular formation (which maintains wakefulness) and on limbic system (thought and mental functions).

The pharmacological effects of alprazolam do not differ appreciably from those of diazepam. However, alprazolam is about 10 times more potent than diazepam.

Following oral administration, alprazolam is readily absorbed. Peak concentration in the plasma occur in one to two hours following administration. Alprazolam and its metabolites are excreted primarily in the urine. Alprazolam is 80% bound to plasma proteins.

Alprazolam has **caused** a lower incidence of drowsiness, light-headedness and depression than diazepam. Alprazolam, like other benzodiazepines, has the potential for the development of tolerance and withdrawal symptoms, although the incidence is lower than that seen with other benzodiazepines. Alprazolam's potential for drug dependence is less in comparison to other benzodiazepines.

It is **used** in the management of generalised anxiety disorder or the short term relief of symptoms of anxiety. It is also indicated for the treatment of panic disorders with or without agoraphobia.

CHLORDIAZEPOXIDE

It is the first benzodiazepine used clinically. **Adverse effects** include nausea, vertigo, headache and skin rash.

It is **indicated** in fear, anxiety, tension, pre and postoperative apprehension behavioural disorders, insomnia and emotional disturbances.

CLONAZEPAM

It **acts by enhancing GABA induced increase in conductance of chloride in neurons**.

After oral administration, over 80 percent of clonazepam is absorbed. It is extensively bound to plasma proteins and is widely distributed. It is metabolised and the metabolites are excreted in urine.

Adverse effects include impaired alertness, amnesia, drowsiness, lethargy, respiratory depression, salivary and bronchial hypersecretion in infants, behavioural problems, muscle weakness, vertigo, ataxia and dizziness.

It is **indicated** in typical and atypical absence seizure, infantile spasms, myoclonic epilepsy, atonic seizures, minor motor seizures of childhood, refractory grandmal epilepsy or temporal lobe epilepsy and seizures not controlled by conventional antiepileptics.

NEWER COMPOUNDS

ZOPICLONE

It is a novel hypnotic belonging to cyclopyrrolone derivative. It is useful in short term management of insomnia and has low abuse potential.

Zopiclone exhibits anticonvulsant, muscle relaxant and hypnosedative properties similar to benzodiazepines.

Zopiclone is rapidly absorbed after oral dosing. Its elimination half-life period is 3.5-6 hours. It is mainly excreted in urine.

Adverse effects include metallic or bitter after-taste, nausea, vomiting, allergic skin reaction, irritability, hallucinations, depression, amnesia and confusion.

It is **indicated** in treatment of transient, situational and chronic insomnia, insomnia secondary to psychiatric disorders.

ZOLPIDEM

Zolpidem is a non-benzodiazepine hypnotic of the imidazopyridine class. It is a $GABA_A$ receptor agonist selective for omega-1 receptor subunit.

Zolpidem is rapidly absorbed and has a quick onset of hypnotic action. Bioavailability is 70 percent following oral administration and the drug demonstrates linear kinetics in the therapeutic dose range. Peak plasma concentration is reached at 0.5 and 3 hours. The elimination half-life is short. It is 92% plasma protein bound and is metabolised in liver to inactive metabolites. It is eliminated in the urine and in the faeces.

Adverse effects include diarrhoea, nausea, vomiting, vertigo, dizziness, headache, drowsiness, nightmares, asthenia, memory disturbances, depression, confusion, diplopia, tremor and ataxia.

It is **indicated** in short term management of insomnia.

ZALEPLON

It is a nonbenzodiazepine hypnotic. Zaleplon interacts and **binds selectively to the brain omega-1 receptor situated on the alpha subunit of the $GABA_A$ receptor complex**.

It is rapidly and almost completely absorbed following oral administration. It undergoes significant presystemic metabolism, all the metabolites are pharmacologically inactive.

Adverse effects include dizziness, amnesia, headache, tremor, nausea, abdominal pain, dyspepsia, anorexia, eye pain, asthenia, malaise and myalgia.

It is **indicated** in short term management of insomnia.

❑❑❑

CHAPTER 2.3

Narcotic Analgesics (Opioids)

Analgesics are the drugs (natural or synthetic origin) which relieve pain by acting on CNS or peripheral pain mechanism without causing loss of consciousness. Dental pain is the initial sign of any dental disease which is usually acute in nature. In dentistry, non-steroidal anti-inflammator drugs (NSAID's) are commonly employed for dental pain and inflammation which may be due to caries, abscess tooth extraction or after any dental procedures. Analgesics can be divided into two main groups:

a. Opioid/narcotic/morphine like analgesics.
b. Nonopioid/nonnarcotic/aspirin like analgesics.

Drugs obtained from morphine are known as opioids or narcotic analgesics.

The opium is obtained from the opium poppy *Papaver somniferum.* It contains two type of alkaloids e.g. phenanthrene derivatives (morphine, codeine & thebaine) and benzyl isoquinoline derivatives (papaverine and noscapine).

The opioid analgesics are classified as in table 2.3.1.

NATURAL COMPOUNDS

MORPHINE

Opium is the milky exudate obtained by incising the unripe seed capsule of the poppy plant *Papaver somniferum* and morphine is the most important alkaloid of opium. Morphine produces analgesia through action in the brain and spinal cord, that contain peptides possessing opioid like pharmacological action. These endogenous substances are known as **endogenous opioid peptides** (earlier known as endorphin & now known as **β-endorphin**).

Morphine and other opioids exert their pharmacological actions by acting on different receptors namely mu (μ), kappa (κ) and delta (δ).

Analgesic, respiratory, depression as well as euphoria produced by morphine result mainly from action at mu receptors. Most of the currently available narcotic analgesics act primarily on the mu receptors.

Table 2.3.1: *Classification of narcotic analgesics.*

I. Natural alkaloids	
Morphine (as sulphate; MORCONTIN)	0.2-0.8 mg/kg BD, IM/SC
Codeine (as phosphate)	20-60 mg/day
II. Semisynthetic compounds	
Pholcodeine (ETHNINE)	10-30 mg/day
Diacetyl morphine (HEROIN)	3-5 mg/day IM/SC
Other semisynthetic agents are hydromorphone, oxymorphone, oxycodone, hydrocodone, dihydrocodeine etc.	
III. Synthetic compounds	
Pethidine (as hydrochloride)	50-100 mg/day IM/SC
Fentanyl (as citrate; FENDROP)	50-100 µg/day IM/IV
Methadone (PYSEPTONE)	5-10 mg/day oral/SC
Dextropropoxyphene (DEXOVON)	65-130 mg/day
Tramadol (TRANDOL)	50-100 mg BD-TDS
Ethoheptazine (EQUAGESIC)	75-150 mg/day
Newer compounds include sufentanil, alfentanil etc.	

Delta and kappa receptors can also contribute to analgesia, particularly at spinal level. Although morphine also acts on kappa and delta sites but it is not clear that up to what level they contribute in its analgesic action.

Pharmacological Actions

Effect on CNS: The main action of morphine is CNS depression which further results in analgesia, depression of respiratory centre, cough centre and sleep. In addition it causes euphoria or dysphoria and dependence.

Analgesia: Morphine produces analgesia by elevation of pain threshold, thereby reducing the perception of pain. It also altered psychic reaction to pain which may be associated with feeling of well being e.g. euphoria. It also produces lethargy and sleep, morphine relieves all types of pain, but dull constant pain is relieved more effectively than sharp intermittent pain and is very effective in visceral pain.

Morphine also produces a sense of anxiety, known as dysphoria. The morphine produces euphoria (which makes morphine as one of the main drugs of abuse) and analgesia by acting on higher centres and spinal cord.

On intrathecal injection, it acts on substantia gelatinosa of dorsal horn of spinal cord and inhibit the release of excitatory transmitters. At supraspinal sites, it acts on medulla, mid brain, limbic and cortical areas.

Action on eye: Morphine causes constriction of pupil (miosis) due to action on oculomotor nerve nucleus.

Action on respiration: Morphine depresses the medullary respiratory centre in medulla oblongata and by reducing the sensitivity of the medullary respiratory centre to increased plasma CO_2. The rise in arterial

CO_2 causes an increase in cerebrospinal fluid pressure.

Action on cough centre: Morphine suppresses cough reflexes, but cough suppression by opioids may allow accumulation of respiratory secretions and may produce airway obstruction.

Chemoreceptor trigger zone (CTZ): Morphine stimulates CTZ and produces nausea and vomiting. These effects are more marked in upright position due to vestibular involvement.

Vagal centre: Morphine stimulates the vagal centre and produces bradycardia.

Effect on GIT: It increases the tone of smooth muscle as well as sphincters but at the same time it decreases the propulsive movements and gastrointestinal secretions are diminished, the overall action is constipation.

Other smooth muscle: Morphine causes bronchoconstriction which is due to histamine release and may be dangerous in patients suffering from bronchial asthma.

Morphine also cause flushing and itching of skin due to histamine release.

Urinary system: Morphine causes spasm of detrusor as well as sphincters of urinary bladder and causes distension, urgency and difficulty in micturition.

Endocrine system: Morphine and other opioid analgesics stimulate the release of vasopressin and prolactin and inhibit the release of luteinizing hormone, ACTH and follicle stimulating hormone.

Metabolism: Morphine decreases the metabolic rate which can lead to decrease in body temperature. It also depresses temperature regulating centre.

Pharmacokinetics

Morphine orally is less effective and absorption is very slow. It has variable and high first pass metabolism when given by subcutaneous route, its analgesic effect starts within 10 minutes which persists for 4 to 5 hours and by IV route, it produces immediate action. In plasma, it binds to plasma proteins (approx. 30%). In liver it is metabolized by conjugation to glucuronic acid to form active and inactive products, which are excreted in urine. It is also excreted though bile and in the faeces.

Adverse Reactions

CNS side effects include confusion, anxiety, lethargy, nausea and vomiting. GIT related effect is constipation. Other side effects are urinary retention, dry mouth, miosis, dysphoria, hypotension, skin rash, itching and urticaria. Tolerance, drug dependence and drug abuse are the main drawbacks of morphine.

Acute Overdose/Toxicity (Morphine Poisoning)

It is characterised by respiratory depression, miosis, cyanosis, reduced body temperature, urinary retention, hypotension, pulmonary edema and coma.

The acute poisoning can be treated by:

- Maintenance of airway and oxygen inhalation. Maintenance of BP.
- Specific antagonists: Naloxone 0.4-0.8 mg IV; alternatively nalorphine (3-5 mg IV) can be given.

- Stomach lavage with potassium permanganate.
- Enhancing excretion of unabsorbed morphine from the intestine.
- Acidify the urine to enhance the renal excretion of morphine.

Contraindications

1. Head injury, because morphine can cause increase in intracranial tension, cause marked respiratory depression and certain physiological signs e.g. miosis and vomiting can interfere with the assessment of clinical progress.
2. Myxoedema patients are more sensitive to morphine.
3. Bronchial asthma: Morphine releases histamine which can trigger bronchoconstriction.
4. In liver damage chance of cumulative toxicity is more.
5. In elderly patients, chances of urinary retention are high.
6. In hypotensive states, more fall in blood pressure occurs due to morphine.

Therapeutic Uses

1. ***Analgesia***: Morphine is used in the following painful conditions:
   - In the treatment of any severe, constant pain.
   - Visceral pain e.g. myocardial infraction, pleurisy, vascular occlusion, renal and biliary colic.
   - Traumatic pain e.g. long bone fractures and burns.
   - Pain of terminal illness e.g. in cancer patients.
   - Postoperative pain.
   - Obstetrical analgesia.
2. In the suppression of cough and dyspnea (due to left ventricular failure and pulmonary edema).
3. For sedation.
4. In the treatment of diarrhoea.
5. As preanaesthetic medication.
6. In the treatment of acute left ventricular failure.
7. Use of opioids in dentistry is very limited.

CODEINE

It is a methyl ester of morphine and less potent analgesic than morphine. It is widely used as antitussive agent. **Pholcodeine** is also used as antitussive agent and causes less constipation (Details are given in chapter 'Drugs acting on respiratory system').

SYNTHETIC COMPOUNDS

PETHIDINE

Pethidine is predominantly a μ agonist and it exerts its action on the CNS and the neural elements in the bowel. In equianalgesic doses, pethidine produces as much sedation, respiratory depression and euphoria as does morphine. A few patients may experience dysphoria.

The analgesic effects of pethidine are detectable about 15 minutes after oral administration, reach a peak in about two hours and subside gradually over several hours. Pethidine is absorbed by all routes of administration, but the rate of absorption is erratic after IM injection. Pethidine crosses the placental barrier.

Pethidine is metabolized chiefly in the liver, to mainly meperidinic acid and minor metabolite norpethidine, which are conjugated with glucuronic acid and excreted in urine. Only a small amount of pethidine is excreted unchanged. Pethidine differs from morphine in that toxic doses sometimes cause CNS excitation, characterized by tremors, muscle twitches and seizures; these effect are largely due to norpethidine.

Adverse effects include nausea, vomiting, respiratory depression, dizziness, dysphoria, constipation, urinary retention. Tolerance develops to some of these effects and it has abuse potential.

It is mainly **indicated** for analgesia, as preanaesthetic medication, for epidural and intrathecal analgesia.

FENTANYL

It is a potent opioid analgesic. Chemically it is N-phenyl-N-propanamide. It interacts predominantly with opioid μ-receptor in human brain, spinal cord and other tissues. It exerts its principle pharmacologic effects on the CNS. It is 80-100 times more potent than morphine, both in analgesia and respiratory depression.

Adverse effects include respiratory depression (death from hypoventilation), dependence, apnoea, muscle rigidity, bradycardia, arrhythmia, chest pain, GI symptoms, haemoptysis, abdominal pain, headache, somnolence, confusion and hallucinations.

It is **indicated** as a narcotic analgesic supplement in general or regional anaesthesia, as an anaesthetic agent with oxygen and skeletal relaxant in selected high risk patients (e.g. open heart surgery).

METHADONE

It is synthetic compound having same or more analgesic activity than morphine. It's pharmacology and side effects are similar to that of morphine. It is **used** in the treatment of visceral pain and as an antitussive. It is also used as substitution therapy of opioid dependence.

DEXTROPROPOXYPHENE

It is dextro isomer of propoxyphene which is an analgesic and possesses antitussive property. It has low analgesic activity even half of codeine. It is metabolized in liver. **Side effects** include vomiting, epigastric distress and sedation. The demethylated metabolite of propoxyphene is cardiotoxic. It is **used** in the treatment of mild type of pain.

TRAMADOL

It is centrally acting synthetic analgesic compound that is not derived from natural sources nor is chemically related to opiates. It acts via opioid receptors in CNS to produce analgesia and has no abuse potential. It **also inhibits the reuptake of noradrenaline and serotonin**.

It causes less respiratory depression, sedation, constipation and urinary retention than morphine. Its hemodynamic effects are minimal.

Side effects include nausea, vomiting and dizziness.

It is **indicated** in moderate to severe, acute or chronic pain and in painful diagnostic procedures and surgery; arthralgia, dental pain, musculoskeletal pain, pain associated with fractures, dislocation and other related type of pain.

ETHOHEPTAZINE

It is orally active analgesic, similar to pethidine with low abuse potential. It is generally **used** in combination with nonsteroidal antiinflammatory drugs for mild to moderate type of pain.

Opioid Agonists/Antagonists

They are classified as in table 2.3.2.

PENTAZOCINE

It is **agonist-antagonist** of morphine and is used as an analgesic. It exerts morphine like action. It is a partial agonist at opioid receptors and is effective in mild to moderate type of pain associated with surgery, trauma, burns, colics, toothache, cancer, in labour and as preanaesthetic medication. It is kappa receptor agonist with weak mu antagonist or partial antagonist properties. It causes tachycardia and rise in BP due to sympathetic stimulation. Tolerance and dependence develops on repeated use. It is effective orally. It is oxidized and glucuronide conjugation occurs in liver and excreted in urine.

NALORPHINE

It is an N-allylnormorphine, semisynthetic congener of morphine. The agonistic actions are produced by kappa receptor activation and antagonistic properties are due to action on mu receptor which antagonizes all morphine actions (mainly reverses the analgesia and respiratory depression). It is **used** mainly in the treatment of acute morphine poisoning.

NALBUPHINE

It is a **strong kappa receptor agonist and mu receptor antagonist**. Its agonistic property is approximately three to four times more than pentazocine and its antagonistic property is approximately 10 times more than pentazocine. It has less abuse liability in comparison to pentazocine. It is **useful** in postoperative pain, myocardial infarction and labour.

BUPRENORPHINE

It is a potent and long acting opioid with **partial mu receptor agonist** property. 25 times more potent than morphine. Effects are similar to morphine but constipation is less marked. It undergoes extensive presystemic elimination and therefore is

Table 2.3.2: *Classification of opioid agonists and/or antagonists.*

I. **Agonists-antagonists**	
Pentazocine (PENTAWIN)	30-60 mg/day IM/SC (used as analgesic; 50-100 mg oral)
Nalorphine (LETHIDRONE)	2-5 mg IM/IV (not used as analgesic)
Nalbuphine	10-20 mg/day SC/IM/IV
The other compounds which are agonist-antagonist are levallorphan and cyclazocine which are not used as analgesics.	
II. **Partial/weak agonists**	
Buprenorphine (TIDIGESIC)	0.2-0.4 mg TDS SL, 0.3-0.6 mg/day IM/slow IV
Butorphanol	1-4 mg/day IM/IV
III. **Pure antagonists**	
Naloxone (NARCOTAN)	0.4-0.8 mg/day IM/IV
Naltrexone (NALTIMA)	50-100 mg/day
Nalmefene	0.1-1.0 mg/day IM/IV

given by parenteral route. It is excreted unchanged in urine. Side effects include dizziness, sedation, miosis, respiratory depression, sweating and vomiting.

It is **indicated** in moderate to severe pain, premedication to surgery, pain due to myocardial infarction and in postoperative pain.

BUTORPHANOL

It is a **kappa agonist**. It produces analgesia equivalent to nalbuphine and buprenorphine but produces more sedation.

It is **used** in postoperative pain and renal colic pain.

NALOXONE

It is N-allyl analogue of oxymorphone, have a **high affinity for mu receptor** and lower affinity at delta and kappa sites. It selectively antagonizes the respiratory depression produced by opioids. After intravenous administration, it antagonizes all actions of morphine. It also **blocks the actions of endogenous opioid peptides**.

It is inactive orally because of high first pass metabolism in liver. Metabolised by glucuronidation in liver. The main **use** of naloxone is in the treatment of acute opioid overdose (acute morphine poisoning). It also precipitates withdrawal syndrome when administered to morphine addicts. The constricted pupils of addicts dilate after administration of naloxone. This has been used as a diagnostic tool for opioid addiction.

NALTREXONE

It is a **pure antagonist** and chemically related to naloxone. It is more potent than naloxone and because of its longer duration of action, it can be **used** as maintenance drug for morphine addicts. It has no euphoric effect and no physical dependence liability. It is effective orally. It is also claimed to be beneficial in decreasing craving for alcohol in alcoholics. **Side effects** include gastrointestinal disturbances and muscular pain.

❑❑❑

CHAPTER 2.4

Non-Narcotic Analgesics (NSAID's)

Non-steroidal antiinflammatory drugs (NSAIDs) are also known as nonopioid analgesics. They relieve pain without interacting with opioid receptors and do not depress CNS and have no drug dependence or drug abuse property and possess antipyretic activity also. They act primarily on peripheral pain mechanisms and also in CNS to raise pain threshold.

They can be classified as in table 2.4.1.

NSAIDs exert analgesic, antipyretic, anti-inflammatory and related effects. During pain, fever and inflammation the arachidonic acid is liberated from the phospholipid fraction of the cell membrane which is then converted to prostaglandins (PGs) via cyclooxygenase pathway (both COX-1 & COX-2). COX-1 is present in kidney, stomach and blood vessels and COX-2 is present in activated leukocytes and other inflammatory cells.

SALICYLATES

Salicylates are esters or salts of salicylic acid. Acetyl salicylic acid (aspirin) is rapidly converted in the body to salicylic acid and produce the pharmacological actions.

Analgesic action: Salicylates relieve pain by both central and peripheral action. The site of action of central analgesia seems to be the hypothalamus. It does not have cortical action on the reaction component of the pain but raises the threshold to pain perception. Unlike morphine, they do not produce sedation and there is no drug tolerance or dependence and are not effective against visceral pain.

The peripheral component of their analgesic **action is due to the inhibition of prostaglandin synthetase and thereby inhibiting the synthesis of prostaglandins (PGs)** which sensitise the pain receptors to mechanical and chemical stimuli. Aspirin inhibits prostaglandin synthesis and blocks the sensitization of pain mechanism.

They are useful in relieving all dull itching, throbbing pain of muscles and joints, dysmenorrhoea, toothache, headache etc. The NSAID's are the mainstay for the management of acute dental pain.

Table 2.4.1: *Classification of non-steroidal antiinflammatory drugs.*

	Drug	Dose
I.	**Salicylates and their congeners**	
	Acetyl salicylic acid (ASPIRIN, DISPRIN)	300-600 mg/day
	Sodium salicylate	1.5-6 g/day
	Salicylamide (SALAMIDE)	300-600 mg TDS-QID
	Diflunisal (DOLOBID)	500 mg BD-TDS
II.	**Pyrazolone derivatives**	
	Phenylbutazone (ZOLANDIN)	200-600 mg/day
	Oxyphenbutazone (SIORIL)	200-600 mg/day
III.	**Indole derivatives**	
	Indomethacin (INDOCAP)	25-50 mg BD-TDS
	Sulindac (CLINORIL)	100-200 mg BD
IV.	**Propionic acid derivatives**	
	Ibuprofen (BRUFEN)	400-800 mg TDS
	Naproxen (NAPRYN)	250 mg BD
	Flurbiprofen (FROBEN)	50-100 mg TDS
V.	**Anthranilic acid derivatives**	
	Mefenamic acid (MEFTAL)	250-500 mg TDS
	Enfenamic acid (TROMARIL)	800 mg BD-TDS
VI.	**Oxicam derivatives**	
	Piroxicam (DOLONEX)	20 mg OD-BD
	Tenoxicam (TOBITIL)	20 mg OD
VII.	**Aryl acetic acid derivatives**	
	Diclofenac (VOVERAN)	50-150 mg BD-TDS, 25-75 mg IM
	Aceclofenac (ACECLO)	100-200 mg BD
VIII.	**Para-aminophenol derivatives**	
	Paracetamol (CROCIN)	0.5-1 g TDS
IX.	**Miscellaneous (newer compounds including selective COX-2 inhibitors)**	
	Nimesulide (NIMULID)	100 mg BD
	Ketorolac tromethamine (KETANOV)	40 mg/day (oral/IM)
	Celecoxib (ZYCEL)	100-200 mg OD-BD
	Nabumetone (NABUFLAM)	1-2 g/day
X.	**Drugs for rheumatoid arthritis**	
	Gold compounds (Auranofin; GOLDAR)	6 mg/day OD-BD
	d-Penicillamine (CILAMIN)	125-250 mg OD then 250 mg BD
	Sulfasalazine (SALAZOPYRIN)	1-3 g/day
	Methotrexate (FOLITRAX)	2.5-15 mg/week
XI.	**Drugs for gout**	
	Colchicine (COLCHICINDON)	0.25 mg to 10 mg (max.)/day
	Allopurinol (ZYLORIC)	200-800 mg/day
	Probenecid (BENCID)	500 mg-1 g BD
	Sulfinpyrazone (ARTIRAN)	200 mg BD (max 800 mg/day)

Combination of two drugs e.g., paracetamol + ibuprofen or diclofenac) also used for its additive effect.

Antipyretic action: Salicylates lower the elevated body temperature. Hypothalamic thermoregulatory centre acts as a thermostat of the body which maintains the balance between heat production and heat loss. Salicylates reset the hypothalamic thermostat which is disturbed during fever. They do not affect the heat production but they increase the heat loss by causing vasodilatation and sweating. The antipyretic action of salicylates is probably due to the inhibition of PG synthesis.

Effect on respiratory system: Salicylates stimulate respiration by increasing the consumption of oxygen primarily by skeletal muscles and this results in increased production of carbon dioxide, which leads to direct stimulation of the respiratory centre in the medulla oblongata producing an increase in the depth and to some extent in the rate of respiration. Toxic doses depress the respiratory centre.

Antiinflammatory and antirheumatic action: Salicylates suppress the clinical signs and symptoms of rheumatoid arthritis and other related inflammatory disorders by inhibiting prostaglandin synthesis, reducing the capillary permeability and inhibition of neutrophil aggregation. Salicylates by inhibiting the prostaglandin synthesis, prevent sensitization of the pain receptors to certain biological amines such as histamine, 5-HT (serotonin) and bradykinin, the chemical mediators of inflammation and pain.

Effect on kidney: In low doses, aspirin inhibits the tubular secretion of uric acid and can cause uric acid retention while in higher dose, it also inhibits tubular reabsorption of uric acid and have beneficial effect in gout by producing uricosuric action.

Acid-base and electrolyte balance: High therapeutic dose especially when used in rheumatic fever, stimulates respiration and causes respiratory alkalosis. Reduction in bicarbonate and potassium level reduces the buffering capacity of the extracellular and intracellular fluid. Hypokalemia may lead to dehydration and hypernatremia. They also interfere with carbohydrate metabolism resulting in accumulation of pyruvic acid and lactic acid.

Effect on GIT: Aspirin and related compounds irritate gastric mucosa which may cause epigastric distress, nausea and vomiting as a result of gastric irritation. The salicylates are unionised at the pH of the stomach and can easily enter the mucosal cell and at the pH of the cell they get ionised thus unable to cross it and accumulate inside the gastric mucosal cell and causing damage to the gastric mucosa and the damaged mucosa permits back flow of H^+ ions which may damage the endothelium of submucosal capillaries and gastric bleeding occurs.

Metabolic effects: Salicylates cause uncoupling of oxidative phosphorylation which leads to conversion of energy into heat and may thus produce hyperpyrexia and increased protein catabolism. Larger dose produces hyperglycemia and glycosuria in normal individual while in diabetic patient it produces hypoglycemia which may be due to an enhanced peripheral utilization of glucose and inhibition of neoglucogenesis induced by salicylates and related compounds. Chronic use can also lead to negative nitrogen balance by increased conversion of protein to carbohydrate.

Effect on blood: Platelets are the important factors in thrombus formation and aspirin has been shown to inhibit platelet aggregation. They reduce the blood prothrombin level by inhibition of prothrombin synthesis and prothrombin time is prolonged. The aspirin suppresses the synthesis of thromboxane (TXA_2) in the platelets. They also prolong the bleeding time due to prevention of platelet aggregation which may be due to inhibition of release of adenosine diphosphate (ADP) from the platelets by salicylates.

Effect of CVS: In therapeutic doses, aspirin has no direct effect on CVS but in larger doses, it can lead to increase in cardiac output to meet increased peripheral oxygen demand and can cause direct vasodilatation.

Endocrine effects: Salicylates decrease the plasma protein bound iodine due to displacement of thyroxine from prealbumin and stimulation of central sympathetic centre causes release of adrenaline from the adrenal medulla.

Pharmacokinetics

Salicylates are well absorbed after oral administration. They are absorbed from the stomach and largely from the upper part of small intestine. After oral administration, appreciable plasma concentrations are found within half an hour, peak plasma level is achieved within two hours and approximately 50 percent of the drug is eliminated within 24 hours and plasma half life is two to eight hours. After absorption, about 80 percent of salicylate is bound to plasma protein (mainly albumin) and rapidly distributed in the tissues. Aspirin is deacetylated to **salicylic acid** which is the major circulating and active form. Salicylates are mainly metabolized in the liver and excreted in urine in the form of conjugates with glycine (mainly) and glucuronic acid.

Adverse Effects

These include nausea, vomiting, gastric irritation and occult blood in stool.

Allergic reactions include urticaria, skin rash, rhinorrhoea, asthmatic attack and anaphylactic reactions.

Prolonged administration of salicylates cause a syndrome called 'salicylism' which is characterized by headache, dizziness, tinnitus, vertigo, difficulty in hearing, dimness of vision, mental confusion, drowsiness, lethargy, hyperventilation and electrolyte imbalance.

Overdose/acute salicylate **poisoning** is characterized by salicylism which consists of tinnitus, vertigo and deafness, hyperthermia, toxic encephalopathy (agitation, confusion and convulsions followed by coma), dehydration (due to hyperpyrexia, sweating and vomiting), disturbances of acid base balance and petechial haemorrhages.

Treatment of Overdose/Toxicity (Salicylate Poisoning)

i. Gastric lavage.
ii. Intravenous fluid to correct dehydration.
iii. Cold water/alcohol sponges for hyperthermia.

iv. To prevent intracellular potassium loss, potassium is given along with sodium bicarbonate.
v. For ketoacidosis and hypoglycemia, glucose may be given.
vi. In severe intoxication, dialysis (peritoneal dialysis and haemodialysis) may be used.

Therapeutic Uses

1. **In Dentistry:** The NSAID's are the most important drugs for the management of acute dental pain. The particular drug may be selected on the basis of severity of pain and presence of other related symptoms e.g. for mild to modrate pain, paracetamol is generally recommended and in accute pain diclofenac alone or combined with paracetamol is generally preferred. But care must be taken when given to patient who is having peptic ulcer, asthama or any hypersensitivty history.
2. **As analgesic-antipyretic:** Salicylates are effective in the treatment of mild to moderate types of pain. They are used in the treatment of headache, bodyache, arthralgias, neuralgias and dysmenorrhoea. They are also effective in fever of any origin.
3. **As an antiinflammatory:** Salicylates are commonly used in the treatment of various inflammatory conditions such as arthritis and fibromyositis.
4. **As antirheumatic:** Salicylates are the drug of choice in the treatment of rheumatoid arthritis. In larger dose they suppress the swelling, immobility and redness of the joints involved. They are also useful in the acute rheumatic fever. They produce relief in pain, swelling and morning stiffness in the rheumatoid arthritis patients.
5. **Treatment of gout:** In large dose, aspirin is effective in the treatment of gout.
6. **As antiplatelet agent:** By inhibiting platelet aggregation aspirin may lower the incidence of reinfarction. It has been used to prevent the formation of platelet-fibrin thrombus in ischemic heart disease patients.

Pyrazolone Derivatives

PHENYLBUTAZONE

It is a potent antiinflammatory agent. It has poor analgesic and antipyretic action. Mechanism of action is similar to other NSAIDs.

It is readily absorbed from the GI tract with peak plasma concentration occurring two hours after ingestion. It is 98% bound to plasma proteins and it is extensively metabolised in the liver by oxidation and by conjugation with glucuronic acid.

Adverse effects include nausea, epigastric distress, aplastic anaemia, vomiting, diarrhoea, peptic ulcer, depression, neutropenia, hypothyroidism, skin rash and urticaria.

It is **indicated** in ankylosing spondylitis, rheumatoid arthritis, rheumatic fever, osteoarthritis, after blunt injuries, fractures, tooth extraction, vasectomy and acute gout.

OXYPHENBUTAZONE

It is a metabolite of phenylbutazone and having similar pharmacodynamic and pharmacokinetic properties and similar therapeutic uses.

INDOLE DERIVATIVES

INDOMETHACIN

It is indole acetic acid derivative possessing potent antiinflammatory property and having a good analgesic and antipyretic action also. Mechanism of action is same as other NSAIDs.

It is readily absorbed from the GI tract, 99% bound to plasma proteins, distributed into synovial fluid, the central nervous system, placenta and breast milk. It is metabolised in the liver to glucuronide conjugates, excretion of metabolites is predominantly in the urine with some amount appearing in the faeces.

Adverse effects include nausea, vomiting, anorexia, gastric bleeding, diarrhoea, dizziness, frontal headache, confusion, depression, psychosis, hallucination, leukopenia, epigastric distress and rarely aplastic anaemia.

It is **used** in rheumatoid arthritis, osteoarthritis, ankylosing spondylitis and gout.

SULINDAC

It is a fluorinated derivative of indomethacin, has longer duration of action and is used orally. It is prodrug, converted to active sulfide metabolite.

PROPIONIC ACID DERIVATIVES

The drugs like ibuprofen, flurbiprofen, ketoprofen etc. possess antiinflammatory property similar to aspirin but toxicity and adverse effects are fewer and of lesser intensity. These preparations alone and in combination with other NSAIDs are used for treatment of inflammatory disorders, muscle spasm and rheumatic disorders.

They are all well absorbed orally and are highly bound to plasma proteins (90-99%). Metabolized largely in liver by hydroxylation and glucuronide conjugation and excreted in urine as well as in bile.

Adverse effects include nausea, vomiting, epigastric discomfort, dizziness, headache, skin rash and thrombocytopenia.

It is **indicated** in rheumatoid and osteoarthritis, ankylosing spondylitis, mild to moderate pain including dysmenorrhoea, soft tissue injuries, fractures and postoperative analgesia.

FLURBIPROFEN

It is NSAID used in musculoskeletal and joint disorders. It acts by inhibition of cyclooxygenase.

It is readily absorbed from GI tract and is 99% bound to plasma proteins. Metabolised mainly by hydroxylation and conjugation and excreted in urine.

KETOPROFEN

It is an inhibitor of cyclooxygenase with analgesic, antiinflammatory and antipyretic properties.

Readily absorbed from the GI tract. Food slows the rate of absorption but not the total bioavailability. Extensively bound to plasma proteins and substantial concentrations are found in synovial fluid. Metabolised mainly by conjugation with glucuronic acid and excreted mainly in the urine.

NAPROXEN

After oral administration, it is fully absorbed. It is 99% bound to plasma proteins and crosses placenta. The metabolites of naproxen are almost entirely excreted in urine. Naproxen is more efficacious and better tolerated. It is also longer acting and has the advantage of twice daily dosing.

Adverse effects include dyspepsia, gastric discomfort, nausea, vomiting, heartburn, dizziness, drowsiness, headache, fatigue, sweating, depression, ototoxicity, pruritus and thrombocytopenia.

It is **indicated** in osteoarthritis, rheumatoid arthritis, musculoskeletal disorders, primary dysmenorrhoea, acute gout, pelvic inflammation, ankylosing spondylitis, tooth extraction, tendinitis, bursitis and juvenile arthritis.

Anthranilic Acid Derivatives

MEFENAMIC ACID

It is an inhibitor of cyclooxygenase with analgesic, antiinflammatory and antipyretic properties.

It is readily absorbed from the GI tract, extensively bound to plasma proteins and excreted mainly in the urine as unchanged drug or conjugated metabolites.

Adverse effects include drowsiness, diarrhoea, rashes (withdraw treatment), thrombocytopenia, haemolytic anaemia, aplastic anaemia. Convulsions may occur in overdosage.

It is **indicated** in muscle, joint and soft tissue pain, dysmenorrhoea, rheumatoid and osteoarthritis, as antipyretic, in dental pain, postoperative or postpartum pain.

Oxicam Derivatives

PIROXICAM

Piroxicam is a new NSAID and has anti-inflammatory, analgesic and antipyretic activity. It provides effective and long-lasting relief of pain and stiffness. Its convenient once daily dosage provides round the clock relief of symptoms.

It acts peripherally by inhibiting the synthesis of prostaglandins by reversible inhibition of cyclooxygenase. Inhibition of the migration of leukocytes to an inflammatory site and inhibition of the release of lysosomal enzymes may also be involved in the antiinflammatory action.

It is well absorbed from the GIT. The rate, but not the extent of absorption is decreased by food and 99% plasma protein bound. Piroxicam is metabolised in liver. Because of long half life single daily administration is sufficient. The half life may be especially prolonged in patients with renal function impairment. Excretion of piroxicam is through renal, fecal and as unmetabolised piroxicam.

Adverse effects include, nausea, vomiting, epigastric distress, skin rash, rarely haematuria, proteinuria, hepatitis and depression.

It is **indicated** in acute or long term use in acute and chronic rheumatoid arthritis and other rheumatic disorders like osteoarthritis, ankylosing spondylitis, cervical spondylosis, acute gouty arthritis and acute musculoskeletal disorders.

Tenoxicam is a congener of piroxicam with similar properties and uses.

ARYL ACETIC ACID DERIVATIVES

DICLOFENAC

It is a NSAID with pronounced antirheumatic, antiinflammatory, analgesic and antipyretic properties. Inhibition of prostaglandin biosynthesis is fundamental mechanism of action. In rheumatic diseases, it leads to marked relief from pain at rest, pain on movement, morning stiffness and swelling of the joints, as well as by an improvement in function.

In posttraumatic and postoperative inflammatory conditions, diclofenac rapidly relieves both spontaneous pain and pain on movement and reduces inflammatory swelling and wound oedema.

It also exerts a pronounced analgesic effect in moderate and severe pain of nonrheumatic origin.

After the passage of the tablet through the stomach, it is completely absorbed. Due to the enteric coating, onset of absorption is delayed. However, once the absorption sets in diclofenac is rapidly absorbed.

Diclofenac enters the synovial fluid, where maximum concentrations are measured two to four hours after peak plasma values have been attained.

Adverse effects include nausea, vomiting, epigastric discomfort, skin rash, peptic ulcer, fluid retention, edema and impairment of hepatic function rarely.

It is **used** in the treatment of inflammatory and degenerative forms of rheumatism, rheumatoid arthritis, ankylosing spondylitis, osteoarthritis and spondyloarthritis, painful syndromes of the vertebral column, non-articular rheumatism and acute attacks of gout,

Also used in posttraumatic and postoperative pain, inflammation and swelling e.g. following dental or orthopaedic surgery, painful and/or inflammatory conditions in gynaecology e.g. primary dysmenorrhoea or adnexitis, in severe painful inflammatory infections of the ear, nose or throat e.g. pharyngotonsillitis, otitis etc.

ACECLOFENAC

It is newer COX-2 inhibitor and is a phenylacetic acid derivative. It also inhibits synthesis of IL-1b and TNF-a, thus inhibiting PGE_2 production. It is rapidly and completely absorbed after oral administration, highly protein bound and bioavailability is almost 100%. It is metabolized to a major metabolite 4'-hydroxyaceclofenac.

It is **indicated** for the relief of pain and inflammation in osteoarthritis, rheumatoid arthritis, ankylosing spondylitis and musculo-skeletal trauma.

Adverse effects include dyspepsia, abdominal pain, nausea and diarrhoea.

PARA-AMINOPHENOL DERIVATIVES

PARACETAMOL

It is a para-amino phenol derivative, acts on CNS to produce analgesia and antipyretic effect. It has negligible antiinflammatory action peripherally in therapeutic uses. It is poor inhibitor of PG synthesis in peripheral tissues, but more active on COX in brain. It also raises the pain threshold.

Paracetamol is given orally and is well absorbed, peak plasma concentration is reached in 30 to 60 minutes. About 1/3rd is bound to plasma proteins and the drug is inactivated in the liver, being conjugated to give the glucuronide or sulphate which are excreted in urine.

Adverse effects include nausea, epigastric distress. Rarely it can cause skin rash. Acute toxicity may result in hepatic failure.

Paracetamol is **used** for the rapid relief of fever, pains and aches such as headache, earache, toothache, fibrositis, myalgia, neuralgia, arthralgia, osteoarthritis and postoperative pain.

Newer Cox-2 Inhibitors

KETOROLAC

Ketorolac is a NSAID chemically related to indomethacin and tolmetin.

Ketorolac has antiinflammatory and antipyretic action that, together with its analgesic effects.

The absorption is rapid with maximum plasma concentration being attained 30 to 40 minutes after oral administration. Highly plasma protein bound and metabolised by glucuronidation. 60% is excreted unchanged in urine.

Adverse effects include, nausea, vomiting, epigastric distress, diarrhoea, drowsiness, dizziness, skin rash etc.

It is **indicated** in short term management of acute pain, pain associated with surgical procedures.

NIMESULIDE

Nimesulide is a NSAID of the sulfonanilide class. Nimesulide has exhibited potency similar to or greater than that of indomethacin, diclofenac, piroxicam and ibuprofen in standard animal models of inflammation.

Oral drug absorption is nearly complete and concomitant administration of food may decrease the rate, but not the extent of absorption. The drug is 99% bound to plasma proteins and metabolised (1 to 3% of a dose is excreted unchanged in the urine) to several metabolites which are excreted mainly in the urine or the faeces.

The **adverse effects** are gastrointestinal disturbances (epigastralgia, heart burns, nausea, diarrhoea and vomiting). It can also lead to rash, pruritus, dizziness, somnolence and headache.

There were reports of hepatotoxicity especially in children, due to which it should not be used in children and in the presence of hepatic dysfunction.

It is **indicated** in the treatment of a variety of painful inflammatory conditions, including osteoarthritis, oncology, postoperatively, trauma, sports injuries, ear, nose and throat disorders, dental surgery, bursitis/ tendinitis, thrombophlebitis, upper airways inflammation and gynaecological disorders. Nimesulide has shown to be well tolerated even by aspirin sensitive asthmatic patients.

CELECOXIB

It is a NSAID which has COX-2 selectivity. It is a diaryl substituted pyrazole.

It exhibits antiinflammatory, analgesic and antipyretic activities which are believed to be due to inhibition of COX-2. At therapeutic concentrations in humans, celecoxib does not inhibit COX-1 enzyme.

After oral administration it is rapidly absorbed from the GI tract and undergoes predominantly hepatic metabolism with little unchanged drug recovered in the urine and faeces. It is widely distributed into tissues. All metabolites are inactive.

Adverse effects include headache, diarrhoea, rhinitis, nausea, sinusitis, dyspepsia, abdominal pain etc.

It is **used** in rheumatoid arthritis, osteoarthritis and other conditions including rheumatic pain, neuralgia, gout and ankylosing spondylitis etc.

NABUMETONE

Nabumetone selectively inhibits COX-2. It is metabolised into 6-methoxy-2-naphthylacetic acid (MNA), that is a potent inhibitor of COX-2. It has no inhibitory effect on COX-1 which is responsible for prostaglandin synthesis in gastric mucosa, thereby minimising the risk of problems like ulcers and hypertension. After oral administration 80% of dose is excreted in the urine. Peak plasma concentration is reached after 2.5 to 4 hours.

Adverse effects include nausea, vomiting, heartburn, diarrhoea, constipation, headache and dizziness.

It is **indicated** in osteoarthritis, rheumatoid arthritis, inflammatory conditions and soft tissue injuries.

DRUGS USED IN RHEUMATOID ARTHRITIS

Rheumatoid arthritis (RA) is an autoimmune chronic inflammatory joint disease. It is a progressive symmetrical, destructive and deforming polyarthritis affecting proximal small joints of hand (usually) and large joints as well. It is also associated with a number of extra-articular and systemic features. There is joint inflammation, synovial proliferation and destruction of articular cartilage by inflammatory cells. There is no single treatment for RA and the principles of treatment are directed towards relief of symptoms and suppression of active and progressive disease with conservation and maintenance of joint function.

Initial treatment consists of NSAIDs, low dose corticosteroids. If the symptoms are not controlled then second line/disease modifying drugs (DMDs) are added. Since it is a progressive disease, spontaneous remissions are rare and joint damage occurs early, DMDs are started early and continued indefinitely with regular monitoring.

The disease modifying drugs (DMDs/DMARDs) used are gold, d-penicillamine, hydroxychloroquine, sulfasalazine and immuno-suppressants like methotrexate, azathioprine, cyclosporin etc.

GOLD COMPOUNDS

It appears to **reduce immune responsiveness.** It **inhibits the migration of mononuclear cells** in area of inflammation. It may **also stabilise lysosomal membrane**, hence damage to cartilage is prevented.

It can be used orally and bioavailability is 25%. After administration it binds extensively to plasma albumin and is distributed to inflamed synovium, liver and kidney.

Adverse effects include diarrhoea, dermatitis, stomatitis, glossitis, pharyngitis, pruritus, exfoliative dermatitis, alopecia, blood dyscrasias including thrombocytopenia, leucopenia, renal and hepatic damage and encephalopathy.

PENICILLAMINE

The exact mechanisms of action of penicillamine in rheumatoid arthritis is not known. After oral administration it is partly metabolised and partly excreted unchanged.

Adverse effects include Gl upset, dose related impairment of taste, thrombocytopenia, aplastic anemia, allergic reactions, skin rash, fever, SLE and proteinuria.

SULFASALAZINE

When taken orally, it liberates 5-ASA (5-aminosalicylic acid) and sulfapyridine in colon. 5-ASA acts locally by inhibiting PG synthesis and provide symptomatic relief in ulcerative colitis. Sulfapyridine is absorbed systemically and inhibits generation of superoxide radicals and cytokine elaboration by inflammatory cells and is responsible for beneficial effects in RA.

METHOTREXATE

It is a dihydrofolate reductase inhibitor immuno-suppressant. Benefit in RA is due to inhibition of cytokine production, chemotaxis and cell mediated immune reaction.

DRUGS FOR GOUT

Gout results from hyperuricemia i.e. increased serum uric acid levels. Normal serum uric acid level is 1-5 mg/dl. Uric acid is formed in the metabolism of purine. When the blood levels of uric acid are high, it precipitates in joints, cartilage, kidney and subcutaneous tissues and leads to various signs and symptoms. Hyperuricemia is also seen in various leukemias, lymphomas (increased production) or is drug induced (due to reduced renal excretion by uric acid).

Drugs used for gout can be divided into two groups:

a. Drugs for acute attack of gout: NSAIDs, colchicine, corticosteroids.
b. Drugs for chronic gout/hyperuricemia: Can be uric acid synthesis inhibitors (allopurinol) and uricosurics (increase renal excretion of uric acids) e.g. probenecid and sulfinpyrazone.

NSAIDS

Drugs useful are indomethacin, piroxicam or naproxen. Their usefulness is due to strong antiinflammatory action and can be continued for 3-4 weeks. They also inhibit chemotactic migration of leukocytes into the affected joint.

CORTICOSTEROIDS

Systemic/intraarticular steroids can be used in those cases not responding to or tolerating NSAIDs/colchicine.

COLCHICINE

It is effective for treatment of acute attacks of gout. It has no effect on renal excretion of uric acid. It **binds to tubulin, it interferes with function of mitotic spindles, causes depolymerization and disappearance of fibrillar microtubules in granulocytes**. In gout, the useful of colchicine is due to the **inhibition of the release of glycoproteins** from granulocytes in inflamed joint thus preventing precipitation of uric acid crystals and release of lysosomal enzymes.

After oral administration it is rapidly absorbed. A major part of the drug is excreted in faeces.

Adverse effects include nausea, vomiting, diarrhoea, abdominal pain, neuropathy, myopathy especially in patients with decreased renal function. Prolonged therapy may lead to aplastic anaemia, agranulocytosis, alopecia and myopathy.

It is **used** in the treatment of acute gout and prophylaxis of gout.

ALLOPURINOL

It **inhibits the terminal steps in uric acid biosynthesis by inhibiting enzyme xanthine oxidase**. During therapy with allopurinol the uric acid plasma levels decline.

After oral intake it is absorbed relatively rapidly. It is converted to alloxanthine which is active and non competitive inhibitor.

Adverse effects include hypersensitivity reactions, maculopapular rash, urticaria, myalgia, malaise fever, transient leucopenia or leukocytosis, hepatic damage, nausea, vomiting, diarrhoea, headache and drowsiness.

It is **indicated** in primary hyperuricaemia of gout, secondary hyperuricaemia due to myeloid metaplasia, radiation, cancer chemotherapy, thiazide diuretics.

PROBENECID

It **increases the excretion of uric acid** (by inhibiting its reabsorption from kidney tubules) and hence **causes reduced serum levels of uric acid**.

After oral administration it is completely absorbed. It is 90% plasma protein bound. It is partly metabolised and excreted in urine. The metabolites also have uricosuric action.

Adverse effects include skin rash, gastro-intestinal irritation. Overdosage may result in convulsions and death due to respiratory failure.

It is **used** in chronic gout and secondary hyperuricaemia.

SULFINPYRAZONE

Pyrazolone derivative related to phenylbutazone. It has uricosuric action. It also inhibits platelet aggregation.

It is well absorbed orally and 98% plasma protein bound. It is excreted by active secretion in proximal renal tubule.

Adverse effects are gastric irritation (most common), hypersensitivity reactions. It is **used** in chronic gout.

❑❑❑

CHAPTER 2.5

Psychotropic Agents

Psychopharmacological agents may be classified into three broad groups used in various states of psychic disorders.

1. **Antipsychotic drugs** or major tranquillizers used in all types of psychosis mainly schizophrenia.
2. **Antianxiety drugs** or minor tranquillizers used in anxiety.
3. **Antidepressants** for minor and major depressive disorders and mood stabilisers (antimanic drugs) for mania.

ANTIPSYCHOTIC DRUGS (MAJOR TRANQUILLIZERS)

They are classified as in table 2.5.1.

Table 2.5.1: *Classification of antipsychotic drugs.*

I. Phenothiazines	
Chlorpromazine (MEGATIL)	100-800 mg/day
Triflupromazine (SIQUIL)	50-200 mg/day
Trifluoperazine (NEOCALM)	5-15 mg BD
II. Butyrophenones	
Haloperidol (HEXIDOL)	5-10 mg/day
Droperidol (DROPEROL)	10 mg IM, 5-15 mg/day IV
Trifluperidol (TRIPERIDOL)	0.5-8 mg/day
III. Other newer compounds	
Loxapine (LOXAPAC)	60-100 mg BD-QID
Clozapine (SIZOPIN)	25-50 mg/day
Pimozide (PIMODAC)	3-4 mg/day
Zuclopenthixol (CLOPIXOL)	20-40 mg IM repeated 2-4 week interval
Molindone	20-200 mg/day
Sulpiride	0.4-2 g/day
Sertindole	4-24 mg/day

PHENOTHIAZINES

PHARMACOLOGICAL ACTIONS

a. **Action on CNS:** Effects differ in normal and psychotic individuals.

1. ***Sedation***: They produce sedation which does not progress to anaesthesia. They decrease the agitation, anxiety and aggressiveness in psychotic patient without affecting wakefulness.

2. ***Antipsychotic effect***: In schizophrenic patients, they improve thought disorders, blunted affect, withdrawal and self centered behaviour. They also improve the hallucinations and delusions.

They produce neuroleptic syndrome which consists of motor retardation and emotional quietening.

In animal studies, they reduce the spontaneous motor activity and produce catalepsy (state of rigidity and immobility).

3. ***Action on CTZ***: Chlorpromazine depresses the chemoreceptor trigger zone (CTZ) and acts as a powerful antiemetic agent.
4. ***Effect on hypothalamus***: They produce hypothermia by acting on temperature regulating centre. They also produce central sympathoplegia resulting in miosis and failure in ejaculation.

They produce parkinsonism like reaction by increasing the spontaneous firing of dopaminergic neurons of basal ganglia.

b. **Effect on CVS:** Chlorpromazine may produce orthostatic hypotension probably due to inhibition of centrally mediated pressor reflexes. It also causes prolongation of QT interval in ECG.
c. **Effect on endocrine system:** They can produce amenorrhoea and galactorrhoea due to increase in serum prolactin level in females. It also blocks the release of growth hormone, ADH and gonadotrophin secretion.
d. **Local anaesthetic:** Chlorpromazine has a potent local anaesthetic action.
e. **ANS:** They have varying degree of a adrenergic blocking activity. They also have weak anti-cholinergic, H_1-antihistaminic and anti 5-HT actions as well.

They also cause blockade of postsynaptic monoaminergic (including 5-HT, noradrenaline and dopamine) transmission in the brain resulting in decrease in central sympathetic activity.

Pharmacokinetics

Phenothiazines are well absorbed after oral and parenteral administration. They are distributed in all the body tissues and metabolised in liver by hydroxylation and glucuronide conjugation and demethylation. The metabolites are excreted in urine and bile for long period of time even after discontinuing the drug.

Adverse Reactions

CNS side effects include lethargy, drowsiness, increase in REM sleep, restlessness, excitement and impaired psychomotor functions.

The other side effects include epileptic seizures, disturbances in body temperature regulation. ANS side effects include tachycardia, difficulty in micturition, inhibition of ejaculation, postural hypotension, blurring of vision (with thioridazine), constipation, nasal stuffiness etc.

Extrapyramidal reactions include parkinsonism, acute muscular dystonias, akathisia, tardive dyskinesia and malignant neuroleptic syndrome. They can also cause hypersensitivity reaction including cholestatic jaundice, skin rash, urticaria, photosensitivity and contact dermatitis. There is also blue pigmentation of skin, lenticular opacities on prolonged use of drug.

Therapeutic Uses

1. Treatment of psychosis (schizophrenia): Schizophrenia is a split mind or splitting of perception from reality. The patient of schizophrenia is dissociated from the world around him and lives in their own world which is characterized by aggression, anxiety, restlessness, hallucinations and delusions. Phenothiazines reduce the hallucinations, aggression, anxiety and make them acceptable and cooperative.
2. In the treatment of manic depressive psychosis (treatment of mania).
3. In alcoholic hallucinosis and Huntington's disease.
4. As an antiemetic in drug and disease induced vomiting. Also useful in morning sickness but are ineffective in motion sickness.
5. In the treatment of intractable hiccough.
6. In the treatment of behavioural disorders in children.
7. As preanaesthetic medication.
8. To produce hypothermia.

TRIFLUOPERAZINE

It is a phenothiazine derivative and is used in hallucination, delusions, agitation, withdrawal and other schizophrenic symptoms in schizophrenia, schizoaffective disorders, mania, hypomania and panic anxiety.

Butyrophenones

HALOPERIDOL

It is a potent antipsychotic drug. It does not cause weight gain. Its pharmacological effects are similar to phenothiazines.

Adverse effects include dystonia, hallucinations, restlessness, nausea, epigastric discomfort, anaemia, blurred vision, hypersensitivity reaction, blood dyscrasia, jaundice, galactorrhoea, gynecomastia and amenorrhoea.

It is **indicated** in acute and chronic schizophrenia, anxiety disorders, acute mania, hypomania and behavioural disorders in children; antiemetic neuroleptanalgesia, Gilles de la Tourette's syndrome and Huntington's disease.

DROPERIDOL

It is a short acting neuroleptic agent **used** in anaesthesia.

TRIFLUPERIDOL

It exerts sedative and tranquillizing effect and it is postulated that it blocks dopamine receptors within CNS. It is **used** in acute and chronic psychoses, anxiety disorders, mania and schizophrenia.

Side effects include nausea, epigastric distress, dry mouth, blurred vision, jaundice, skin rash and photosensitivity.

Newer Compounds

LOXAPINE

It is the antipsychotic agent resembling chlorpromazine in pharmacological actions.

It is **used** in manifestation of psychotic disorders, acute and chronic paranoid schizophrenia.

CLOZAPINE

It is an atypical neuroleptic drug. It interferes with binding of dopamine at D1 and D2 receptors in CNS. It produces few extrapyramidal symptoms.

After oral administration it is rapidly and almost completely absorbed. The absorption is not affected by food and it is almost completely metabolised in liver. The metabolites are much less potent and less toxic.

Adverse effects include nausea, vomiting, heartburn, constipation, diarrhoea, agranulocytosis, eosinophilia, postural hypotension, tachycardia, angina, headache, sedation, dizziness, syncope, seizures, hyperthermia, neuroleptic malignant syndrome, weight gain and sexual dysfunction. May lead to myocarditis.

It is **indicated** in all types of schizophrenia including resistant cases not responding to conventional antipsychotics and chronic schizophrenia.

PIMOZIDE

It is a diphenylbutylpiperidine derivative. Pimozide causes low incidence of dystonic reactions.

It acts by blocking dopaminergic receptors and has weak a-adrenergic and cholinergic blocking activity. It has long duration of action (several days) after a single dose.

Adverse effects include mania, insomnia, nervousness, fatigue, drowsiness, nausea, extrapyramidal reactions and irritability.

It is **used** in the treatment of acute and chronic schizophrenia and manic excitement.

ZUCLOPENTHIXOL

Zuclopenthixol is a thioxanthene of high potency with general property similar to the chlorpromazine. It has a piperazine side-chain.

Adverse effects include extrapyramidal symptoms and on prolonged administration, occasionally tardive dyskinesia, hypothermia (occasionally pyrexia), drowsiness, apathy, pallor, nightmares, insomnia, depression, agitation, EEG changes, endocrine effects such as menstrual disturbances, galactorrhoea, gynaecomastia, impotence and weight gain, alterations in liver function.

It is **used** in the maintenance therapy of schizophrenia.

ANTIANXIETY DRUGS (MINOR TRANQUILLIZERS)

Anxiety is a emotional feeling of fear along with discomfort and uneasiness. Antianxiety drugs are used to control the symptoms of anxiety without affecting the other mental and physical functions of the body. They are classified as in table 2.5.2.

BENZODIAZEPINES

The detailed pharmacology of all the benzodiazepines used in anxiety disorders

Table 2.5.2: *Classification of antianxiety drugs.*

I. **Benzodiazepines**	
Diazepam, lorazepam, oxazepam, alprazolam. Details are already given in chapter 'Sedative and hypnotics' along with trade name and dose also.	
II. **Azapirones**	
Buspirone (BUSPIDAC)	5-15 BD-TDS
III. **Others**	
Hydroxyzine (ATARAX)	25-100 mg TDS-QID
Meprobamate	
Beta blockers e.g. propranolol.	

is discussed in chapter 'Sedative and hypnotics'.

They have selective action on limbic system and have little effect on other body systems. They help in improving the anxiety and stress related symptoms. They are widely used because of lower dependence producing liability and wide margin of safety.

AZAPIRONES

BUSPIRONE

It belongs to azapirones which is chemically and pharmacologically distinct class. It acts as a partial agonist at serotonin and dopamine receptors and having no hypnotic and sedative action. It does not interact with benzodiazepine receptor or modify GABA-ergic transmission.

It is rapidly absorbed and undergoes extensive first pass metabolism and excreted through kidney and faeces.

It is **used** in short-term management of anxiety disorders and relief of symptoms of anxiety with or without accompanying depression.

Adverse effects include headache, excitement, tachycardia, palpitation (may raise BP in patients on MAO inhibitors), nervousness, dizziness, drowsiness, confusion, fatigue, sweating etc.

OTHER COMPOUNDS

HYDROXYZINE

It is antihistaminic agent having antiemetic, sedative, anticholinergic and local anaesthetic property. **Used** in anxiety, pruritus and dermatoses; as an adjunct therapy in acute/ chronic alcoholism.

Side effects include epigastric distress, nausea and impaired alertness.

BETA BLOCKERS

Beta blockers provide symptomatic relief by decreasing the symptoms due to sympathetic overactivity e.g. palpitation, tremors, rise in BP, etc. They may be **used** as adjuvant to benzo-diazepines.

ANTIDEPRESSANTS

They are classified into two main categories e.g. MAO inhibitors and tricyclic/tetracyclic antidepressants as in table 2.5.3.

MAO INHIBITORS

Monoamine oxidase (MAO) is an intracellular enzyme and metabolizes intracellu-

Table 2.5.3: *Classification of antidepressant drugs.*

I. **MAO inhibitors**	
i. ***Non-selective***	
Phenelzine	
Isocarboxazid	
Pargyline	
ii. ***Selective***	
Moclobemide (RIMAPREX)	150-600 mg/day
II. **Tricyclic and related compounds**	
i. ***Tricyclic antidepressants***	
Imipramine (DEPSONIL)	50-200 mg/day
Amitriptyline (AMIXIDE)	150-225 mg/day
Nortriptyline (PRIMOX)	50-150 mg/day
Trimipramine (SURMONTIL)	50-150 mg/day
Doxepin (DOXIN)	25-150 mg/day
Dothiepin (EXODEP)	75-150 mg/day
ii. ***Tetracyclic antidepressants***	
Mianserin (SERIDAC)	30-100 mg/day
Mirtazapine (MIRTAZ)	15-45 mg/day
III. **Serotonin reuptake inhibitors**	
Sertraline (SERNATA)	50-200 mg/day
Citalopram (CITADEP)	20-40 mg OD
Paroxetine (PAROTIN)	20-50 mg/day
Fluoxetine (FLUDAC)	20-60 mg/day
IV. **Mood stabilizers (Antimania drugs)**	
Lithium carbonate (LITHOSUN)	600-1000 mg/day

lar catecholamines present in the non-granular cytoplasmic pool. It also causes oxidative deamination of 5-hydroxytryptamine. Their antidepressant action may be related to increase in the brain catecholamines content.

MAO inhibitors increase the catecholamine content of various organs so that more catecholamine is to be released by indirectly acting sympathomimetic amines.

Adverse effects include tremor, insomnia, delirium, convulsion, postural hypotension, dry mouth, constipation, difficulty in micturition, impotence, constipation. The serious side effects include peripheral neuropathy and jaundice due to hepatocellular injury.

Interaction with Other Drugs and Foods

1. Hypertensive crisis: MAO inhibitors with ingestion of tyramine containing food e.g. cheese, beer, red wine or fermented food can cause intracranial haemorrhage due to hypertensive crisis because of release of noradrenaline from adrenergic nerve endings by unmetabolised tyramine.

2. MAO inhibitors along with barbiturates, alcohol, narcotic analgesic can enhance and prolong the action of these drugs.
3. Potentiate the toxic effects of tricyclic antidepressants.
4. It's use with anticholinergic antiparkinsonian drugs can lead symptoms similar to atropine poisoning.

Because of their toxic effects and serious interactions, they are not commonly used. However, a new selective inhibitor is used clinically.

MOCLOBEMIDE

It is a reversible and selective MAO-A inhibitor used in the major depression. It is devoid of anticholinergic, sedative and cardiovascular effects of TCAs.

Side effects include sleep disturbances, dizziness, nausea, headache, restlessness, agitation, confusion state and nausea.

Tricyclic Antidepressants

Tricyclic antidepressants are the most commonly used drugs. They produce antidepressant effect by blocking the neuronal uptake of noradrenaline and exert anti-cholinergic activity. They also inhibit neuronal uptake of 5HT and dopamine. The exact mechanism of action is not known. The antidepressant effect is noticed after three to four weeks of drug administration.

TCAs lower seizure threshold and overdose leads to convulsions. The side effects are due to anticholinergic effect leading to dry mouth, blurring of vision, constipation, urinary hesitancy and tachycardia. They also lead to postural hypotension due to a_1 blockade and inhibition of cardiovascular reflexes. They also produce T wave suppression or inversion. Oral absorption is good and they are highly bound to plasma proteins. They are extensively metabolized in liver and metabolites are excreted in urine.

IMIPRAMINE

It is an efficacious drug in alleviating depression. When the drug is given to depressed patients, elevation of mood occurs in about three weeks. Tolerance to anticholinergic effects occurs with continued use of imipramine.

It is highly protein bound and is metabolized to pharmacologically active metabolite. It crosses placental barrier.

Adverse effects include dry mouth, tachycardia, palpitation, impotence, constipation, difficulty in accommodation, rarely hyperpyrexia and paralytic ileus; lethargy, headache, drowsiness, tremors, ataxia, sweating, convulsion, urticaria, skin rash, pruritus, cholestatic jaundice, cardiac arrhythmias, orthostatic hypotension, agranulocytosis, gynaecomastia, galactorrhoea and dependence; loss of weight or gain.

It is **indicated** in all types of depression, nocturnal enuresis, intractable chronic pain, narcolepsy, chorea, cachexia, mood disturbances and sleep apnoea syndrome.

AMITRIPTYLINE

It causes sedation and after oral administration it is metabolised to nortriptyline which is active form.

Adverse effects include epigastric distress, sedation, drowsiness, orthostatic hypotension, palpitation, dry mouth, urinary retention, blurred vision, confusion and lowering of seizure threshold.

It is **indicated** in depression, illness accompanied by anxiety, agitation, restlessness and disturbances of sleep; masked depression; dysphoria and depression in alcoholics; childhood bed wetting. It is also useful for prophylaxis of migraine.

NORTRIPTYLINE

It is same as amitriptyline and its antidepressant effect may persist up to six weeks.

Adverse effects include dry mouth, constipation, nausea, epigastric discomfort, sedation, confusion, arrhythmias, altered vision, skin rash, jaundice and impaired alertness.

It is **indicated** in neurotic, reactive, masked endogenous, recurrent depression; depression with insomnia, depression, enuresis, panic disorder, neurogenic pain, urticaria and nausea and vomiting during chemotherapy; maniac depressive psychosis in depressive phase.

TRIMIPRAMINE

It has more sedative effect than other tricyclic antidepressants and is suitable for patients showing depression with agitation and anxiety.

DOTHIEPIN

The mechanism of action is same as of tricyclic antidepressant and used in depression and anxiety associated with depression.

Adverse effects include dry mouth, tachycardia, palpitation, impotence, constipation, difficulty in accommodation, rarely hyperpyrexia and paralytic ileus. Lethargy, headache, drowsiness, tremors, ataxia, sweating, convulsion, urticaria, skin rash, pruritus, cholestatic jaundice, cardiac arrhythmias, orthostatic hypotension, agranulocytosis, gynecomastia, galactorrhoea and dependence are also seen.

TETRACYCLIC ANTIDEPRESSANTS

MIANSERIN

It exerts potent presynaptic central a_2, adrenergic blocking activity which may cause increased noradrenaline release. It does not effect noradrenaline or 5-HT uptake in CNS.

Adverse effects include hypersensitivity reaction, nausea, drowsiness, jaundice, may precipitate seizures, blood dyscrasias, lethargy and tremors.

It is **used** in psychotic and neurotic depression and obsessive compulsive neurosis.

MIRTAZAPINE

It acts as an antagonist at central presynaptic a_2 inhibitory adrenergic auto-receptors and hetero-receptors. This results in an increase in central noradrenergic and serotonergic activity. Mirtazapine is a potent antagonist of 5-HT_2 and 5-HT_3 receptors.

Adverse effects include asthenia, flu like syndrome, back pain, dry mouth, increased appetite, constipation, weight gain, peripheral edema, myalgia, somnolence, dizziness, abnormal dreams, abnormal thinking, tremor, confusion, dyspnea and urinary frequency.

Selective Serotonin Reuptake Inhibitors

Selective serotonin reuptake inhibitors (SSRI) are currently used group of drug in treatment of depression. These have a faster onset of action and are better tolerated.

SERTRALINE

Sertraline is a potent and selective inhibitor of neuronal serotonin (5-HT) reuptake. It has only a weak effect on neuronal uptake of norepinephrine and dopamine. Sertraline's inhibition of serotonin reuptake enhances serotonergic transmission.

It has a wide therapeutic index and can be administered in elderly patients and those with underlying cardiovascular disorders.

Adverse effects include nausea, headache, diarrhoea, insomnia, dry mouth, tremor and fatigue.

It is **indicated** for the treatment of symptoms of depressive illness including accompanying symptoms of anxiety. It is also indicated in preventing relapse of the initial episode of depression or recurrence of further depressive episodes including accompanying symptoms of anxiety.

It is indicated in the treatment of obsessions and compulsions in patients with obsessive compulsive disorder.

It is also indicated for the treatment of panic disorder with or without agoraphobia.

CITALOPRAM

It is orally active SSRI. The mechanism of action is due to potentiation of serotonergic activity in the CNS resulting from its inhibition of CNS neuronal reuptake of serotonin (5-HT).

Following a single oral dose of citalopram, peak blood levels occur at about four hours.

Adverse effects include activation of mania/hypomania, dizziness, insomnia, agitation, nausea and vomiting, dry mouth, diarrhoea, tachycardia, postural hypotension, cardiac failure, MI, arthralgia, myalgia, arthritis, purpura, anaemia, leukocytosis, decreased or increased weight, thirst, ejaculation disorder, impotence, dysmenorrhoea, decreased or increased libido, coughing, epistaxis, bronchitis, rash, pruritus, photosensitivity reaction, urticaria, acne, abnormal accommodation, conjunctivitis, eye pain, fatigue and fever.

It is **indicated** in the treatment of depression.

PAROXETINE

It is an orally administered SSRI.

Paroxetine is readily absorbed from the GIT with peak plasma concentration occurring within about five hours. It is widely distributed throughout body tissues and is about 95% bound to plasma proteins. Excretion is via the urine and the faeces, mainly as metabolites.

Adverse effects include asthenia, sweating, nausea, decreased appetite, somnolence, dizziness, insomnia, tremor, nervousness, constipation, ejaculatory disturbance and impotence.

It is **indicated** in the treatment of depression, obsessive compulsive disorder and panic disorder.

FLUOXETINE

A potent antidepressant drug, it does not cause sedation. In CNS it inhibits the neuronal uptake of 5-HT. It shows negligible binding to histaminergic, muscarinic, α_1 adrenergic receptors, so it is devoid of anticholinergic and hypotensive side effects.

After oral administration the drug is converted to norfluoxetine which has a very long lasting biological activity.

Adverse effects include drowsiness, skin rash, insomnia, anxiety, weakness, fatigue, nausea, anorexia, epigastric distress, diarrhoea, tremor and sweating.

It is **used** in the treatment of depression where sedation is not required and for prophylaxis of recurrent depression.

MOOD STABILIZERS (ANTIMANIC DRUGS)

LITHIUM CARBONATE

It has narrow therapeutic index and treatment requires facility for therapeutic monitoring of serum lithium levels.

Exact mechanism of action is unknown. It brings the patient of mania towards normal. Lithium decreases the neuronal uptake of dopamine and noradrenaline and their synthesis. It increases the rate of 5-HT synthesis in brain. On continuous therapy cyclic mood changes are prevented.

It also inhibits ADH action on distal tubules (diabetes insipidus like state), also has insulin like action on glucose metabolism and decreases thyroxine synthesis by interfering with iodination of thyroxine.

After oral administration it is well absorbed and is not protein bound. It not metabolised and is excreted mainly in urine and it inhibits the reabsorption of sodium in renal tubules. It has narrow margin of safety.

Adverse effects include nausea, vomiting, epigastric distress, polydipsia, polyuria, diarrhoea, dizziness, ataxia, nystagums, hyper-reflexia, arrhythmias, skin rash, glycosuria and blurred vision.

It is **indicated** in acute hypomania, mania, recurrent mania, depression – cyclic and recurring, unipolar depression, bipolar depression, schizoaffective psychosis, mental depression, cluster headache, chemotherapy induced leukopenia and agranulocytosis.

❑❑❑

CHAPTER 2.6 Antiepileptic Agents

Epilepsy is a neurological disorder characterized by short, recurrent and periodic attacks of motor, sensory or psychological malfunction. It is associated with paroxysmal abnormal electrical discharge in the brain. According to Jackson, epilepsy is due to sudden, excessive and rapid discharge in the grey matter of the brain. Anti-epileptic drugs inhibit the spread of abnormal electrical discharge in the brain with minimal general depressant action on the central nervous system.

The antiepileptic drugs belong to following groups as classified in table 2.6.1.

BARBITURATES

PHENOBARBITONE

Phenobarbitone **raises the threshold of electro-shock seizures and modifies maximal electro-shock seizures and abolish the tonic phase** thus useful in the treatment of grandmal epilepsy. The threshold of pentylenetetrazol induced convulsion is slightly raised and has less usefulness in the treatment of petitmal epilepsy.

Phenobarbitone has long plasma half-life but slow oral absorption, is metabolized in liver as well as excreted unchanged in urine.

Phenobarbitone is **useful** in grandmal, focal and temporal lobe epilepsy and sometimes petitmal also. It is also useful in the treatment of febrile convulsions.

Phenobarbitone is cheap and produces less **side effects** which include sedation, behavioural abnormalities, mental confusion, impairment of learning and memory and hyperactivity in children.

MEPHOBARBITONE

It is N-methylphenobarbitone. It is more expensive than phenobarbitone and requires double dose compared to phenobarbitone. It probably offers no advantage over phenobarbitone.

PRIMIDONE

Chemically it is deoxybarbiturate (carbonyl oxygen of urea moiety in phenobarbitone is changed by two hydrogen atoms) and is twice as active as phenobarbitone in modify-

Table 2.6.1: *Classification of antiepileptic drugs*

	Drug	Dose
I.	**Barbiturates**	
	Phenobarbitone (PHENOBARB)	60 mg OD-TDS
	Primidone (MYSOLINE)	250-500 mg BD
II.	**Hydantoins**	
	Diphenylhydantoin (Phenytoin; EPTOIN)	100-200 mg BD
	Mephenytoin (MESANTOIN)	50-200 mg TDS
III.	**Iminostilbene derivatives**	
	Carbamazepine (TEGRETAL)	200-400 mg. TDS
	Oxcarbazepine (OXYTEL)	600-1200 mg BD
IV.	**Succinimides**	
	Ethosuximide (ZARONTIN)	250-500 mg TDS
	Methsuximide	300 mg OD-TDS
V.	**Oxazolidinediones**	
	Trimethadione (TROXIDONE)	300-600 mg TDS
VI.	**Aliphatic carboxylic acid**	
	Valproic acid (Sodium valproate; EPIVAL)	200-800 mg TDS
VII.	**Benzodiazepines**	
	Clonazepam (EPITRIL)	0.5-4 mg TDS
	Diazepam (CALMPOSE)	0.2-0.5 mg/kg IV
	Clobazam (CLODUS)	20-60 mg OD-BD
VIII.	**Phenyltriazine derivative**	
	Lamotrigine (LAMEPIL)	300-500 mg BD
IX.	**Newer compounds**	
	Felbamate	2-4 g/day
	Topiramate (TOPEX)	200-400 mg BD
	Tiagabine	16-56 mg/day

ing electroshock seizures in the rats. It is effective against all type of seizures e.g. grandmal epilepsy, psychomotor epilepsy, focal and myoclonic epilepsy. It is not effective in petitmal epilepsy.

It is **converted into phenobarbitone and phenylethyl malonamide** in the liver, which actually produces the antiepileptic actions. The common **side effects** are anorexia, drowsiness, nausea, leukopenia, osteomalacia and megaloblastic anaemia.

HYDANTOINS

DIPHENYLHYDANTOIN (PHENYTOIN)

In epileptic patients there is repetitive detonation of normal brain cells during the depolarisation shift and consists of synchronous and unusually large depolarisation on which action potentials are superimposed. **Phenytoin prevents repetitive detonation of these normal brain cells as it has a stabilizing influence on the neuronal membrane**. It is achieved by prolonging the inactive state of voltage sensitive neuronal Na^+ channels & governs the refractory period of a neurone.

After oral administration peak plasma concentration of phenytoin usually takes 2 to 4 hours with a second peak at 10 to 12 hours. When administered intramuscularly, phenytoin is eventually absorbed completely, the drug first crystallises out at the injection site and then slowly redissolves in tissue fluids before entering into the circulation. As a result absorption of phenytoin by IM route is too slow to produce a reliable effect. In contrast a phosphate prodrug, **fosphenytoin**, is more soluble and is well absorbed after IM administration.

In liver it is extensively biotransformed by oxidation, with less than 5 percent of the dose excreted unchanged in urine. Majority of dose is excreted in urine with up to 15 percent of the dose is eliminated in the faeces.

Adverse effects include gum hypertrophy, hirsutism, hypersensitivity reaction, megaloblastic anemia, osteomalacia and hyperglycemia.

During pregnancy produces foetal hydantoin syndrome. At higher concentration produces ataxia, vertigo, diplopia, nystagmus, behavioural alteration and mental confusion.

It is **used** in prophylactic treatment of all varieties of partial epilepsy whether or not seizure becomes secondarily generalised. It is also used in prophylactic treatment of generalised convulsive seizures and treatment of status epilepticus; prophylactic management of certain forms of supraventricular cardiac arrhythmia as it has an ability to selectively inhibit high frequency firing; prophylactic management of certain varieties of migraine (particularly childhood, basilar artery and hemiplegic migraine) and in treatment of myotonia.

IMINOSTILBENE DERIVATIVES

CARBAMAZEPINE

It is structurally and chemically related to tricyclic antidepressant drug imipramine and pharmacologically it is similar to diphenyl hydantoin sodium. It is **effective** in grandmal and psychomotor epilepsy and also in the treatment of **trigeminal neuralgia** (a condition characterized by paroxysms of intense pain of stabbing nature within the area of distribution of trigeminal nerve without sensory loss).

It also exerts antidiuretic action by enhancing ADH action on renal tubules.

Carbamazepine, because of its poor water solubility has slow oral absorption. It is metabolized in the liver to an active metabolite, (10-11 epoxy carbamazepine) by oxidation as well as by hydrolysis and conjugation to inactive forms.

Adverse effects include sedation, ataxia, dizziness and extrapyramidal side effects, dry mouth, blurred vision and urinary retention; hepatic damage, bone marrow depression, hypertension, left ventricular failure and cardiovascular collapse in toxic doses.

OXCARBAZEPINE

It is a keto analog of carbamazepine. **It produces blockade of voltage sensitive sodium channels**, leading to stabilisation of hyperexcited neural membranes, inhibition of repetitive neuronal firing and diminution of propagation of synaptic impulses.

Oxcarbazepine is completely absorbed following oral administration and is extensively metabolised to its pharmacologically active 10-monohydroxy metabolite.

Adverse reactions include dizziness, diplopia, fatigue, nausea, vomiting, dyspepsia, ataxia, abnormal vision, tremor etc.

SUCCINIMIDES

ETHOSUXIMIDE

Ethosuximide is most commonly used antiepileptic agent in the treatment of petitmal epilepsy. It acts on thalamocortical system by selectively suppressing T current without affecting other types of Ca^{2+} or Na^{+} currents. It is completely absorbed from gastrointestinal tract and present in plasma in free form and approximately 20% is excreted unchanged in urine and remaining portion is metabolized in liver.

Adverse effects include anorexia, nausea, vomiting, drowsiness, dizziness, agitation, skin rashes and blood dyscrasias and rarely cause systemic lupus erythematosus.

METHSUXIMIDE

It is similar to ethosuximide and used along with the other drugs in the treatment of temporal lobe epilepsy.

ALIPHATIC CARBOXYLIC ACID

SODIUM VALPROATE (VALPROIC ACID)

Sodium valproate **increases the levels of GABA in the brain and increases the responses to GABA in the postsynaptic neurons**. Also sodium valproate affects potassium flow across the neurons. The result of these effects is inhibition of initiation as well as spread of epileptic activity in the neurons.

Valproate has antiepileptic efficacy in different types of epilepsy. It is therefore sometimes called the *broad range antiepileptic drug*. It has no significant hypnosedative effects nor does it have respiratory depressant activity. In addition it does not have undesirable effects on blood pressure, heart rate, kidney function and body temperature.

Absorption is rapid and complete. Protein binding is between 80 to 95 percent and the elimination half life is 8 to 22 hours. It is metabolised in the liver and is excreted by the kidney. There is no presystemic metabolism.

Adverse effects include anorexia, nausea, vomiting, diarrhoea and/or constipation, weight gain, skin rash; hair loss, neutropenia, tremors and ataxia are occasionally reported. Valproic acid is **contraindicated** in liver disease, especially cirrhosis, pregnancy and hypersensitivity.

BENZODIAZEPINES

CLONAZEPAM

It is a benzodiazepine useful in the treatment of petitmal epilepsy, myoclonic seizures and infantile spasms. It is **used** in the treatment of petitmal epilepsy not responding to ethosuximide and sodium valproate. Clonazepam and diazepam **act by increasing the effectiveness of the inhibitory neurotransmitter GABA**, within the central nervous system.

Clonazepam is well absorbed orally and approximately 85 percent is bound with plasma proteins, completely metabolized in liver and excreted through kidney.

Adverse effects include sedation, lack of concentration, irritability, ataxia and behavioural abnormalities.

The detailed pharmacology of diazepam is discussed in chapter 'Sedative and hypnotics'.

CLOBAZAM

It is 1, 5 benzodiazepine with a chemical structure slightly different from that of diazepam and clonazepam. This change in structure results in less sedative and psychomotor retardation. Though introduced as an anxiolytic it has been found to be useful in treatment of patients with refractory epilepsy.

Its antiepileptic activity results from its binding to one or more specific GABA receptors increasing GABA mediated inhibition.

Adverse reactions include drowsiness, hangover effects, dizziness, weight gain, headache, dry mouth and orthostatic hypotension etc.

PHENYLTRIAZINE DERIVATIVE

LAMOTRIGINE

It is phenyltriazine compound, chemically unrelated to existing antiepileptic drugs. It acts primarily via a **dose dependent blockade of voltage sensitive sodium channels** in their slow inactivated state, thus stabilizing the presynaptic neuronal membrane **inhibiting release of** excitatory neurotransmitters mainly **glutamate**.

Lamotrigine is almost completely absorbed after oral administration and metabolized completely in liver.

The **adverse effects** include headache, rash, nausea, dizziness, somnolence and insomnia.

It is mainly **used** as adjunctive therapy in patients for simple partial seizures, complex partial seizures, secondary generalised tonic and clonic seizures.

NEWER COMPOUNDS

TOPIRAMATE

It is used as adjunctive treatment of seizures including refractory seizures, simple and complex partial seizures.

It **acts by reducing epileptiform discharges generated by blocking the sensitive sodium channel and enhancing the activity of GABA receptors**.

It is rapidly absorbed after oral administration and is unaffected by presence of food and excreted mainly through kidney.

Adverse effects include abdominal pain, anorexia, weight loss, impaired concentration, confusion, mood disorders, ataxia, dizziness, drowsiness, fatigue and psychotic symptoms.

GABAPENTIN

It is a new anticonvulsant drug and is a structural analogue of GABA. **It increases the release of GABA** by unknown mechanism. It modifies maximal electroshock as well as inhibits pentylenetetrazol induced convulsions.

After oral administration, it is rapidly absorbed and widely distributed into all tissues. It readily crosses blood brain barrier and is not bound to plasma proteins. It is excreted unchanged in urine. It is mainly **used** as adjunctive therapy in treatment of partial seizures with or without secondary generalization in adults.

Adverse effects include sedation, dizziness, diplopia, ataxia and fatigue.

VIGABATRIN

It is an **inhibitor of GABA transaminase which degrades GABA**. It suppresses maximal electroshock and kindled seizures and is used in partial seizure with or without generalization.

It is well absorbed after oral administration and excreted unchanged in urine.

Adverse effects include drowsiness, dizziness, agitation and amnesia.

❑❑❑

CHAPTER 2.7

Muscle Relaxants

Skeletal muscle relaxants act peripherally at the neuromuscular junction or centrally in the cerebrospinal axis to reduce muscle tone.

Skeletal muscle relaxation can be achieved by following group of drugs as in table 2.7.1.

Neuromuscular Blockers

D-TUBOCURARINE

It is an dextrorotatory quarternary ammonium alkaloid obtained from *Chondrodendron tomentosum* plant. It initially produced motor weakness followed by flaccid paralysis after parenteral administration. The paralysis occurs in following order e.g. paralysis of fingers, toes, eyes, ears producing diplopia, speech slurring, difficulty in swallowing; the muscles of neck, limb, trunk, paralysis of diaphragm and death occur due to hypoxia.

In higher doses, d-tubocurarine can produce blockade of autonomic ganglia. It

Table 2.7.1: *Classification of skeletal muscle relaxants.*

I. Neuromuscular blockers	
d-Tubocurarine	0.2-0.4 mg IV
Atracurium	10-15 mg IV
Pancuronium	40-100 μg/kg IV
Vecuronium	0.08-0.1 mg/Kg IV
Succinylcholine	30-50 mg IV
Benzoquinonium	10-15 mg IV
Dantrolene	25 to 100 mg/day
II. Centrally acting muscle relaxants	
Mephenesin	
Chlorzoxazone (MOBIZOX)	250 mg TDS
Methocarbamol (FLEXINOL)	0.l5-1 g/day oral, 100-200 mg IM/IV
Carisoprodol (CARISOMA)	350 mg TDS
Orphenadrine (ORPHIPAL)	100-300 mg/day
Tizanidine (CITANZ)	2-6 mg/day
Baclofen (LIORESAL)	30-75 mg/day
Metaxalone (FLEXURA)	400-800 mg TDS-QID

can also produce release of histamine and can cause bronchospasm and increase other body secretions.

d-Tubocurarine is not absorbed orally and after intravascular administration, it is widely distributed in tissue. As it does not cross blood brain barrier it has no effect on CNS.

Adverse effects include hypoxia, respiratory paralysis, decreased blood pressure, bronchospasm etc.

d-Tubocurarine is not used now due to its prominent histamine releasing and ganglionic blocking effect.

PANCURONIUM

Pancuronium is a synthetic steroidal compounds and approximately five times potent than d-tubocurarine. **Vecuronium** is congener of pancuronium with short duration of action.

Atracurium is bisquarternary competitive blocker similar to pancuronium in properties and duration of action.

SUCCINYLCHOLINE

It is a quarternary ammonium compound with a structure similar to acetylcholine (Details are discussed in chapter 'Cholinergic agents').

Therapeutic uses

- As a adjuvant to general anaesthesia (specially in major surgical procedures e.g. abdominal and thoracic surgery, orthopaedic procedures, intubation etc).
- Succinylcholine is used for surgical procedure of brief duration (endotracheal intubation, bronchoscopy, esophagoscopy, laryngoscopy etc).
- Succinylcholine is used to avoid convulsion and coma from electroconvulsive therapy.
- In the treatment of tetanus and emergency of epilepsy (status epilepticus).
- As a diagnostic tool for myasthenia gravis.

CENTRALLY ACTING MUSCLE RELAXANTS

These agents reduce skeletal muscle tone by a selective action on cerebrospinal axis without affecting consciousness.

Mephenesin was the first drug used as muscle relaxant but due to its serious side effects e.g. haemolysis, hypotension and thrombophlebitis, it is not clinically used now.

CHLORZOXAZONE

It is mephenesin related skeletal muscle relaxant. After oral administration, it is rapidly and completely absorbed. It is metabolized in liver and excreted in urine primarily as the glucuronide. **Adverse reactions** include gastric irritation, nausea, lethargy, headache.

It is **used** in painful skeletal muscle spasm and is used in combination with paracetamol and diclofenac.

METHOCARBAMOL

It causes skeletal muscle relaxation by preferential blockade of polysynaptic spinal reflexes.

It is rapidly absorbed from the GI tract, metabolised in the liver and excreted in urine as the glucuronide and sulphate conjugates of its metabolites. Small amount is excreted in faeces.

Adverse effects include nausea, anorexia, skin rash, vertigo, drowsiness, headache and fever.

It is **indicated** in skeletal muscle spasm, in surgery, orthopaedic procedures, neurological diseases and tetanus.

CARISOPRODOL

It is used for the treatment of muscle spasm. It has antipyretic and weak antiadrenergic activity.

It is absorbed from the GI tract, metabolised in the liver and excreted in urine as metabolites including meprobamate.

It is **used** in musculoskeletal disorders. **Adverse reactions** include nausea, rash, headache, drowsiness, constipation and dizziness.

ORPHENADRINE

It is a centrally acting, anticholinergic muscle relaxant drug.

With administration of 100 mg of orphenadrine, peak plasma concentration are achieved within two hours. Half-life is 14 hours for the parent drug and 2 to 25 hours for the metabolites. Excretion is via urine and faeces.

It is **used** in musculoskeletal disorders, trauma, sports injuries, low backache, tension headache, sprains and strains, parkinsonism including the drug induced.

Adverse effects include dry mouth, blurred vision, nausea, restlessness, dizziness etc.

TIZANIDINE

Tizanidine is an α_2-adrenergic receptor agonist at supraspinal and spinal levels. This effect results in inhibition of spinal polysynaptic reflex activity. It presumably reduces spasticity by increasing presynaptic inhibition of motor neurons. Tizanidine has no direct effect on skeletal muscle, the neuromuscular junction or on monosynaptic reflex activity.

In humans, tizanidine reduces pathologically increased muscle tone, including resistance to passive movements and alleviates painful spasms and clonus.

Adverse effects include nausea, sedation, dry mouth, dizziness, hypotension, headache, palpitation. Other rarely produced side effects include hallucinations, bradycardia etc.

It is **indicated** in spasticity due to neurological disorders e.g., multiple sclerosis, chronic myelopathy, degenerative diseases of the spinal cord, cerebrovascular accidents and cerebral palsy; painful muscle spasm associated with static and functional disorders of the spine (cervical and lumbar syndromes); painful muscle spasm following surgery e.g., for herniated intervertebral disc or for osteoarthritis of the hip.

BACLOFEN

It is beta-4 (chlorophenyl)-gamma aminobutyric acid. It is a **powerful neuronal depressant**. It reduces the release of excitatory transmitter and is antinociceptive in animal studies. It inhibits monosynaptic and polysynaptic reflex transmission at spinal level, probably by stimulating the $GABA_B$

receptors which in turn inhibit the release of glutamate and aspartate.

After oral administration, it is rapidly and completely absorbed and eliminated from the body by kidney in unchanged form.

Adverse effects include weakness, fatigue, dizziness, headache, insomnia, hypotension, confusion, skin rash, constipation, nausea, anorexia, dry mouth and taste disturbance etc.

It is mainly **used** in the treatment of spasticity in multiple sclerosis, spastic spinal paralysis etc. It is also used in the treatment of trigeminal neuralgia.

METAXALONE

It is a skeletal muscle relaxant, oxazolidinone derivative used in conjunction with other therapeutic agents to treat and discomfort associated with acute musculoskeletal conditions. Mechanism of action is not known, however, it is thought that the skeletal muscle relaxation is due to its central nervous system depressant action. It probably acts by inhibiting polysynaptic pathways but has no effect on monosynaptic pathways.

It is well absorbed from GIT and mostly metabolised in liver and excreted in urine. Peak plasma levels are reached at two hours and onset of action occurs within one hour.

Adverse effects include blurred or double vision, dizziness, drowsiness, abdominal cramps, confusion, headache, hiccups, anaemia etc.

It is mainly **used** to relieve pain and discomfort caused by strains, sprains and other painful muscular conditions in which muscles are in spasm i.e. fibromyalgia, dislocations and fractures.

❑❑❑

CHAPTER 2.8 Local Anaesthetics

Local anaesthetics reversibly block impulse conduction in a restricted area of the body where it is applied by topical application or local injection. They are classified as in table 2.8.1.

All the local anaesthetics possess varying degree of water and lipid solubility. Both the properties are essential for a local anaesthetic, lipid solubility helps in migration of active drug into the neuronal fibre and water solubility is essential to get the drug to site of action from the site of administration.

Local anaesthetics are employed routinely in dentistry by nerve block or by infiltration and/or regional block techniques to cary out varous operative procedures.

Local anaesthetics can also be classified into two categories based on their chemical structure:

a. **Ester linked local anaesthetics** e.g. cocaine, procaine, tetracaine, benzocaine, chloroprocaine.
b. **Amide linked local anaesthetics** e.g. lidocaine, bupivacaine, dibucaine, prilocaine, ropivacaine.

Table 2.8.1: *Classification of local anaesthetics.*

I.	**Used topically**	
	Lignocaine (XYLOCAINE)	1-5% (as ointment, jelly & topical solution)
	Benzocaine (MANDELAY)	5% ointment
	Tetracaine (ANETHANE)	0.25-0.5% (powder & ointment)
	Dibucaine (NUPERCAINAL)	1% ointment
	Oxethazaine (MUCAINE GEL)	2% suspension
II.	**Used parenterally**	
	Procaine (NOVOCAINE)	0.5-2% inj
	Lignocaine (XYLOCAINE)	0.5-2% inj, 5% for spinal anaesthesia
	Tetracaine (ANETHANE)	0.25-0.5%
	Bupivacaine (SENSORCAINE)	0.25-0.5% inj, 0.5-0.75% for spinal anaesthesia
	Dibucaine (NUPERCAINE)	0.1-0.5%, 0.25-0.50% for spinal anaesthesia
	Newer compounds are prilocaine, ropivacaine, etidocaine etc.	

Local anaesthetics block both the generation and conduction of the nerve impulse.

Pharmacological Actions

Action on CNS: Local anaesthetics stimulate CNS and produce restlessness, tremor, mental confusion, convulsion. In toxic doses, it causes respiratory depression, coma and death. Cocaine is a powerful stimulant while procaine and other agents produce less CNS stimulant effect.

Action on CVS: Local anaesthetics are myocardial depressant and decrease heart rate and amplitude of myocardial contraction. In high doses, they produce changes in the ECG and may precipitate ventricular fibrillation. Bupivacaine is more cardiotoxic and can produce ventricular tachycardia or fibrillation.

Local anaesthetics also produce decrease in blood pressure which may be due to sympathetic blockade. Only cocaine has the property to raise the BP due to its sympathomimetic property.

Pharmacokinetics

Local anaesthetics are readily absorbed through mucous membranes and damaged skin. These are weak bases and at tissue pH diffuse through the connective tissue and cellular membranes to reach the nerve fibres where ionization can occur. Amide type local anaesthetics (lignocaine, bupivacaine) are metabolised in the liver and in some cases the kidneys. These are considerably protein bound. For certain procedures the duration of action is prolonged by adding adrenaline 1 in 2,00,000. In dentistry, where the total dose is small higher concentration such as 1 in 80,000 may be used.

Adverse Effects

CNS side effects include dizziness, mental confusion, tremors, twitching, visual disturbances, convulsion and respiratory depression. CVS toxicity includes hypotension, cardiac arrhythmias and bradycardia. Other side effects include allergic dermatitis, asthma, anaphylactic shock etc.

Therapeutic Uses

Local anaesthetics are used for

- Surface anaesthesia.
- Spinal anaesthesia.
- Infiltration anaesthesia.
- Nerve block or conduction block and
- For systemic use in the treatment of cardiac arrhythmias (Details are given in chapter 'Antiarrhythmic agents').
- Dental anaesthesia—The total amount of local anaesthetics injected is much smaller (20-80 mg of lignocaine) than that used for othr purpose. Lignocaine (2%) with adrenaline (1:80,000) is the standard local anaesthetic preparation used in dentistry which produces good soft tissue and pulpal anaesthasia and also reduce postextraction bleeding.

LIGNOCAINE

Mechanism of Action

Lignocaine stabilizes the neuronal membrane by inhibiting ionic fluxes required for initiation and conduction of impulses thereby affecting local anaesthetic action.

Pharmacokinetics

Lignocaine is completely absorbed following parenteral administration, its rate of absorption depending upon various factors such as site of administration and the presence or absence of vasoconstrictor agent.

Lignocaine is metabolised rapidly by the liver and metabolites and unchanged drug are excreted by the kidneys. Approximately 90% of lignocaine administered is excreted in the form of various metabolites and less than 10% is excreted unchanged.

The elimination half-life of lignocaine following an intravenous bolus injection is 1.5 to 2.0 hours.

Adverse Effects

CNS manifestations are excitatory and/or depressant and may be characterised by light-headedness, nervousness, apprehension, euphoria, confusion, dizziness, drowsiness, tinnitus, blurred or double vision, vomiting, sensation of heat, cold or numbness, twitching, tremors, convulsions, unconsciousness, respiratory depression.

Drowsiness following the administration of lignocaine is usually an early sign of a high blood level of the drug and may occur as a consequence of rapid absorption.

Cardiovascular manifestations are usually depressant and are characterised by bradycardia, hypotension and cardiovascular collapse, which may lead to cardiac arrest.

Allergic reactions are characterised by cutaneous lesions, urticaria, edema or anaphylactoid reactions may occur as a result of sensitivity to local anaesthetic agent.

Indications

Lignocaine injections are indicated for production of local or regional anaesthesia by infiltration techniques such as percutaneous injection, peripheral nerve block, spinal or subarachnoid block.

Lignocaine (2%) with adrenaline (1:80,000) is mostly used local anaesthetic in dentistry which produces good soft tissue and pulpal anaesthesia and also reduces post extraction bleeding. The pulpal anaesthesia is obtained within 2-3 minutes after injection and lasts for about on hour.

BENZOCAINE

It is a local anaesthetic belonging to the ester group. It inhibits conduction of nerve impulses from sensory nerves. This action is a result of alteration of cell membrane permeability to ions. It is poorly absorbed from the intact epidermis.

Benzocaine has been termed by the FDA as 'one of the most widely used and safest external analgesic and that the incidence of sensitivity of benzocaine is quite low'. It's male genital desensitizing product has been termed as premature ejaculation remedy. Benzocaine when applied on the penis aids in temporarily slowing the onset of ejaculation.

DIBUCAINE

It is another local anaesthetic with longer action but most toxic. It is **used** for surface anaesthesia.

BUPIVACAINE

It is a potent and long acting local anaesthetic used for spinal, infiltration, epidural anaesthesia and nerve block.

Side effects include cardiac arrest, cardiac arrhythmias and respiratory failure.

Bupivacaine (0.5%) with adrenaline (1:2,00,000) is less frequently used in dentistry because of its poor penetration into bone.

BENOXINATE

It is a surface anaesthetic used in eye for producing corneal anaesthesia for tonometry and does not cause mydriasis or any corneal damage.

OXETHAZAINE

A potent local anaesthetic used for anaesthetizing gastric mucosa. Along with antacid in suspension form it is **used** in gastritis, gastric irritation and gastroesophageal reflux. **Side effects** include drowsiness and dizziness.

ROPIVACAINE

Newer compound, long acting local anaesthetic which produces less cardiotoxicity. It is used mainly for nerve block and in post-operative pain. It is occasionally used in dentistry.

❑❑❑

CHAPTER 2.9

CNS Stimulants

These are the group of drugs which are used to stimulate the central nervous system. Some of them are also known as analeptics, but they are not much useful clinically due to non-selectivity of action.

They are classified as in table 2.9.1.

ANALEPTICS

These drugs stimulate respiration in coma or fainting but because of its narrow margin of safety, they are occasionally used. Nikethamide is no longer used. Doxapram stimulates respiration and raises the blood pressure.

Table 2.9.1: *Classification of CNS stimulants.*

I.	**Analeptics**	
	Nikethamide (CORAMINE)	25% solution oral/IM/IV
	Doxapram	40-80 mg IM/IV
II.	**Psychostimulants**	
	Amphetamine, dexamphetamine, methamphetamine etc.	
	Methylphenidate (RETALIN)	5-10 mg BD
	Methylxanthines: Theophylline, caffeine etc.	
III.	**Convulsants**	
	Strychnine, picrotoxin, pentylenetetrazol etc.	
IV.	**Cerebroactive drugs**	
	Pyritinol (ENCEPHABOL)	100-200 mg TDS, 200-400 mg IV
	Piracetam (CERECETAM)	50 mg/kg TDS
	Dihydroergotoxine (HYDERGINE)	3-6 mg/day
	Nicergoline (SERMION)	30 mg OD-BD
	Piribedil (TRIVASTAL)	50 mg OD-BD
	Nimodipine (NIMODIP)	2 mg/hr IV infusion

PSYCHOSTIMULANTS

Amphetamines (dexamphetamine, methamphetamine etc.) are central sympathomimetics. These are drugs of abuse and repeated use can cause long lasting behavioural abnormalities and can precipitate psychosis. The detail is discussed in chapter 'Adrenergic drugs'.

Methylphenidate is chemically and pharmacologically similar to amphetamine. Both act by releasing norepinephrine and dopamine in brain. Both produce increased mental activity with little action on central and peripheral functions. It is well absorbed orally, metabolized and excreted in urine.

CONVULSANTS

Strychnine (alkaloid obtained from the seeds of *Strychnos nux vomica*) was used earlier due to its convulsant properties. It acts by blocking the postsynaptic inhibition produced by inhibitory transmitter glycine. It acts at Renshaw cell-motor neurone junction in spinal cord through which inhibition of antagonistic muscles is achieved. **Picrotoxin** (obtained from fish berries) is a potent convulsant. It acts by blocking presynaptic inhibition mediated through GABA by preventing Cl^- channel opening. It is not used now-a-days. **Bicuculline** is a synthetic convulsant and possessing picrotoxin like action. **Pentylenetetrazol** is a CNS stimulant, acting by direct depolarization of central neurons.

But none of these compounds are now used therapeutically and used in laboratories only as a research tool.

CEREBROACTIVE DRUGS

In this category, some of the compounds are used in the treatment of dementia and other related cerebral disorders.

PYRITINOL

It enhances cholinergic transmission and improves cerebral microcirculation in ischemic regions. It protects the neurons against hypoxia & disturbance of glucose metabolism.

Adverse effects include anorexia, epigastric distress, vomiting, fatigue, headache, sleep disturbances, skin rash, pruritus and increased excitement.

It is **indicated** in organic brain syndrome, intellectual impairment of senility, encephalitis, alcohol withdrawal state and perinatal distress, cerebrovascular accidents, and organic psychosyndrome.

PIRACETAM

It improves the functioning of the brain involved in cognitive processes e.g. memory, thought, learning in normal and in subnormal conditions. It is categorized as nootropic agent (cognition enhancers).

The beneficial effects are due to improved microcirculation, promotes the metabolism and modulates neurotransmission.

Adverse effects include nausea, epigastric distress and skin rash.

It is **indicated** in mental retardation and learning problems in children, confusional state in old age, cerebrovascular accidents, senile dementia, cerebral insufficiency and behavioural problem in elderly.

The other drugs in this category are aniracetam, oxiracetam, fosracetam, nefiracetam, nebracetam and pramiracetam.

DIHYDROERGOTOXINE

It increases cerebral blood flow by blocking alpha adrenergic receptors.

Adverse effects include nausea, epigastric distress, headache, dizziness, nasal congestion, skin rash and orthostatic hypotension.

It is **indicated** in arteriosclerotic dementia, primary progressive dementia, Alzheimer's dementia, multiinfarct dementia and primary progressive dementia.

NICERGOLINE

It is an ergot derivative with activity similar to that of dihydroergotoxine.

Adverse effects include GI disturbances, malaise, dizziness, agitation and hot flushes.

It is **indicated** in cognitive, behavioural and somatic symptoms associated with cerebral decay, parkinson's disease, memory disorders, apathy, asthenia, anorexia, dizziness and tinnitus.

PIRIBEDIL

It is a dopaminergic agonist and improves memory, concentration and vigilance in older individuals.

NIMODIPINE

It is a calcium channel antagonist. It enters the brain and acts by blocking the entry of extracellular calcium in smooth muscle cells and neurons.

Adverse effects include nausea, epigastric distress, hypotension and flushing.

It is **indicated** in prevention and treatment of ischaemic neurological deficit following subarachnoid haemorrhage.

Some of the plant preparations containing *Ginkgo biloba* are used in cerebral impairment due to organic degeneration of cortex, multiple vascular infarcts, in psychobehavioural symptoms, certain syndrome of vertigo, dizziness and tinnitus etc. Benefit is due to ginkgoflavin glycosides which has PAF antagonistic action.

DRUGS USED IN ALZHEIMER'S DISEASE (AD)

It is progressive neurodegenerative disorder and mainly affects older individuals. It is the most common cause of dementia which is a impairment of intellect, memory and personality in the absence of gross clouding of motor involvement.

The drugs used in AD are:

- **Centrally acting ChE inhibitor:** Tacrine, donepezil.
- **ChE inhibitors:** Metrifonate, rivastigmine, epastigmine, galantamine.
- **Cholinergic agonists:** Milameline, xanomeline.

TACRINE

It is the first centrally acting anti-ChE used in mild to moderate cases of AD. **Side**

effects include diarrhoea, abdominal cramps, polyuria etc. The major side effect is rise in serum transaminase and hepatitis.

DONEPEZIL

It is another predominant centrally acting ChE inhibitor and does not cause hepatotoxicity. It is given in dose of 5-10 mg OD HS.

RIVASTIGMINE

It is given in a dose 6-12 mg/day for six months and has been shown to improve cognitive functions in patients of AD and it has central ChE inhibitory action.

GALANTAMINE

It acts by dual mechanism i.e. inhibition of central ChE and as an agonist on central acetylcholine nicotinic receptors.

Other drugs which may have beneficial property in the AD are antioxidants, beta blockers and drugs from natural origin e.g. *Ginkgo biloba*.

❑❑❑

CHAPTER 2.10 Drugs Used in Parkinsonism

Parkinsonism is an extrapyramidal motor disorder, characterized by akinesia, rigidity and tremor with secondary manifestations such as excessive salivation, seborrhoea, mood changes (especially depression) and in certain patients, liver damage has been reported. It was first described by James Parkinson in 1817.

In parkinsonism, there is a degeneration of dopaminergic nerve endings of the basal ganglion (neurons in substantia nigra and the nigrostriatal tract), which results in deficiency of dopamine and cholinergic overactivity. This imbalance between the dopamine deficiency and overactivity of cholinergic system gives rise to this motor disorder. Thus, the rational approach to the therapy of parkinsonism would be either to increase the central dopaminergic activity or to decrease the central cholinergic activity.

The drugs used in the treatment of parkinsonism can be classified as in table 2.10.1.

LEVODOPA

Levodopa is the most effective drug available for the treatment of parkinsonism and used in combination with peripheral dopa decarboxylase inhibitors. Levodopa as such is inactive but it is the immediate precursor of the transmitter dopamine. When administered orally, 95 percent of the dose is decarboxylated in the peripheral tissues (mainly in liver). Dopamine thus formed in peripheral system act on CVS and other peripheral tissues and produce the unwanted effects. Dopamine, as such, can not be used to treat parkinsonism as it does not cross the blood brain barrier. However, the precursor of dopamine i.e. dopa crosses the blood brain barrier and is converted to dopamine in the brain and is released as a neurotransmitter.

Pharmacological Actions

1. **CNS:** Levodopa does not produce any significant action in normal individual. In parkinsonism patient, it improves all manifestations of parkinsonism. Akinesia responds first, followed by rigidity and tremor. Other symptoms such as seborrhoea, sialorrhoea and aphonia also improve. The drug also improves mood, memory and patients

Table 2.10.1: *Classification of antiparkinsonism agents.*

I.	**Drug acting on central dopaminergic system**	
i.	***Precursors of dopamine***	
	Levodopa (LEVOPA)	0.5-3.0 g/day
ii.	***Dopaminergic agonists***	
	Bromocriptine (PROCTINAL)	10-40 mg/day
	Lisuride	2-5 mg/day
	Pergolide	2-4 mg/day
	Ropinirole (ROPARK)	0.25 mg TDS, increased each week by 0.25 mg (max 24 mg/day)
iii.	***Drugs facilitating dopaminergic transmission***	
	Amantadine	100 mg BD
	Selegiline	5-10 mg/day
iv.	***Peripheral dopa-decarboxylase inhibitors***	
	Carbidopa (used with levodopa; 25 mg carbidopa + 100 mg levodopa; TIDOMET PLUS)	20-100 mg/day
	Benserazide (used with levodopa; BENSPAR)	50-250 mg/day
II.	**Drug acting on central cholinergic system**	
i.	***Anticholinergics***	
	Trihexyphenidyl (Benzhexol; PACITANE)	2 mg OD-QID
	Procyclidine (KEMADRIN)	2.5-5 mg OD-TDS
	Biperiden (DYSKINON)	1-4 mg TDS oral/IM/IV
	Benztropine (COGENTIN)	1-2 mg OD-TDS
ii.	***Antihistaminics***	
	Promethazine (PHENERGAN)	10-25 mg TDS
	Orphenadrine (DISIPAL)	50-100 mg BD-TDS
	Diphenhydramine (BENADRYL)	50-100 mg/day

become more alert and interested in life and surroundings.

2. **CVS:** The levodopa produces its CVS effect by being converted into dopamine. It acts by stimulating alpha adrenergic receptors in blood and produce vasoconstriction and may raise the blood pressure. It also acts by stimulating betaadrenergic receptors in heart and produce tachycardia and increase force of myocardial contraction (positive inotropic action).
3. **Endocrine system:** Dopamine inhibits prolactin release in human being. It also acts on somatotrophs to increase growth hormone release.
4. **Miscellaneous actions:** Peripherally formed dopamine (converted peripherally after levodopa therapy) gains access to the CTZ (chemoreceptor trigger zone) causing nausea and vomiting.

Pharmacokinetics

Levodopa is rapidly absorbed when given orally and peak plasma level is reached at 30 minutes to 2 hrs and plasma half life is 1 to 3 hours. More than 95 percent of oral dose is rapidly decarboxylated peripherally mainly in GIT, liver and other tissues to dopamine and very little (less than 5%) is left to enter the central nervous system. Hence, levodopa is given along with peripheral dopa decarboxylase inhibitors (i.e. carbidopa, benserazide) so that more and more levodopa enters into CNS and is converted into dopamine in CNS.

Levodopa is excreted in the urine as conjugated metabolites and its main metabolite is homovanillic acid (HVA).

Adverse Effects

Nausea and vomiting because of CTZ stimulation, which can be minimized by starting with a lower dose. It also causes confusion, hallucinations, delusions and other behavioural effects. Certain cardiovascular effects such as palpitation, postural hypotension, sinus tachycardia and ventricular arrhythmias have also been reported.

On prolonged administration, grimacing facial tics and choreoathetoid movements of limbs have been reported.

Drug Interaction with Levodopa

- Levodopa with MAO inhibitors may precipitate severe rise in blood pressure (MAO inhibitors should be stopped at least two weeks before levodopa therapy).
- Methyldopa intensifies the adverse effects of levodopa.
- Pressor agents (catecholamines such as adrenaline and isoprenaline) should be avoided in patients on levodopa therapy.
- Pyridoxine accelerates the peripheral dopadecarboxylation of levodopa.

PERIPHERAL DECARBOXYLASE INHIBITORS

CARBIDOPA AND BENSERAZIDE

Carbidopa and benserazide are peripheral decarboxylase inhibitors used in combination with levodopa. They do not penetrate blood-brain barrier and do not inhibit the conversion into dopamine from levodopa in brain.

They make more of levodopa available to cross blood-brain barrier where levodopa is converted into dopamine and reach at the site of action.

When used along with levodopa, the plasma half life of levodopa is prolonged and dose may be markedly reduced. Also the most common side effect i.e. nausea and vomiting are not prominent and cardiac complications are minimized. It has no effect on involuntary movements, behavioral abnormalities and postural hypotension.

DOPAMINERGIC AGONISTS AND OTHER DRUGS

BROMOCRIPTINE (Bromoergocriptine)

It is an ergot preparation which has a specific dopamine receptor agonist action (**acts mainly on D_1 receptors**) and capable of crossing the blood brain barrier. It is less active than levodopa and used only in late cases as a supplement to levodopa. **Adverse effects** are vomiting hallucinations, hypotension, nasal stuffiness.

AMANTADINE

It is an antiviral compound and also improves akinesia, rigidity and tremor in parkinsonism. It is more effective than atropine like drugs but it is less effective than levodopa. Its effect on tremors is less than on rigidity. It **acts by releasing dopamine from the neuronal storage sites**. The drug is well absorbed orally and excreted unchanged in urine and drug is tolerated well and cause fewer adverse effects. In toxic dose, it causes convulsions and mania and should be used cautiously in epileptic patients.

SELEGILINE

It is a selective MAO-B inhibitor, which is predominant in brain and blood platelets. It retards intracerebral degradation of dopamine. It is used with levodopa in early cases of parkinsonism. It prolongs levodopa action, attenuates motor fluctuations and decreases wearing off effect. But clinical benefits are short lived (6-24 months).

Adverse effects are postural hypotension, nausea, confusion, increased levodopa induced involuntary movements and confusion.

Drugs Acting on Central Anticholinergic System

The cholinergic neurons are immediately distal to dopaminergic fibres in the caudate nucleus in brain. They are excitatory and in parkinsonism, there is a degeneration of inhibitory dopaminergic neurons and thus, there is increased cholinergic activity (preponderance of cholinergic system) which results in the symptoms of parkinsonism.

The central anticholinergic drugs having a higher central versus peripheral cholinergic action ratio are useful. The drugs like atropine are much less effective than levodopa but they are used when levodopa is not tolerated or contraindicated or the patient is not benefitted by levodopa or drug induced parkinsonism.

Atropine like drugs antagonize the rigidity and akinesia and cause reduction in the intensity of tremors. They act by reducing the unbalanced cholinergic activity in parkinsonism. **Benzhexol** is most commonly used and effective drug among the atropine substitutes used in parkinsonism.

Atropine like drugs cause several side effects such as dry mouth, blurred vision, urinary retention, mental confusion, hallucinations etc.

Antihistaminics are better tolerated by elderly patients who do not tolerate anticholinergics. Antihistaminics do not cause blurring of vision and xerostomia and also possess some central anticholinergic properties.

Newer Drugs

ROPINIROLE

Ropinirole is a non-ergot dopamine agonist with high relative *in vitro* specificity and full intrinsic activity at the D_2 and D_3 dopamine receptor subtypes, binding with higher affinity to D_3 than to D_2 or D_4 receptor subtypes. Ropinirole is more specific than dopamine agonists, bromocriptine and pergolide. The relevance of D_3 receptor binding in Parkinson's disease is unknown.

Ropinirole is rapidly and well absorbed from the GIT with maximum plasma concentration achieved within one to two hours after single oral dose.

Adverse effects include nausea, vomiting, drowsiness, fainting, fatigue, dyspepsia, abdominal pain, constipation, pharyngitis, abnormal vision, confusion and hallucinations.

It is **indicated** for the treatment of signs and symptoms of idiopathic Parkinson's disease.

Pramipexole has preferential affinity for D_3 family of receptors.

❑❑❑

Section 3

Drugs Acting on ANS

CHAPTER 3.1

Sympathomimetics

(Adrenergic Agents)

The sympathomimetic or adrenergic or adrenomimetic drugs mimic the effects of adrenergic sympathetic nerve stimulation. These are the important group of therapeutic agents which may be used to maintain blood pressure and in certain cases of severe bronchial asthma.

The sympathomimetics are classified as in table 3.1.1.

Mechanism of Action and Adrenoceptors

The catecholamines produce their action by direct combination with receptors located on the cell membrane. In 1948, Ahlquist divided the adrenergic receptors into two main groups – alpha and beta. The alpha receptor stimulation produces excitatory effect and beta receptor stimulation usually produces inhibitory effect.

Adrenergic receptors: These are membrane bound G-protein coupled receptors which function primarily by increasing or decreasing the intracellular production of second messengers cAMP or inositol triphosphate (IP_3)/diacylglycerol (DAG). Adrenergic receptors are classified into two main groups α and β.

Alpha receptors: There are two major groups of alpha receptors, α_1 and α_2. Activation of postsynaptic α_1 receptors increases the intracellular concentration of calcium by activation of a phospholipase C in the cell membrane via G protein. α_2 receptor is responsible for inhibition of renin release from the kidney and for central a-adrenergically mediated blood pressure depression.

Beta receptors: On the basis of the relative selectivity and potency of both agonists and antagonists, three types of beta receptors can be distinguished.

a. **Beta$_1$ receptors** have approximately equal affinity for adrenaline and noradrenaline and are responsible for myocardial stimulation and renin release.

b. **Beta$_2$ receptors** have a higher affinity for adrenaline than for noradrenaline. and are responsible for bronchial muscle relaxation, skeletal muscle vasodilatation and uterine relaxation.

Dopamine receptors: The D_1 receptor is typically associated with the stimulation of

Table 3.1.1: *Classification for sympathomimetics (adrenergic drugs).*

I. **Pressor agents**	
Noradrenaline (Norepinephrine)	2-4 μg/min IV infusion
Ephedrine	30-60 mg oral, 15-30 mg IM/IV
Dopamine (DOPAT)	2-50 μg/kg/min IV infusion
Phenylephrine (FRENIN)	0.5-1 mg IV, 5-10 mg IM
II. **Cardiac stimulants**	
Adrenaline (EPINEPHRINE)	0.2-0.5 mg SC/IM
Isoprenaline (Isoproterenol; ISOPRIN)	10-20 mg SL, 1-2 mg IM
III. **Bronchodilators**	
Adrenaline	0.2-0.5 mg SC/IM, 0.5% aerosol
Salbutamol (ASTHALIN)	2-4 mg TID-QID oral, 0.25-0.50 mg IM/SC, 100-200 mcg (1-2 puffs) TDS-QID aerosol inhalation
Isoprenaline (ISOPRIN)	10-20 mg SL, 1-2 mg IM, 0.4-0.8 mg aerosol (AUTOHALER)
Orciprenaline (ALUPENT)	20 mg Q1D, 0.75-1.5 mg (1-2 puffs; max. of 9 mg daily)
Terbutaline (BRICANYL)	2.5-5.0 mg TDS, 250-500 μg QID SC/IM, 250-500 μg (1-2 puffs) TDS-QID
Bambuterol (ROBUROL)	10-20 mg OD
Salmeterol (SEROBID)	25 μg BD (aerosol)
Other agents are isoetharine, fenoterol, rimeterol etc.	
IV. **Nasal decongestants**	
Ephedrine	0.5-2% topical solution, 0.75% nasal drops
Phenylephrine (ANDRE)	0.125-5% topical, 5-10% eye drops, 0.25% nasal drops
Pseudoephedrine (SUDAFED)	60 mg oral
Oxymetazoline (NASIVION)	0.025-0.05% nasal drops
Xylometazoline (OTRIVIN)	0.05-0.1% nasal drops
Naphazoline (PRIVINE)	0.1% nasal drops
V. **CNS stimulants**	
Ephedrine	30-60 mg oral
Dexamphetamine (DEXEDRINE)	5-10 mg oral
VI. **Uterine relaxants and vasodilators**	
Isoxsuprine (DUVADILAN)	5-10 mg oral/IM 4-6 hourly
Nylidrin (ARLIDIN)	3-12 mg oral, 5-10 mg IM
Ritodrine	0.1-0.35 mg /min IV infusion
Orciprenaline	2-8 μg/min IV infusion
Terbutaline	1-8 μg/min IV infusion
VII. **Anorectics**	
Fenfluramine (FLABOLIN)	20-40 mg/day
Dexfenfluramine (ISOMERIDE)	15 mg BD
Sibutramine (OBESTAT)	10-15 mg OD

adenylyl cyclase. The important agonist of dopamine receptors is fenoldopam (D_1) and bromocriptine (D_2) and antagonist is clozapine (D_4).

These receptors are distinct from alpha and beta receptors and are particularly important in the brain.

Adrenergic drugs can also be classified into:

a. **Direct sympathomimetics:** These act directly on a or/and b adrenoceptors e.g. adrenaline, noradrenaline, isoprenaline, phenylephrine, methoxamine, salbutamol etc.
b. **Indirect sympathomimetics:** They act on adrenergic neurones to release noradrenaline e.g. tyramine.
c. **Mixed action sympathomimetics:** They act directly as well as indirectly e.g. ephedrine, amphetamine, mephentermine etc.

Pharmacological Action of Sympathomimetics (Particularly adrenaline and noradrenaline)

Heart: Direct effects on the heart are determined largely by β_1 receptors. Adrenaline increases the heart rate, force of myocardial contraction and cardiac output which is associated with increased metabolism by the myocardium, increased oxygen consumption and thus decreasing cardiac efficiency.

Blood vessels: Adrenaline and noradrenaline constrict the blood vessels of skin and mucous membranes. Constriction predominates in cutaneous and mucous membranes which occur through both α_1 and α_2 receptors. Adrenaline also dilates the blood vessels of the skeletal muscles on account of the preponderance of β_2 receptors.

Blood pressure: Because of vasoconstriction (α_1) and vasodilatation (β_2) action of adrenaline, the net result is decrease in total peripheral resistance. Although adrenaline increases the systolic blood pressure but simultaneously lowers the blood pressure by its peripheral action. The rise in systolic blood pressure is often followed by decrease in blood pressure, adrenaline in such doses activates both a and b receptors. But mean blood pressure rises with increase in pulse pressure.

Noradrenaline causes rise in systolic, diastolic and mean blood pressure and does not cause vasodilatation (because of no action on β_2 receptors) and increase in peripheral resistance due to its a action.

Isoprenaline causes rise in systolic blood pressure (because of β_1 cardiac stimulant action) but marked fall in diastolic blood pressure (because of b_2 vasodilatation action) but mean blood pressure generally falls.

GIT: Adrenaline causes relaxation of smooth muscles of GIT and reduce its motility. Relaxation of smooth muscles of GIT can be brought about by both alpha and beta stimulants. It decreases the tone, frequency and amplitude of contraction of smooth muscles.

Respiratory system: The presence of β_2 receptors in bronchial smooth muscle causes relaxation and activation of these receptors by β_2 agonists cause bronchodilatation. Among catecholamines, adrenaline and isoprenaline are potent bronchodilators due to its β_2 action but not noradrenaline.

Uterus: The response of the uterus to the catecholamines varies according to species and absence or presence of pregnancy. In rats both pregnant and nonpregnant uterus, relaxation is produced while in rabbits both pregnant and nonpregnant uterus is contracted. In human beings, nonpregnant uterus is contracted while pregnant uterus is relaxed in the last month of pregnancy.

Eye: Mydriasis occur due to contraction of radial muscles of iris, intraocular tension is lowered due to less production of the aqueous humor secondary to vasoconstriction and conjunctival ischemia due to constriction of conjunctival blood vessels.

Action on other smooth muscles & other miscellaneous actions:

a. **Urinary bladder:** Detrusor is relaxed (b) and trigone is constricted (a) and both the actions tend to inhibit micturition.
b. **Spleen:** In animals, it causes contraction (due to its a action) of the splenic capsule resulting in increase in number of RBCs in circulation.
c. It also cause contraction of retractor penis, seminal vesicles and vas deferens.
d. Adrenaline causes lacrimation and salivary glands are stimulated.
e. Adrenaline increases the blood sugar level by enhancing hepatic glycogenolysis and also by decreasing the uptake of glucose by peripheral tissues. Adrenaline inhibits insulin release by its a-receptor stimulant action whereas it stimulates glycogenolysis by its b receptor stimulant action.
f. Adrenaline produces leucocytosis and eosinopenia and accelerates blood coagulation and also stimulates platelet aggregation.

Action on CNS: Catecholamines do not produce any marked CNS effects because they do not cross blood brain barrier satisfactorily. However, adrenaline may produce restlessness, apprehension, excitement and tremors on intravenous or intracarotid injection.

Pharmacokinetics

Catecholamines are absorbed from the intestines, but are rapidly degraded in gut and liver by enzymes MAO and COMT. Thus they are inactive on oral administration.

Adverse Effects

Restlessness, anxiety, tremor, headache. Both adrenaline and noradrenaline cause sudden increase in blood pressure, precipitating sub-arachnoid haemorrhage and occasionally hemiplegia, and ventricular arrhythmias. May produce anginal pain in patients with ischemic heart disease.

Contraindications

a. In patients with hyperthyroidism.
b. Hypertension.
c. During anaesthesia with halothane and cyclopropane.
d. In angina pectoris.

Therapeutic Uses

Allergic reaction: Adrenaline is drug of choice in the treatment of various acute allergic disorders by acting as a physiological antagonist of histamine (a known mediator of many hypersensitivity reactions). It is used in bronchial asthma, acute angioneurotic edema, acute hypersensitivity reaction to drugs and in the treatment of anaphylactic shock.

Bronchial asthma: When given subcutaneously or by inhalation, adrenaline is a potent drug in the treatment of status asthmaticus.

Cardiac uses: Adrenaline may be used to stimulate the heart in cardiac arrest. Adrenaline can also be used in Stokes-Adam syndrome, which is a cardiac arrest occurring at the transition of partial to complete heart block. Isoprenaline or orciprenaline may be used for the temporary treatment of partial or complete AV block.

Vascular uses: Pressor agents like adrenaline (more appropriate dopamine or dobutamine) may be useful in hypotensive crisis.

Adrenaline along with local anaesthetics may be used for infiltration, nerve block and spinal anaesthesia for prolonging the action and to reduce the systemic toxicity of local anaesthetics.

Adrenaline may be useful in control of haemorrhage from the skin and mucous membrane such as epistaxis and after tooth extraction.

Also used as nasal decongestant.

Miscellaneous uses:

a. Phenylephrine is used in fundus examination as mydriatic agent.
b. Amphetamines are sometime used as adjuvant and to counteract sedation caused by antiepileptics.
c. Anoretic drugs can help the obese people.
d. Amphetamine may be useful in nocturnal enuresis in children.
e. Isoxsuprine (uterine relaxant) has been used in threatened abortion and dysmenorrhoea.

DOPAMINE

It is an immediate metabolic precursor of noradrenaline. It activates D_1 receptors in several vascular beds, which causes vasodilatation. It acts on dopaminergic and other adrenergic receptors (α & β_1).

Pharmacological Actions of Dopamine

The actions of particular sympathomimetic amine depend on its relative activity at different types of adrenergic receptors. The overall actions are:

Cardiovascular system:

a. **Blood vessels:** D_1 receptors promote vasodilatation of renal, splanchnic, coronary and cerebral arteries. Activation of the D_1 receptors in the renal vasculature may play a major role in the natriuresis induced by pharmacologic administration of dopamine.
b. **Heart:** In the heart, intraventricular pressure rises and falls more rapidly, and ejection time is decreased. These direct effects are easily demonstrated in the absence of reflexes evoked by changes in blood pressure, e.g. in isolated myocardial preparations and in patients with ganglionic blockade. In the presence of normal reflex activity, the direct effects on heart rate may be

dominated by a reflex response to blood pressure changes.

c. **Blood pressure:** The enhanced arterial constriction may lead to a marked rise in blood pressure. In the presence of normal cardiovascular reflexes, the rise in BP elicits a baroreceptor mediated increase in vagal tone with slowing of the heart rate.

Eye: The radial pupillary dilator muscle of the iris contains *alpha-receptors;* activation by drugs causes mydriasis.

***Respiratory tract*:** The blood vessels of the upper respiratory tract mucosa contain α_1-receptors; the decongestant action of alpha stimulants is clinically useful.

***Gastrointestinal tract*:** Relaxation of GIT smooth muscle can be brought about by both α and β stimulant agents. Alpha stimulants especially α_2 selective agonists, decrease muscle activity indirectly by presynaptically reducing the release of catecholamines. α_2-receptors may also decrease salt and water flux into the lumen of the intestine.

***Effect on endocrine function*:** Catecholamines are important endogenous regulators of hormone secretion from a number of glands. Insulin secretion is stimulated by beta receptors and inhibited by α_2-receptors. Similarly, renin secretion is stimulated by β_1 and inhibited by α_2 receptors; indeed, beta-receptor antagonists may lower plasma renin at least part by this mechanism.

Adverse effects of dopamine include nausea, vomiting, ectopic beats, anginal pain, tachycardia, palpitation and widened QRS.

Contraindications are atrial or ventricular tachyarrhythmias, hyperthyroidism and pheochromocytoma.

It is **indicated** in shock syndrome due to MI, trauma, septicaemia, heart surgery, renal failure and chronic cardiac failure.

DOBUTAMINE

It is a derivative of dopamine and has relatively β_1-selective action and it also activates α_1 receptors and do not have D_1 or D_2 receptor agonistic property. It increases the force of myocardial contraction and cardiac output without significant change in heart rate, blood pressure and peripheral resistance. It is **used** as inotropic agent and for short term management of CHF and also in patients who are unresponsive to digitalis.

EPHEDRINE

Ephedrine is an alkaloid obtained from '*Ephedra vulgaris*' plant. It act indirectly and directly on α and β receptors. It increases blood pressure both by peripheral vasoconstriction and by increasing the cardiac output. Ephedrine also relaxes the bronchial smooth muscles.

Ephedrine stimulates CNS and produces restlessness, insomnia, anxiety and tremors. Ephedrine produces mydriasis on local as well as systemic administration.

Ephedrine is **useful** for the treatment of chronic and moderate type of bronchial asthma, used as nasal decongestant and as a mydriatic without cycloplegia. It is also useful in preventing ventricular asystole in Stokes Adams syndrome. It is also used in narcolepsy, however amphetamines are the drug of choice.

PSEUDOEPHEDRINE

Pseudoephedrine appears to have less pressor activity and weaker central nervous system effects than ephedrine. It has agonist activity at both β_1 and β_2 adrenoceptors, leading to increased cardiac output and relaxation of bronchial smooth muscle.

It is readily and completely absorbed from the GIT following oral administration with no presystemic metabolism.

Pseudoephedrine is rapidly absorbed throughout the body. It is eliminated largely unchanged in urine by N-demethylation.

It is excreted in breast milk at concentration constantly higher than those in maternal plasma. The elimination of pseudoephedrine is reduced in renal impairment. Hepatic dysfunction is unlikely to affect the pharmacokinetics of the drug.

Adverse effects include excessive tiredness, restlessness, nervousness, tremors, headache, palpitation, elevation in BP, vomiting, anorexia, constipation, nausea and convulsions.

It is **contraindicated** in cardiovascular disease causing hypertension, angina pectoris etc., endocrine disorders like hyperthyroidism, diabetes mellitus, prostate enlargement and concurrent use of MAO inhibitors.

It is **indicated** in symptomatic relief from stuffed nose, respiratory tract congestion, bronchospasm associated with asthma, bronchitis and other similar disorders.

OXYMETAZOLINE

It is a directly acting sympathomimetic amine used in symptomatic relief in nasal congestion which increases mucosal secretion.

Local vasoconstriction is normally achieved within 5 to 10 minute of intranasal administration. Oxymetazoline enters tissues rapidly and is released slowly. The plasma half life is 5-8 days. 30% of absorbed drug is eliminated in the urine and approximately 10% in the faeces.

It is used:

1. As a nasal decongestant in allergic rhinitis, with or without the addition of antazoline or sodium chromoglycate.
2. As a nasal decongestant in sinusitis, in otitis media where there is evidence of obstruction of the eustachian tube especially in subacute serous otitis media and otitic barotrauma.
3. As an ocular decongestant in allergic conjunctivitis.
4. To 'whiten' an inflamed (red) eye caused by a local irritant such as dust or following the removal of a foreign body.

Adverse effects include local stinging or burning, sneezing, dryness of mouth and throat. Prolonged use may cause rebound congestion and drug induced rhinitis, headache, tachycardia may occur.

Compounds like naphazoline and xylometazoline are relatively selective α_2 agonists, which on topical application produce local vasoconstriction. They are used as nasal decongestants and have longer duration of action. Prolonged use can produce atrophic rhinitis and anosmia.

ISOPRENALINE

It is beta-receptor stimulant, which stimulates the heart and causes tachycardia. It relaxes the smooth muscles particularly the bronchial and GIT. It is mainly used in bronchial asthma, in the treatment of shock and as a cardiac stimulant in heart block.

ORCIPRENALINE

Is a potent β-adrenergic agonist. Receptor sites in the bronchi and bronchioles are more sensitive to the drug than those in the heart and blood vessels.

It decreases reversible bronchospasm associated with chronic bronchitis, pulmonary emphysema, bronchial asthma, silicosis, tuberculosis and sarcoidosis. The resultant decrease in airway obstruction may relieve the dyspnea associated with bronchospasm.

It is effective both by oral route as well as inhalation.

There is more rapid onset of action following inhalation administration.

Absorption via the bile is 45 percent of renal excretion. Bioavailability of the active substance is 33% owing to a first pass effect.

It is **indicated** in bronchial asthma and reversible bronchospasm associated with chronic bronchitis and pulmonary emphysema, including bronchospasm due to the use of b-blocking agents.

Can be used as a supportive therapy with antibiotics, secretomucolytics, corticosteroids, physiological saline and disodium chromoglycate.

Side effects such as palpitation, restlessness and finger tremor may occur; in isolated cases, flushing, headache, sleep disturbances, nausea, ventricular disturbances or angina pectoris and allergic skin reactions have been observed.

The injection or infusion of high doses may also cause tachycardia, arrhythmia and a decrease in blood pressure.

AMPHETAMINE

It is a synthetic compound with structural similarity to ephedrine and is available in racemic and dextro isomers. It increases the systolic and diastolic blood pressure. Amphetamine is a potent CNS stimulant and causes alertness, insomnia, increased concentration, euphoria or dysphoria and increased work capacity. Amphetamine produces wakefulness and improved physical performance. It contracts the sphincter of the bladder and relaxes the bronchial smooth muscle in large doses. Amphetamines are **drugs of abuse** and can produce behavioural abnormalities and can precipitate psychosis. It can produce psychological but no physical dependence.

Because of its misuse especially by teenagers, its use is limited to the treatment of Attention Deficit Hyperactivity Disorder (ADHD) and narcolepsy.

PHENYLEPHRINE

It is a vasopressor agent with some structural similarity to adrenaline and has a powerful alpha$_1$ receptor stimulant action. The pressor response is accompanied by reflex bradycardia. It is **used** as a nasal decongestant and mydriatic agent and also in the treatment of paroxysmal supraventricular tachycardia.

UTERINE RELAXANTS (TOCOLYTICS)

These are the agents which decrease uterine motility and have been used to delay or postpone labour and to arrest threatened abortion which is needed to allow fetus to mature.

ISOXSUPRINE

Both nylidrin and isoxsuprine have got beta receptor stimulant action and is **used** in the treatment of peripheral vascular diseases. But nylidrin is not used clinically.

Isoxsuprine has a potent inhibitory effect on vascular and uterine smooth muscle and has been **used** in the treatment of dysmenorrhoea, threatened abortion, premature labour and peripheral vascular diseases. **Adverse effects** include nausea, tachycardia, flushing and dizziness.

RITODRINE

It is β_2 selective agonist with uterine relaxant property and preferred to suppress premature labour and delay delivery of fetus. But, use of ritodrine in suppressing labour has been found to increase maternal morbidity and neonate may develop hyperglycemia. So it should not be used if mother has a history of diabetes, heart disease or is on β-blocker or steroid therapy.

Certain other drugs also having uterine relaxant property are calcium channel blockers, prostaglandin synthesis inhibitors, progesterone, nitrites, anticholinergics, ethyl alcohol etc.

FENFLURAMINE

It is a sympathomimetic amine. the mechanism of action is related to brain levels (or turnover rates) of serotonin or to increase glucose utilization. Its antiappetite effect is suppressed by serotonin blocking drugs. Its use in clinical practice is recently banned in 'India' because of severe toxicity.

❑❑❑

CHAPTER 3.2 Treatment of Shock & Vasopressor Agents

Shock is a clinical syndrome in which profound and widespread reduction in the effective delivery of oxygen and other nutrients to the tissues. In shock condition, the individual is weak, anxious with coldness of extremeties, sweeting and marked fall in arterial pressure. Physiologic mechanisms can effect the arterial pressure by acting on one or more of two variables i.e. preload, impedance to blood flow (after load) and myocardral contractility. These machanisms include:

- Local release of vasodilater metabolits e.g. adenosine
- Release form the endothelium of substances that relax (e.g. endothelium derived relax factor, nitric oxide) or contract (e.g. endothelium)
- Activity of autonomic nervous system and the modulation of this activity by baroreceptor reflexes and vasomotor centre in the brainstem.
- The release of epinephrine or norepinephrine by adrenal medulla and sympathetic nerve endings.
- Release of vasopressin.
- Release of vasodilators, including kinin and prostaglandins.
- Two activity of renin-angiolension system

All these mechanism can affect the arterial pressure by altering the vascular resistance and/or cardiac output.

FORMS OF SHOCK

The classification of shock is based on the cause which is as under:

I Cardiogenic shock

- Myopathic
- Arrhythmic
- Mechanical

II Oligemic shock or hypovolaemic shock

- Haemorrhage
- Fluid depletion

III Extracardiac obstructive shock

- Constrictive pericarditis
- Pulmonary embolism

- Severe pulmonary hypertension
- Percardial tamponade
- Coarctation of aorta

IV **Distributive shock**

- Anaphylaxis
- Septic shock
- Neurogenic shock
- Endocrinologic shock
- Due to toxic products e.g. overdose

TREATMENT

CARDIOGENIC SHOCK

It is characterized by severe, persisting pain, shock and hypotension with possible development of arrhythmias and is due to severe depression of systolic cardiac performance, systolic arterial pressure is below 80 mm Hg, low cardiac index, ventricular filling pressure is elevated and pulmonary edema may or may not be evident. The most frequent cause is infarction involving more than fourty percent of the left ventricular myocardiam, leading to a severe reduction in left ventricular contractility contradictively and failure of the left ventricular pump.

Acute myocarditis and depression of myocardial contractility following cardiac arrest and prologed cardiac surgery also the causes of cardiogenic shock.

Cardiogenic shock is also caused by mechanical abnormalities of the ventricle. Acute mitral or ventricular aneurysm, usually caused by acute myocardial infarction, can cause a severe reduction in forward cardiac output and thereby result in cardiogenic shock.

The management of cardiogenic shock when it is due to myocardial infarction (after mechanical causes have been excluded), the therapy should be directed toward reducing ischemia and salvaging severely, ischemic but reversibly damaged myocardium at the infart border. This may also be supported by administration of oxygen and nitrates, intraaortic balloon pumping and depending upon the specific condition, thrombolytic agents may be added.

The repaired myocardium may be treated by combination of intraaoritc balloon couterpulsation and sympathomimetics amines e.g. dopamine, dobutamine, etc.

In other conditions of cardrogenic shock (due to mechanical abnormalities) e.g. acute mitral regurgitation or ventricular septal defect, surgical correction is usually required.

OLIGEMIC OR HYPOVOLEMIC SHOCK

It occur due to haemorrhage or a large loss of body fluids secondary to diarrhoea, vomiting, burn or dehydration leads to inadequate ventricular filling i.e. to decreased preload severely, decreased right and left ventricular end-diastolic volumes and pressures. These changes leads to oligemic shock by causing an inadequate stroke volume and inadequate cardiac output.

Oligemic shock may be managed by rapid infusion of blood plasma or plasma substitutes/expanders and simultaneously the source of blood / fluid loss in identified and corrected.

EXTRACARDIAC OBSTRUCTIVE SHOCK

Pericardial temponade is the main cause of extracardric obstructive shock, which is the inability of the ventricle of fill during diastole markedly limiting the stroke volume and cardiac output. Another cause is massive pulmonary embolism

In pericardial temponade, administration of sympathomimetic amines e.g. norepinephrine and/or dopamine may improve haemodynamics temporarily and surgical pericardial drainage is the only effective treatment.

DISTRIBUTIVE SHOCK

Anaphylactic, septic and neurogenic shock are the examples of distributive shock and all of which usually cause profound decrease in periperal vascular resistance.

In anaphylactic shock, when a sensitized person is re-exposed to the specific antigen and due to antigen-antibody reaction there is large amount of histamine release along with other mediators of anaphylaxis, resulting in fall in blood pressure with savere allergic reaction and bronchospasm. Penicillin is the common example of anaphylactic shock in sensitized individuals. Epinephrine is a life saving drug of choice in this type of case. Dopamine may be given in severe vasomotor collapse. Septic shock is characterized by a low systemic vascular resistance and an elevated cardiac output and it usually begins with a nidus of infection that releases microbes and/or one or more mediators e.g. histamine, kinine, prostaglandins, endorphins, TNF, interlukin 1 & 2 etc. into the blood stream which produce vascular dilatation and vasoconstriction (some PG's & leukotrienes). The peripheral vasodilatation result in a reduced systemic vascular resistance and high cardric output.

Management of septic shock may be carried out in three simultaneous ways, firstly, the nidus of infection must be identified and eliminated, using surgical drainage and antimicrobial therapy. Sacondly, using cardiovascular monitoring and support, adequate organ system perfusion and function must be maintained. Thirdly, to interrupt the pathogenic sequence leading to septic shock.

Neurogenic shock is generally occur in abdominal trauma, spinal anasthesia, spinal cord injury and is managed by vasopressor agents e.g. dopamine.

❑❑❑

CHAPTER 3.3

Sympatholytics

(Antiadrenergic Agents)

These are the agents, which block the action of adrenaline and noradrenaline. They block either alpha or beta or both adrenergic receptors. They are classified as in table 3.3.1 and 3.3.2.

General Characteristics of Alpha Blockers

Alpha blockers are the drugs which block the pressor response to noradrenaline and

Table 3.3.1: *Classification for alpha adrenergic blocking agents.*

A. **Non-equilibrium**	
Phenoxybenzamine (FENOXENE)	20-60 mg orally, 1 mg/kg IV infusion
B. **Equilibrium**	
I. ***Nonselective (α_1+α_2 blockers)***	
i. *Ergot alkaloids*	
Ergotamine (GYNERGEN)	1-3 mg oral, 0.25-0.5 mg IM/SC
Dihydroergotamine	2-6 mg oral, 0.5-1 mg IM
Dihydroergotoxine (HYDERGINE)	1.5 mg oral TDS, 0.15-0.6 mg IM
ii. *Imidazolines*	
Phentolamine mesylate (FENTANOR)	50 mg QID
Tolazoline (PRISCOL)	25-50 mg TDS
iii. *Phenothiazines*	
Chlorpromazine (LARGECTIL)	25-50 mg oral/IM
II ***α_1 Selective***	
Prazosin (MINIPRESS)	0.5-1.0 mg TDS
Terazosin (OLYSTER)	2-10 mg/day, 1 mg HS
Triamazosin	25-200 mg TDS
Doxazosin (DOXACARD)	1-4 mg/day
Tamsulosin (DYNAPRES)	0.4-0.8 mg OD
III. ***α_2 Selective***	
Yohimbine	2-4 mg TDS

convert adrenaline induced stimulation response to depressor response. Blockage of vasoconstrictor receptors reduces peripheral resistance, venous return and cardiac output leading to fall in blood pressure. The decrease in blood pressure by alpha blockers can reduce renal blood flow, which can lead to reduction of glomerular filtration rate and more reabsorption of sodium and water in the tubules and ultimately sodium retention and increase in blood volume.

Positive inotropic and chronotropic effects of catecholamines are not blocked by alpha blockers, but these drugs can block catecholamine induced cardiac arrhythmias.

Certain stimulant actions of catecholamines on various smooth muscles are blocked by alpha blockers such as uterine contraction of certain species, contraction of vas deferens and retractor penis, stimulation of seminal vesicles and vas deferens. Alpha blockers can inhibit ejaculation and produce impotence. Salivary secretion and sweat formation induced by catecholamines is blocked by alpha blockers.

Alpha blockers also produce certain metabolic effects such as inhibitory action of adrenaline on insulin secretion is blocked and adrenaline induced rise in blood potassium level is also blocked.

Miosis and nasal stuffiness can occur with alpha blockers by acting on radial muscles of iris and nasal blood vessels. Diarrhoea may occur due to increase in intestinal motility.

The common **adverse effects** with alpha blockers are palpitation, nasal stuffiness, postural hypotension, retention of fluid, diarrhoea, inhibition of ejaculation and impotence.

PHENOXYBENZAMINE

It is a potent alpha-adrenergic blocking agent and only haloalkylamine used clinically. It effectively prevents the responses mediated by alpha receptors and diastolic blood pressure tends to decrease. It interferes with the reflex adjustment of blood pressure and produces postural hypotension. It increases the cardiac output and decreases the total peripheral resistance. It also antagonizes cardiac arrhythmias provoked by catecholamines. Apart from these effects, phenoxybenzamine has other actions also e.g. antagonism of acetylcholine, histamine, 5-hydroxytryptamine (serotonin). However, the vasodilatation produced by phenoxybenzamine is because of alpha blockage. **Adverse reactions** are miosis, dryness of mouth, inhibition of ejaculation, palpitation, nasal stuffiness and in higher doses, postural hypotension and reflex bradycardia.

It is **used** in the management of pheochromocytoma and also to treat peripheral vasospastic conditions e.g. Raynaud's disease and shock syndrome.

Phentolamine, another alpha blocker is exclusively used for the diagnosis of pheochromocytoma and for the prevention of abrupt rise in blood pressure during surgical removal of adrenal medulla tumors.

ERGOT ALKALOIDS

Ergot is a parasitic fungus (*Claviceps purpurea*). It contains different alkaloids of complex chemical structure. The amino acid ergot alkaloids are ergotamine, ergocristine, ergocornine, ergosine, ergocryptine and their dehydrogenated derivatives can block the alpha receptors. Ergotamine is an important alkaloid that possesses both vasoconstrictor and alpha-receptor blocking activity. Both ergotamine and dihydroergotamine are used in the treatment of migraine.

MIGRAINE

Migraine is a severe episodic throbbing or dull pain in head, may be lateralized or generalised associated with anorexia, nausea, vomiting, photophobia and blurring of vision. The pain of migraine and vascular headaches are associated with vasodilatation, edema and visible pulsations of the extracranial blood vessels. The 5-HT plays a pivotal role in pathophysiology of migraine.

DRUG THERAPY OF MIGRAINE

a. Simple analgesics (aspirin or paracetamol), NSAIDs and antiemetics are useful in mild attacks of migraine.

b. Moderate and severe attacks of migraine besides NSAIDs need specific drugs like ergot alkaloids, sumatriptan and methysergide along with antiemetics.

METHYSERGIDE

It is a 5-hydroxytryptamine antagonist ($5HT_{2A/2C}$). It is effective in preventing an attack of migraine. **Adverse effects** include nausea, abdominal pain, diarrhoea and nervousness.

SUMATRIPTAN

It is a potent selective 5-HT_{1D} receptor agonist used in the treatment of migraine. The $5HT_{1D}$ receptor is found dominantly in cranial blood vessel. It activates other subtype of 5-HT_1 receptor at very high concentration.

Oral bioavailability is only 15% but after SC injection absorption is rapid and complete. It is metabolized by MAO-A isoenzyme and metabolites are excreted in urine. **Adverse effects** include tightness in head and chest, paresthesia in limb, dizziness, rise in BP and bradycardia. Rarely seizures and hypersensitivity reactions occur.

Dose: SUMINAT; 25-100 mg/day, 6 mg SC.

Drugs useful in prophylaxis of migraine are β-adrenergic blockers (usually propranolol), methysergide, calcium channel blockers.

OTHER α-INHIBITORS

PRAZOSIN

It is an piperazinyl quinazoline effective in the management of hypertension. It is highly selective for α_1 receptors. It also reduces the venous return and cardiac output. It is used in essential hypertension, benign prostatic hypertrophy and in Raynaud's syndrome. Prazosin lowers blood pressure in human beings by relaxing both veins and resistance vessels but it dilates arterioles more than veins.

It has variable absorption from GIT and has about 50% hepatic first pass metabolism. It is highly bound to plasma proteins.

Adverse effects include orthostatic hypotension, dizziness, headache, drowsiness, weakness, palpitation and impotence.

TERAZOSIN

It is similar to prazosin but has higher bioavailability and longer plasma t½.

It is another α_1-selective blocker used in hypertension and benign prostatic hypertrophy.

DOXAZOSIN

It is another potent and selective α_1-adrenoceptor antagonist and quinazoline derivative. It's antihypertensive effect is produced by a reduction in smooth muscle tone of peripheral vascular beds.

Doxazosin is well absorbed after oral administration and approximately two third of the dose is bioavailable.

TAMSULOSIN

It is uroselective α_{1A} blocker and has been found effective in improving BPH symptoms.

Adverse effects include dizziness and retrograde ejaculation.

YOHIMBINE

It is an alkaloid obtained from an African plant *Yohimbehe.* Chemically it is an indolealkylamine related to reserpine. It has selective α_2 blocking property with short duration of action and also blocks 5-hydroxytryptamine receptors. It produces increase in heart rate and blood pressure due to increase in noradrenaline release. It does not have any role in clinical practice.

Therapeutic Uses of Alpha Blockers

1. ***Diagnosis and treatment of pheochromocytoma:*** Phenoxybenzamine is used in the treatment of inoperable pheochromocytoma. **Phentolamine test** is used for the diagnosis of pheochromocytoma.
2. ***Hypertension:*** The selective α_1 blockers such as prazosin, terazosin, doxazosin etc. are used in the management of essential hypertension.
3. ***Congestive heart failure:*** The selective α_1 blocker affords symptomatic relief in congestive heart failure in short term.
4. ***Peripheral vascular disease:*** In Raynaud's phenomenon, the drugs like prazosin, phenoxybenzamine produce a symptomatic relief.
5. Alpha blockers can be used in secondary shock due to any blood/ fluid loss accompanied by reflex vasoconstriction.
6. ***Benign prostate hypertrophy:*** Alpha receptor blockers increase urinary flow rate and causing more complete emptying of urinary bladder in benign prostate hypertrophy patients.
7. ***Migraine:*** Ergotamine is used in the treatment of migraine.
8. ***Erectile dysfunction:*** Injection of papaverine with or without phentolamine in the corpus cavernosum has been found to be effective in erectile dysfunction of penis.

Other drugs used for erectile dysfunction

Sildenafil: It is orally active selective inhibitor of phosphodiesterase type 5 useful in treatment of erectile dysfunction. It results in reduced breakdown of cyclic guanosine monophosphate (cGMP) which is responsible for nitric acid (NO) mediated vasodilatation in corpora cavernosa. Thus inducing an erectile response to sexual stimulation. It has no direct relaxant effect on smooth muscle of corpus cavernosa and has no effect in absence of sexual stimulation.

It is rapidly absorbed after oral administration with 40% bioavailability. It is metabolised in liver by cytochrome P450 to a less active metabolite which is predominantly excreted in faeces (80%) and in urine (13%).

It is **useful** in erectile dysfunction of any etiology.

Adverse effects include headache, flushing, dyspepsia, nasal congestion, abnormal vision (mild and transient), diarrhoea, dizziness, angina pectoris, AV block, palpitation, postural hypotension, priapism etc.

Dose: VIAGRA; 25-100 mg/day.

The newer drug of same category are **alprostadil, vardenafil** and **tadalafil** which are recently introduced for erectile dysfunction in man. **Apomorphine** is recently introduced for erectile dysfunction with proven efficacy and safety, given sublingually and acts within 20 minutes in a dose of 2-3 mg.

BETA ADRENERGIC BLOCKERS

These are the agents which block the action of sympathetic nerve stimulation and circulating sympathomimetic amines on the beta adrenergic receptors. At the cellular level, they inhibit the activity of the membrane cAMP. The main effect is to reduce cardiac activity by diminishing β_1 receptor stimulation in the heart. This decreases the rate and force of myocardial contraction of the heart, and decreases the rate of conduction of impulses through the conduction system. They are classified as in table 3.3.2.

Table 3.3.2: *Classification for beta adrenergic blocking agents.*

A. **Non-selective (β_1+β_2)**	
Propranolol (CIPLAR)	10-80 mg TDS, 2-8 mg IV
Sotalol (SOTAGARD)	80-480 mg/day
Nadolol	40-240 mg OD
Timolol (TIMOPRESS)	5-20 mg BD, 0.25-0.5% topical (eye)
Alprenolol	200-800 mg/day
Pindolol (VISKEN)	10-30 mg/day
With additional alpha blocking activity	
Labetalol (LOBATE)	100-200 mg TDS, 50 mg IV
Carvedilol (CARDIVAS)	12.5-50 mg BD
B. **β_1 Selective (cardioselective)**	
Metoprolol (BETALOC)	100-450 mg/day
Atenolol (BETACARD)	50-100 mg/day
Bisoprolol (CONCOR)	5 mg OD-BD
Celiprolol (CELIPRESS)	100-200 mg/day
C. **β_2 Selective**	
Butoxamine	

PROPRANOLOL

Propranolol is an optically active compound. The β-adrenergic receptor blocking activity resides entirely in the L-isomer, although the D-isomer has equivalent membrane stabilising activity. L-propranolol is a competitive antagonist at both β_1 and β_2 receptor. It is not cardioselective although it has slightly greater activity at the β_1 than at β_2 receptor. It has no agonist activity but has membrane stabilizing activity at concentration exceeding 1 to 3 mg, though such concentrations are rarely achieved during oral therapy.

If adrenaline is administered to an animal which has been pretreated with propranolol the pressor action is potentiated because the α-adrenergic vasoconstriction is not affected but the β_2 vasodilator action is blocked.

Pharmacokinetics

Propranolol is well absorbed after oral administration. Peak concentration occurs after 1-3 hrs after administration. Propranolol undergoes extensive hepatic first pass metabolism. The proportion of drug, reaching the systemic circulation increases as the dose is increased when the hepatic circulation may become saturated. It is rapidly distributed because it is lipid soluble. It can readily cross blood brain barrier (BBB).

It is highly bound to plasma protein (90% to 95%). The major binding protein is α_1-acid glycoprotein. Plasma half life is 3 to 6 hrs, and excreted through urine (95%) breast milk & 5% in faeces as glucuronide metabolites.

Therapeutic Uses

1. ***Hypertension:*** Propranolol is antihypertensive. Propranolol suppresses the activation of heart by blocking the β_1 receptor. They reduce the work of heart by decreasing the cardiac output and causing a slight decrease in blood pressure.
2. ***Glaucoma:*** Timolol and other ocular β-blockers are used to treat glaucoma. Propranolol is effective in diminishing intraocular pressure in glaucoma. This occurs by decreasing the secretion of aqueous humor by ciliary epithelium. It neither affects the ability of eye to focus for near vision, nor changes pupil size. Used in chronic cases only.
3. ***Migraine:*** Effective in reducing migraine episodes due to blockade of catecholamine induced vasodilatation in the brain vasculature. Propranolol decreases the incidence and severity of the attack.
4. ***Hyperthyroidism*:** Propranolol blocks the peripheral conversion of thyroxine to triiodothyronine. It controls palpitation, nervousness, tremor & sweating etc.
5. ***Angina pectoris:*** Propranolol decreases O_2 requirement and work of heart muscle and therefore is effective in reducing the chest pain on exertion which occurs in angina.
6. ***Myocardial infarction:*** It blocks the action of circulating catecholamines which would increase the oxygen demand in already ischemic heart muscle thereby limiting the infarct size.
7. ***Anxiety:*** Exerts an antianxiety effect during nervousness and panic attacks.

8. *Cardiac arrhythmias:* It is life saving in protecting against serious cardiac arrhythmias. It suppresses tachycardia.
9. *Pheochromocytoma:* Propranolol is used.
10. *Hypertrophic obstructive cardiomyopathy:* Propranolol inhibits the inotropic effect of sympathetic stimulation and may reduce intraventricular pressure gradient.
11. *Essential tremor:* Non selective β blockers are useful.

Adverse Reactions & Contraindications

1. *II or III degree heart block:* Cardiac arrest may occur.
2. *Bronchial asthma:* An immediate contraction of bronchiolar smooth muscle prevents air from entering the lungs. Bronchospasm may occur in patient with obstructive pulmonary diseases.
3. *Bradycardia:* If it taken, resting heart rate reduces to 60/min or less.
4. *In digitalis and verapamil therapy:* Severe bradycardia may occur. Both verapamil and propranolol are negative inotropic agents.
5. *Cardiac failure:* Beta blockers depress myocardial contractility and may precipitate cardiac failure & bradycardia.
6. *Cardiogenic shock.*
7. Carbohydrate tolerance may be impaired in prediabetics.
8. *Hypoglycemia.*
9. Rebound hypertension & angina can occur on abrupt withdrawal of propranolol.
10. *Metabolic acidosis.*
11. *Cold hand & feet.*
12. *Severe haemorrhage.*
13. Tiredness & reduced exercise capacity.
14. Can precipitate CHF by blocking sympathetic support to the heart.

OTHER BETA BLOCKERS

SOTALOL

It is **nonselective (β_1+β_2) blocking agent** with lower lipid solubility with additional potassium channel blocking activity.

NADOLOL

It is another **nonselective beta blocker** with longer duration of action and mainly used in hypertension. It is excreted largely in urine and does not cross blood-brain barrier and has no central side effects.

TIMOLOL

It is **nonselective agent** with no local anaesthetic activity and having **excellent ocular hypotensive effect** preferred for ophthalmic use. It is useful in chronic wide-angle and aphakic glaucoma. **Levobunolol** and **betaxolol** are other agents used as ophthalmic preparation used in glaucoma.

PINDOLOL

It is a **nonselective beta blocker** with marked intrinsic sympathomimetic activity. It has advantage over propranolol that it produces less bradycardia and rebound hypertension. **Oxprenolol** resembles propranolol and is short acting with mild intrinsic sympathomimetic activity. **Alprenolol** is similar to pindolol and oxprenolol.

BETA BLOCKERS WITH ADDITIONAL ALPHA BLOCKING ACTIVITY

LABETALOL

It is a **adrenergic antagonist** which can **block both alpha and beta receptors.** It is non-selective ($\beta_1+\beta_2$) and selective (α_1) receptor blocker. Labetalol is five times more potent in blocking beta than alpha receptors. Both alpha and beta blocking actions of labetalol contribute to a decrease in blood pressure in hypertensive patients. It is effective in mild to moderate hypertension, pheochromocytoma and clonidine withdrawal hypertension. The most serious **side effect** is postural hypotension because of alpha blocking activity. Other side effects include sexual dysfunction, failure of ejaculation, depression etc.

CARVEDILOL

It is **beta ($\beta_1+\beta_2$) and alpha (α_1) blocking agent** with additional antioxidant property. It is mainly **used** in hypertension and in CHF as cardioprotective agent.

Carvedilol significantly reduces systemic blood pressure, pulmonary artery pressure, right atrial pressure, systemic vascular resistance, and heart rate, while stroke volume index is increased.

Carvedilol is a dualaction cardiovascular agent with non selective beta blocking, α_1 antagonistic vasodilating properties and is devoid of intrinsic sympathomimetic activity.

Carvedilol is well absorbed after oral administration with peak serum levels occurring after one hour. Excretion is primarily in bile and significant accumulation of carvedilol or its active metabolites is unlikely in patients with renal impairment.

Carvedilol is **indicated** for the management of essential hypertension. It can be used alone or in combination with other anti-hypertensive agents. It is effective also in CHF.

Carvedilol may be used in patients unable to tolerate an ACE inhibitor. Carvedilol may be used in patients who are not receiving digitalis, hydralazine and nitrate therapy.

Adverse effects include symptomatic postural hypotension, dizziness, headache, fatigue, gastrointestinal upset and bradycardia.

CARDIOSELECTIVE/β_1 BLOCKERS

METOPROLOL

It is **cardioselective beta blocking agent** and is devoid of intrinsic sympathomimetic activity. It reduces plasma renin activity in hypertensive patients. Metoprolol may be preferred to a nonselective agent in asthmatics and patients prone to develop hypoglycemia. Its antianginal action is comparable to that of propranolol. It is metabolised by hydroxylation and excreted.

ATENOLOL

It is **cardioselective beta$_1$ blocking agent** with low lipid solubility, generally administered once daily because of its longer duration of action. Most commonly **used** in hypertension and angina pectoris.

BISOPROLOL

Another cardioselective beta$_1$ blocking agent devoid of intrinsic sympathomimetic activity given once daily in the treatment of hypertension and angina pectoris.

CELIPROLOL

It is **beta$_1$ selective blocker** with a modest capacity to activate beta$_2$ receptors also. It is **used** in treating hypertension and angina pectoris.

NEBIVOLOL

Nebivolol is a **new selective β_1-adrenergic blocking agent** that possesses a unique pharmacodynamic profile, by which it differs from traditional β_1-blockers.

Nebivolol is quite safe and is well tolerated. The most common **adverse effects** are dizziness, headache and fatigue. Owing to its combined dual mechanism of action, nebivolol leads to a unique haemodynamic and therapeutic profile by which it may be advantageous in essential hypertension, ischemic heart disease and congestive heart failure.

β_2 Selective Blockers

BUTOXAMINE

It is **selective beta$_2$ blocker**, but does not have any efficacious role in clinical practice.

THERAPEUTIC USES OF BETA BLOCKERS

1. Hypertension.
2. Ischemic heart disease, angina pectoris.
3. Cardiac arrhythmias.
4. Hypertrophic cardiomyopathy.
5. Congestive heart failure.
6. Myocardial infarction.
7. Pheochromocytoma.
8. Hyperthyroidism.
9. Neurologic diseases: Migraine, anxiety, essential tremor.
10. Glaucoma.

❑❑❑

CHAPTER 3.4

Parasympathomimetics

(Cholinergic Agents)

These are the drugs which stimulate the parasympathetic system and mimic the action of acetylcholine. The acetylcholine receptor stimulants and cholinesterase inhibitors together comprise a large group of drugs that initiate the action of acetylcholine. They belong to the various groups (Table 3.4.1).

Table 3.4.1: *Classification of cholinergic agents.*

I. Choline esters	
Acetylcholine	
Methacholine (Acetyl-β-methylcholine)	5-10 mg SC
Carbachol (Carbamocholine)	1-4 mg oral, 0.25-0.5 mg SC and 0.75-3.0% topical (eye).
Bethanechol (Carbamoyl-β-methylcholine; UROCONTIN)	10-40 mg oral, 2.5-5.0 mg SC
II. Naturally occurring alkaloids	
Pilocarpine (PILOCAR)	1, 2, 4% topical (eye)
III. Anticholinesterases (Cholinesterase inhibitors)	
i. Reversible	
Physostigmine (BIO-MIOTIC)	0.5-1 mg oral/IM, 0.1-1.0% topical (eye)
Neostigmine (PROSTIGMIN)	15-30 mg TDS oral, 0.5-5.0 mg IM/SC, 3-5% topical (eye)
Pyridostigmine (MYESTIN)	60-180 mg oral, 1-5 mg IM/SC
Edrophonium	1-10 mg IV
Distigmine	5 mg oral, 0.5 mg IM
Rivastigmine, Donepezil, Tacrine etc. (used in Alzheimer's disease).	
ii. Irreversible	
Diisopropyl fluorophosphate (DFP; DYFLOS)	0.025% topical (eye)
Hexaethyl tetraphosphate (HETP)	
Certain insecticides such as parathion and malathion.	

ACETYLCHOLINE

Acetylcholine (ACh) is an ester of choline and acetic acid available in powder form as chloride or bromide salt. It is extremely hygroscopic and rapidly undergoes hydrolysis in a neutral or alkaline medium.

It is synthesized within the cholinergic neurons by the transfer of an acetyl group from acetyl coenzyme A to the organic base choline. The specific enzyme 'choline acetylase' is essential for this reaction. Coenzyme A is widely distributed in the body and choline acetylase is synthesized in the cell bodies of the cholinergic neurons.

ACh is produced throughout the neurone and is stored in synaptic vesicles at the nerve endings.

There are two types of esterases found in animal tissues. **True cholinesterase** which is found in neural structures, RBC and placenta and is concerned with destruction of acetylcholine released at the nerve endings. The second type is **'pseudocholinesterase'** (non-specific cholinesterase) is found in blood serum, intestines, liver and skin and is responsible for the hydrolysis of benzoylcholine and does not hydrolyse methacholine. **Cholinesterase** hydrolyses acetylcholine into choline and acetic acid.

Pharmacological Actions

Stimulation of the parasympathetic nervous system modifies the organ functions by two main pathways. Firstly, the acetylcholine released from parasympathetic nerves can activate **muscarinic receptors** which are present in gland cells (sweat glands), smooth muscles and heart. The muscarinic action of acetylcholine are stimulated by muscarine and are blocked by atropine. Second, by its **nicotinic action** on autonomic ganglia, motor end plates of skeletal muscles and adrenal medulla etc. The action of acetylcholine on autonomic ganglia can be blocked by ganglion blocking agents such as hexamethonium and action on myoneural junction can be antagonised by d-tubocurarine.

Muscarinic Actions

Cardiovascular system: Acetylcholine decreases the contractility (negative inotropy) and decreases the conduction velocity (negative dromotropy) of the atria. It depresses the sinoauricular node, decreases the heart rate (negative chronotropy) and may cause cardiac arrest.

In isolated heart preparation, acetylcholine reduces the cardiac rate and in the presence of atropine, it can stimulate the heart causing ventricular arrhythmias.

Acetylcholine dilates all blood vessels causing flushing and fall in blood pressure. The vasodilatation is mediated through the release of endothelium dependent relaxing factor (EDRF). The fall in blood pressure is because of decrease in total peripheral resistance and cardiac output in anaesthetized animals.

Effect on smooth muscles: Acetylcholine causes increase in tone, amplitude of contractions, peristalsis and secretory activity of the gastrointestinal tract. It causes contraction of smooth muscles of gall bladder and relaxation of sphincters of gastrointestinal and biliary tract.

It also causes contraction of detrusor resulting in decrease in the capacity of the bladder and increase in the frequency of ureteral peristaltic waves.

Acetylcholine causes bronchoconstriction and increase in bronchial secretion and can precipitate the bronchial asthma.

Effect on secretions: Acetylcholine increases the salivary, sweat, lacrimal, nasopharyngeal, gastric and bronchial secretions. All these secretory effects are blocked by atropine and enhanced by cholinesterase inhibitors e.g. physostigmine.

Effect on eye: After intraconjunctival instillation, acetylcholine causes miosis, due to contraction of circular muscles of the iris and fall in intraocular tension.

Nicotinic Actions

Effect on autonomic ganglia: It can cause stimulation of sympathetic and parasympathetic ganglia and stimulation of adrenal medulla, which leads to rise in arterial blood pressure due to peripheral vasoconstriction.

Effect on myoneural junction: Acetylcholine cause stimulation of skeletal muscles and in larger concentration at the myoneural junction can produce paralysis of skeletal muscles.

Effect on CNS: Acetylcholine when injected parenterally does not cross blood brain barrier being a quarternary ammonium compound and does not have any central action.

Therapeutic Uses

Because of nonselective actions, acetylcholine can not be used for any therapeutic purpose.

CHOLINOMIMETIC DRUGS

METHACHOLINE

It is effective orally and resistant to pseudo-cholinesterase and possesses longer duration of action. Its nicotinic action is less than acetylcholine and actions are more marked on CVS as compared to GIT and urinary system. Earlier it was used for CVS disorders such as peripheral vascular disease and paroxysmal supraventricular tachycardia. But now, it is rarely used in therapeutics.

CARBACHOL

It is resistant to both true and pseudo-cholinesterase and is more potent than methacholine and action is more prolonged. It is used topically for ophthalmic purpose.

BETHANECHOL

It is resistant to hydrolysis by both true and pseudocholinesterase and has mainly muscarinic actions. It has been used in postoperative and postpartum non-obstructive urinary retention and gastroesophageal reflux.

PILOCARPINE

It is a natural alkaloid obtained from leaves of *Pilocarpus microphyllus* and *Pilocarpus jaborandi*. Pilocarpine is direct acting muscarinic agonist. It acts on M_3 receptor. It produces contraction of iris to produce miosis. It also stimulates ciliary muscle resulting in increased accommodation and improved outflow of aqueous humor. As a result of miosis the pressure on canal of Schlemm is reduced and hence improves drainage and thus reduces intraocular pressure. Thus it is useful in treatment of glaucoma.

Pilocarpine when given IV increases the flow from salivary gland and other exocrine glands. Bronchial smooth muscle and intestinal smooth muscle contract. Small doses generally cause fall in BP, but higher doses elicit rise in BP and tachycardia (which is due to ganglionic stimulation).

Therapeutic Uses

a. Open angle glaucoma.
b. Angle closure glaucoma.
c. Ocular surgery.
d. To counteract mydriasis.
e. Diagnosis of Adie's tonic pupil.
f. Accommodative esotropia.

Adverse Reactions

1. **Potentially life threatening effects:** Some commercially available preparation of pilocarpine contain sodium bisulphite which may cause allergic reactions including anaphylaxis and severe asthmatic episode.
2. **Acute overdosage:** The clinical symptoms may include nausea, vomiting, diarrhoea, abdominal pain. In addition frequent urination, excessive salivation, lacrimation, sweating, bronchoconstriction, nasal congestion. Severe pilocarpine toxicity may produce tremors, muscle weakness, bradycardia, cardiac arrhythmia, hypotension etc.
3. **Severe or irreversible adverse effect:** Some patient with peripheral retinal degeneration may develop retinal detachment. A sudden drop of intraocular pressure indicates that retinal detachment has occurred.
4. **Symptomatic adverse effects:** Topical pilocarpine therapy produces blurred vision or myopia, poor vision in dim light or sometime painful spasm. Many patients on pilocarpine may experience ciliary or conjunctival congestion, headache, photophobia. Some patient may develop pupillary dilatation following use of pilocarpine.

Ibopamine (2% eye drop) is recently introduced newer compound, producing dose dependent mydriasis endowed with very interesting characteristics: rapid onset, marked pupil dilatation and rapid return to normal pupillary diameter. This rapid return to normal pupillary diameter after its diagnostic application in eye offers significant advantages compared to other currently available mydriatics. Ibopamine is well absorbed through the cornea, it is rapidly hydrolyzed by esterases to epinine and the mydriatic effect is correlated with the concentration of epinine in the aqueous humor.

It is approved for mydriasis in ocular examination and surgery and for the early diagnosis of glaucoma.

ARECOLINE

It is obtained from the betel nut *'Areca catechu'* and has got muscarinic and weak nicotinic actions. It has no therapeutic value except for chewing to promote salivary secretion and in pan masala etc.

ANTICHOLINESTERASES

These are the drugs which act by inhibiting the enzymes true and pseudocholinesterase and thereby produce an accumulation of acetylcholine at the various cholinergic sites. The released acetylcholine from the nerve endings is quickly destroyed by the enzyme cholinesterase. Anticholinesterase inhibit this enzyme which results in accumulation of acetylcholine and continuous stimulation of muscarinic and nicotinic receptors.

As given in classification, these agents are of two type e.g. reversible and irreversible. The **reversible anticholinesterases** have a structural resemblance to acetylcholine, are capable of combining with anionic and esteratic sites of cholinesterase as well as with acetylcholine receptor. The complex formed with the esteratic site of cholinesterase is less readily hydrolyzed than the acetyl esteratic site complex formed with acetylcholine. Edrophonium forms reversible complex with the anionic site and has shorter duration of action. Also, neostigmine and edrophonium have a direct stimulating action at cholinergic sites.

Irreversible cholinesterases are mostly organophosphorus compounds and combine only with esteratic site of cholinesterase and that site gets phosphorylated. The hydrolysis of phosphorylated site produces irreversible inhibition of cholinesterase. And, because, of this property, the therapeutic usefulness is very limited. Most of the compounds are used as insecticides e.g. parathion, malathion and war gases e.g. tabun, sarin, soman etc.

REVERSIBLE ANTICHOLINESTERASE

PHYSOSTIGMINE

It is a tertiary ammonium alkaloid obtained from the Calabar bean, the dried ripe seed of '*Physostigma venenosum*', which is indigenous to tropical west Africa.

The pharmacological actions of physostigmine are similar to those of cholinergic drugs. Topical instillation into the eye produces miosis, spasm of accommodation and decrease in intraocular pressure. Physostigmine is well absorbed after oral as well as parenteral administration and also produces central cholinergic actions because of penetration into blood brain barrier.

The main **therapeutic use** of physostigmine is as miotic to treat glaucoma and also to reverse the mydriatic effect of atropine and its analogues used in refraction of the eye. It is also used in the treatment of atropine intoxication and poisoning with phenothiazines. It is also used in primary stages of Alzheimer's disease.

NEOSTIGMINE

It is a synthetic quarternary ammonium compound, similar to physostigmine and rapid onset of action and can inhibit both true and pseudocholinesterases.

It increases the tone and motility of the gut and enhances the gastric juice production and also promotes the propulsion of intestinal contents.

At the neuromuscular junction, it produces the contraction of skeletal muscle by its direct action and by inactivation of anticholinesterase and has got anticurare action. By virtue of its structural similarity to acetylcholine, it acts as partial agonist on motor end plate.

Neostigmine, by its peripheral vasodilatation action reduces the blood pressure and heart rate.

On local ophthalmic administration, it

produces miosis, spasm of accommodation and reduction in intraocular tension.

Neostigmine does not cross blood-brain barrier, hence has no significant central action.

Neostigmine is a drug of choice in the treatment of **myasthenia gravis**, a chronic disease characterized by muscular weakness and rapid fatiguability of the skeletal muscles due to impaired neuromuscular transmission. The defect may be presynaptic or postsynaptic.

Apart from neostigmine, pyridostigmine and ambenonium are the other standard drugs used in the treatment of myasthenia gravis.

Neostigmine preceded by atropine to block muscarinic effects rapidly reverses muscle paralysis induced by competitive neuromuscular blockers (decurarization).

Neostigmine is also useful in postoperative paralytic ileus/urinary retention.

PYRIDOSTIGMINE

It structurally and pharmacologically resembles neostigmine but has longer duration of action and less potent than neostigmine and better tolerated by myasthenia gravis patients.

EDROPHONIUM

It is a quarternary ammonium anticholinesterase and structurally related to neostigmine but has got weak anticholinesterase activity as compared to neostigmine. It is mainly **useful** as diagnostic agent for myasthenia gravis and for postoperative decurarization.

DISTIGMINE

It is a longer acting neostigmine analogue and is **used** to treat atony of the bladder and intestine and its action lasts for 24 hours. It is given daily before breakfast.

IRREVERSIBLE ANTICHOLINESTERASES

The organophosphorus cholinesterase inhibitors like diisopropyl fluorophosphate, phospholine, parathion, malathion etc. are highly toxic compound and cause irreversible inhibition of both true and pseudocholinesterases. They are highly lipid soluble compound and can easily cross the blood-brain barrier.

DIISOPROPYL FLUOROPHOSPHATE (DFP)

The pharmacological effects are those of acetylcholine. It produces prolonged inhibition of true and pseudocholinesterases. They are inactivated in the body completely by oxidation and hydrolysis and excreted in urine.

The are mainly **used** for the treatment of glaucoma, especially when other miotic agents fail.

❑❑❑

CHAPTER 3.5

Parasympatholytics

(Anticholinergic Agents)

Anticholinergic or cholinergic blocking agents are the agents which block the action of acetylcholine at the postganglionic parasympathetic nerve endings. They are also termed as antimuscarinic or muscarinic blockers and atropine is the classical antagonist which blocks the effect of acetylcholine on muscarinic receptors. The nicotinic antagonists also block certain actions of acetylcholine and are termed as ganglion blocking agents.

The anticholinergics can be classified as in table 3.5.1.

The cholinergic blocking agents which mainly include atropine and related alkaloid are obtained from the plant *Atropa belladonna* (deadly nightshade), *Atropa acuminata, Hyoscyamus niger* (black henbane) and *Datura stramonium* (datura) and semisynthetic atropine/hyoscine analogues and synthetic compounds.

The two important alkaloids of belladonna are atropine and hyoscine (scopolamine).

ATROPINE

The alkaloids namely atropine, hyoscyamine and scopolamine are obtained from *Atropa belladonna.* Atropine is dl-hyoscyamine, and, l-isomer is more potent than d-form both peripherally and centrally. Atropine blocks the muscarinic effects of acetylcholine, the antagonism between acetylcholine and atropine is of competitive type.

Pharmacological Actions

Pharmacological actions of atropine are due to equal blockade of M_1, M_2 and M_3 muscarinic receptors.

Effect on cardiovascular system: Atropine initially decrease the heart rate due to stimulation of vagal centre followed by tachycardia due to peripheral vagal block on SA node. It also shortens effective refractory period of AV node and facilitates AV conduction. In therapeutic doses, atropine completely blocks the peripheral vasodilatation and decrease in blood pressure produced by cholinergic agents.

Table 3.5.1: *Classification of anticholinergic agents.*

I. Natural alkaloids	
Atropine (used as sulphate; ATRO)	0.5-2 mg IM/IV, 1-2% topical (eye)
Hyoscine (Scopolamine; BELLADENAL)	0.3-0.5 mg oral/IM
II. Semisynthetic compounds	
Homatropine (HOMARIN FORTE)	1-3% topical (eye)
Atropine methonitrate (SPASMOLYSIN)	2.5-10 mg oral/IM
as inhalant (BROVON INHALANT)	0.1-0.2% inhalation
Hyoscine methylbromide	2.5 mg oral/IM
Ipratropium bromide (IPRAVENT)	40-80 µg inhalation
III. Synthetic compounds	
i. Used as mydriatics	
Cyclopentolate (CYCLATE)	0.5-2% topical (eye)
Tropicamide (ITROP PLUS)	0.5-1% topical (eye)
ii. Used as antisecretory-antispasmodics	
Glycopyrrolate (GLYCO)	1-2 mg oral, 0.1-0.3 mg IM
Pipenzolate methylbromide (PIPTAL)	5-10 mg/day
Isopropamide (STELABID)	5 mg/day
Mepenzolate methylbromide	30-60 mg/day
Dicyclomine (CATASPA)	10-20 mg/day TDS
Pirenzepine	100-150 mg/day
Flavoxate (URIPAS)	100-200 mg/day TDS-QID
Mebeverine (COLOSPA)	135 mg TDS-QID before meals
Drotaverine (DOVERIN)	40-80 mg TDS
Valethamate (VALOSIN)	10-20 mg BD-TDS
iii. Used as antiparkinsonian agents	
Trihexyphenidyl (PACITANE)	2 mg OD-QID
Procyclidine (KEMADRIN)	2.5-5 mg TDS
Biperiden (DYSKINON)	2-10 mg oral/IM/IV
Benztropine (COGENTIN)	1-2 mg oral/IM OD-TDS
Cycrimine (PAGITANE)	2.5-5 mg OD-TDS

In higher doses, atropine produces dilatation of the cutaneous blood vessels which may be due to paralysis of vasomotor centre.

Effect on central nervous system: In therapeutic doses, atropine causes stimulation of medullary vagal nuclei and higher cerebral centres and may produce bradycardia and increase in rate & depth of respiration. By depressing vestibular excitation, it has antimotion sickness property. It also decreases tremors and rigidity in parkinsonism by blocking relative cholinergic overactivity in basal ganglia. Scopolamine also stimulates the respiratory and vagal centres. Toxic doses of atropine may lead to CNS excitatory effects e.g. restlessness, anxiety, insomnia, delusions and hallucinations etc. It also cause medullary paralysis (respiratory paralysis) in still higher dose.

Both atropine and scopolamine induce sleep like pattern of EEG, it also cause rise in body temperature due to its action on temperature regulating centre in hypothalamus and also inhibits sweating.

Effect on gastrointestinal system: Atropine decreases the tone and motility of all parts of gastrointestinal tract. It also decreases the amplitude of contraction and frequency of peristaltic wave of stomach and intestines. Atropine also exerts a weak antispasmodic action on biliary tract and gall bladder.

Effect on other smooth muscles: Atropine relaxes the smooth muscles of bronchi and bronchioles which results in widening of the airways. It is effective in relieving bronchospasm produced by cholinergic agents.

Atropine also produces reduction in normal and drug induced ureteral peristalsis. It also tends to reduce the tone of the fundus of urinary bladder and enhances the tone of trigonal sphincter and may cause of retention of urine.

Effect on secretions: Atropine reduces the various body secretions e.g. sweat, salivary, bronchial and lacrimal etc. It also reduces the volume and total acidity of gastric secretion and, reduce the secretion of mucin and enzymes in the gastric secretions induced by cholinergic drugs.

It has no significant effect on intestinal and pancreatic secretions.

Effect on eye: Atropine produces mydriasis by blocking the cholinergic nerves supplying the smooth muscles of sphincter of the iris on local administration into the eye. It also produces paralysis of accommodation or **cycloplegia** (the condition in which, one can see things clearly only at a long distance and can not constrict the pupil for viewing the near objects clearly). Atropine induced mydriasis can be distinguished from the mydriasis produced by sympathomimetic amines as the latter do not produce cycloplegia.

Pharmacokinetics

All the belladonna alkaloids are well absorbed from the GIT, from the site of injection and the mucous membrane. They are distributed throughout the body and cross the blood-brain barrier. About 50% of the atropine is metabolized in liver and remaining portion is excreted unchanged in urine. Atropine cross the placental barrier and is secreted in milk and saliva.

Adverse Reactions

The adverse reactions are due to the peripheral muscarinic blockade and central actions. The general side effects include dry mouth, difficulty is swallowing, thirst, dry skin, skin rash, flushed skin etc. It also produces constipation, urinary retention, impotence, difficulty in micturition, tachycardia, palpitation, postural hypotension, dilatation of pupil, photophobia, blurred vision, dizziness, fatigue, anxiety and tremors etc.

Toxic doses can gives rise to **acute belladonna poisoning** which is characterized by depression of vasomotor centre, vasomotor collapse, coma and depression of respiratory centre.

Acute belladonna poisoning can be treated by administering universal antidote before gastric lavage, physostigmine in the dose of 1-4 mg SC can be administered after a interval of one to two hours until a satisfactory response is obtained. For urinary retention catheterization can be done and patients is kept in dark room to alleviate photophobia.

Therapeutic Uses

1. **Gastrointestinal colic (as antispasmodic):** Belladonna alkaloids relax the spasm of smooth muscles of intestinal, urinary and biliary tract. They are also effective in functional and drug induced diarrhoea, to relieve urinary urgency and frequency and enuresis in children. They are also used to reduce gastric secretion in peptic ulcer patients. Also, used to reduce the excessive sweating in tuberculosis and sweating and salivation in parkinsonian patients.
2. **CNS disorders:** Scopolamine and hyoscine are effectively used in the treatment of nausea, vomiting and motion sickness. Centrally acting anticholinergic/ antihistaminics e.g. trihexyphenidyl are used in parkinsonism.
3. **Pre-anaesthetic medication:** These agents reduce the salivary and respiratory secretion and are administered half an hour before general anaesthesia. They also prevent laryngospasm. Atropine is given in combination with morphine as a preanaesthetic medication to antagonize the central depressant action of morphine on respiration.
4. **In organophosphorus poisoning:** Atropine is used in mushroom poisoning due to muscarine.
5. **On CVS:** Atropine is used for counteracting bradycardia and partial heart block in some patients of myocardial infarction.
6. **As mydriatic and cycloplegic agent:** Atropine is used to produce mydriasis and cycloplegia for testing errors of refraction. Mydriasis is required for fundoscopic examination and in the treatment of iritis and keratitis.

ANTIMUSCARINICS (SEMISYNTHETIC AND SYNTHETIC)

HOMATROPINE

More potent than atropine. Used in eye and onset of mydriasis and cycloplegia is similar to that of atropine but homatropine is not much used for producing cycloplegia.

CYCLOPENTOLATE

It is more potent and rapidly acting as compared to homatropine for producing mydriasis and cycloplegia especially in children. It is also used in iritis.

TROPICAMIDE

It is used for refraction testing in adults and as mydriating agent for fundoscopy. It has **quickest** and **briefest action**.

ATROPINE METHONITRATE

It is used for abdominal colic and in aerosol form it is used in bronchial asthma.

IPRATROPIUM BROMIDE

It is a valuable drug used in the treatment of chronic obstructive pulmonary disease

(COPD) by inhalation route. **Titropium bromide** is congener of ipratropium bromide producing long lasting bronchodilatation.

DICYCLOMINE

It has got antispasmodic with direct smooth muscle relaxant action. It is used in morning and motion sickness.

GLYCOPYRROLATE

Rapidly acting antimuscarinic lacking central effects. Used for preanaesthetic medication.

ISOPROPAMIDE

Indicated in hyperacidity, dyspepsia, irritable bowel syndrome.

Propantheline, oxyphenonium, panthienate are useful in peptic ulcer and gastrointestinal hypermotility.

Pipenzolate and **mephenzolate** are useful in dyspepsia and infantile colics.

MEBEVERINE

It shows effect on colonic muscle activity. It is indicated in smooth muscle spasm.

PIRENZEPINE

Selective M_1 muscarinic receptor blocker. It inhibits gastric secretion. Thus is effective in peptic ulcer patients and promotes ulcer healing. It does not produce atropinic side effect (due to blockade of M_2 and M_3 receptors).

Only 20-30% oral bioavailability and is excreted unchanged in urine.

FLAVOXATE

It produces direct relaxant action on smooth muscle with analgesic and anaesthetic action and used in the treatment of dysuria, nocturia and urinary urgency and frequency associated with cystitis and urethritis.

❑❑❑

Section 4

Drugs Acting on Cardiovascular & Urinary System

CHAPTER 4.1

Cardiotonics

(Cardiac Glycosides)

Congestive heart failure (CHF) is a clinical syndrome with multiple causes and involve the right or left ventricle or both and in CHF, cardiac output is usually below the normal range. This ventricular dysfunction may be systolic, which leads to inadequate force generation to eject blood normally and diastolic, which leads to inadequate relaxation to permit normal filling. Systolic dysfunction, with decreased cardiac output and significantly reduced ejection fraction is typical of acute heart failure, especially that resulting from myocardial infarction.

Cardiac Glycosides

There are the drugs having cardiac inotropic property. They increase myocardial contractility and cardiac output in a hypodynamic heart without increase in oxygen consumption and overall myocardial efficiency is increased.

The cardiac glycosides are mainly obtained from plants e.g. digitalis, stropanthus and squill species and also present in certain other plants and animals. In 1776, William Withering, a Birmingham physician and botanist identified digitalis and other ingredients, which was found useful in the treatment of dropsy. In 1911, Mackenzie and Cushney studied the effect of digitalis on heart and its use in congestive heart failure.

The important cardiac glycosides are listed in table 4.1.1.

Pharmacological Actions

Effect on Heart

Contractility: Digitalis increases the force of myocardial contraction without causing corresponding increase in the oxygen consumption. This pharmacological action forms the basis of its use in treatment of CHF. In a patient of CHF, force of contraction of the heart at a given fibre length is decreased, thus the stroke volume is decreased. As digitalis increases the force of contraction of the heart and subsequently, it increases the cardiac output, increase in circulating velocity, residual volume is decreased, diastolic volume is decreased and size of heart is decreased but these effects are noticed secondary to increase in

Table 4.1.1: *Classification of cardiac glycosides.*

I	**Natural glycosides**	
	Digitoxin (DIGITALIN)	0.05-0.2 mg/day
	Digoxin (LANOXIN)	0.125-0.5 mg/day oral
		0.25-1.0 mg slow IV
	Lanatoside-C (CEDILANID)	0.25-1.0 mg/day
	Stropanthin-K (STROPHOSID)	0.25-0.5 mg IV
	Stropanthin-G (OVABAIN)	0.25-0.5 mg IV
	Proscillaridin-A	0.3-1.0 ml (Tr. Scilla)
	Cavallotoxin	
	Thevetin	
	Bufotoxin	
II.	**Semisynthetic**	
	Acetyl digoxin (ACYLANID)	0.2-0.5 mg/day oral/IV
	Desacetyl lanatoside-C (DESLANOSIDE)	0.25-1 mg IV
	Acetyl stropanthidin (diagnostic use)	0.25 mg IV

contractility and are not the primary effects of digitalis.

Cardiac output: Digitalis increases the cardiac output in CHF patients by increasing the force of myocardial contraction. It also increases the contractility of normal heart but cardiac output remains unchanged or is slightly decreased. In normal individuals, it increases the tone of arteries as well as that of the veins.

Heart rate: In CHF patients, the heart rate is decreased. Digitalis produce a decrease in heart rate by stimulation of vagus. The 'vagal effect' is probably evoked by sensitization of carotid baroreceptors, and by direct stimulation of vagal centre. The vagal action can be blocked by atropine but after full digitalising dose the effect can not be blocked by atropine and it is due to its direct cardiac action. In CHF patients, the sympathetic activity is increased as a compensatory phenomenon which leads to tachycardia. Digitalis decreases the sympathetic tone and thus reducing the heart rate.

Refractory period: It is a period after onset of depolarization during which a stimulus can not evoke a propagated action potential. In atrium, refractory period is shortened by vagal action and increased by direct action.

SA node: Digitalis sensitizes the SA node to normal vagal impulse resulting in bradycardia. In a patient suffering from paroxysmal supraventricular tachycardia, it decreases the heart rate due to vagal action on SA node which is associated with decrease in the slope of slow diastolic depolarisation and increase in the transmembrane negativity and, also lower the SA rate by antiadrenergic action.

Automaticity: It is the ability to generate propagated impulse. Digitalis increases the ability of the Purkinje cell and the ventricular muscle to initiate impulses.

Conductivity: Conduction through AV node is depressed whereas conduction is slightly increased in the auricle and ventricles.

ECG changes: Digitalis, in therapeutic doses causes inversion of T wave, sagging of S-T segment and shortening of Q-T internal (shortening of systole). In toxic dose, it causes prolongation of P-R interval (slowing of AV conduction), atrial arrhythmias (atrial tachycardia and atrial fibrillation) with AV block and ventricular arrhythmias.

Extracardiac Actions

- Digitalis produces diuresis in CHF patients, it increases excretion of sodium and water by the kidney which may be due to decrease in the venous pressure bringing about shifting of edema fluid into the circulation and also improves the renal circulation.
- Digitalis can produce nausea and vomiting which is probably due to the chemoreceptor trigger zone (CTZ) stimulation.
- Digitalis has mild vasoconstrictor action increasing the peripheral resistance. But in CHF patients peripheral resistance decreases due to withdrawal of reflex sympathetic overactivity. Venous tone improves in normal as well as CHF patients. It has no significant effect on coronary circulation.

Mechanism of Action of Digitalis

Digitalis acts by interfering with the sodium and potassium transport across the cell membrane and by increasing the amount of coupling calcium i.e. making more calcium available for excitation-contraction coupling.

Cardiac glycosides inhibit Na^+ K^+-ATPase by competing with potassium and may probably explain reversal of toxic effects of digitalis by potassium. Inhibition of the Na^+ K^+-ATPase leads to increase in intracellular sodium and decrease in potassium.

Calcium also forms a link between the electrical events in the membrane and contractile proteins. Digitalis makes more calcium available for excitation-contraction coupling and increasing cardiac contractility.

Digitalis also exerts some indirect action on heart mainly by increase in vagal activity which ultimately influences activity of AV node, SA node and auricles.

Pharmacokinetics

Among the cardiac glycosides, digitoxin is absorbed rapidly and completely from the gastrointestinal tract with oral absorption of approximately 90 to 100 percent with plasma protein binding of approx. 95 percent with plasma half life of 5 to 7 days. It enters the liver cells where it is metabolised to epidigitoxigenin and is excreted in bile and urine.

Adverse Effects

It includes anorexia, vomiting which may be of central origin. Headache, visual disturbance, xanthopsia (yellow vision), white vision, diplopia, drowsiness, disorientation, delirium and psychotic behaviour. Cardiac related effects include cardiac arrhythmias e.g. tachyarrhythmias, ventricular arrhythmias, supraventricular arrhythmia, AV block and bradycardia.

Treatment of Digitalis Induced Arrhythmias

Tachyarrhythmias

K^+ tends to antagonise digitalis induced enhanced automaticity and decreases binding of the cardiac glycosides to Na^+ K^+-ATPase. Infuse KCl 20 mmol/hr intravenously or orally depending upon the case.

Supraventricular Arrhythmias

Can be treated by beta blockers e.g. propranolol 10-40 mg every 6 hourly orally or 0.5-1 mg IV.

Ventricular Arrhythmias

Lignocaine (1-2 mg/kg IV) is the drug of choice. Phenytoin is also useful (250 mg IV) and has the added advantage of countering the depression of AV conduction by digitalis.

AV Block and Bradycardia

Can be treated by atropine (0.6-1.2 mg IM).

Therapeutic Uses

Digitalis is used therapeutically in the treatment of:

Congestive Heart Failure

Digitalis increases stroke volume and cardiac output. Digitalis by increasing the cardiac output, brings about more complete emptying of the ventricles during systole. This reduces the pulmonary congestion and edema and decrease in systemic venous pressure. The cardiac glycosides primarily correct systolic dysfunction.

The dosing schedule is dependent on the desired speed of action and urgency. Like other drugs having a longer duration of action the treatment is initiated with a loading dose which is followed by maintenance dose for achieving a rapid onset of action and to avoid cumulative toxicity.

The maintenance dose is the amount required to maintain the therapeutic effect and is equal to the amount eliminated during the day.

Methods of Digitalization

1. *Intravenous digitalization* is done in emergency conditions of CHF or in atrial fibrillation. Digoxin 0.25 mg followed by 0.1 mg hourly be given by slow IV route with close monitoring of cardiac function.
2. *Oral digitalization:* Digoxin 0.5-1.0 mg stat and followed by 0.25 mg 6 hourly with monitoring of toxicity.
   - Digitoxin 1.2 mg is administered as a single dose. This can be given in divided dose also, in 8 hours interval.
3. *Maintenance dose method:* Administration of a daily maintenance dose (0.5 mg) of digoxin will digitalise the patient within a week.

Atrial Fibrillation

Digitalis is the drug of choice in atrial fibrillation for controlling ventricular rate. Its effect is due to the prolongation of the refractory period of the conducting tissue. The dose in so adjusted as to maintain the ventricular rate of 60 to 80 beats per minute at rest and approximately 100 beats per minute during light exercise.

Atrial Flutter

The reversal to normal rhythm is because digitalis converts flutter into fibrillation. Digitalis enhances the AV block and reduces the ventricular rate.

Paroxysmal Supraventricular Tachycardia

Its effects is due to vagomimetic activity, generally one fourth total IV digitalizing dose in given. In this condition, drugs like verapamil is more effective.

Left Ventricular Failure

Digitalis is used in chronic pure, left ventricular failure with hypertension and ischemic heart disease.

Other Positive Inotropic Drugs Used in CHF

BIPYRIDINE COMPOUNDS

AMRINONE

It is a relatively selective inhibitor of cyclic GMP, cyclic AMP-PDE (phosphodiesterase) type III family. It causes vasodilatation with a consequent decrease in systemic vascular resistance. It increases both the force of contraction and velocity of relaxation of cardiac muscles. It is administered IV 0.75 mg/kg/min as a bolus dose followed by 5-10 μg/kg/min IV infusion and total dose not to exceed 10 mg/kg.

Side effects include nausea, abdominal pain, diarrhoea, fever, thrombocytopenia (transient and dose related) and hepatotoxicity.

MILRINONE

It is relatively selective inhibitor of peak III cyclic AMP phosphodiesterase isoenzyme in cardiac and vascular muscle. In patients with CHF, it produces dose related and plasma concentration related increase in the maximum rate of increase of left ventricular pressure. Milrinone has a direct inotropic and direct arterial vasodilator activity. It is administrated by IV infusion 0.50 mg/kg over 10 min with a maximum daily dose of 1.13 mg/kg.

Side effects include ventricular arrhythmias, sustained ventricular tachycardia, angina, ventricular fibrillation, headache and hypokalemia.

Both the compounds are **indicated** in short term management of CHF in patents unresponsive to digitalis, diuretics or vasodilators.

❑❑❑

CHAPTER 4.2

Antihypertensive Agents

Hypertension is the most common cardiovascular disease and pathophysiologically hypertension can be classified into two main groups.

a. **Essential** or **primary hypertension**, where the cause for rise in blood pressure is not known. Responsible for majority of cases.
b. **Secondary hypertension**, where rise is due to renal disease e.g. chronic diffuse glomerulonephritis, pyelonephritis; due to some vascular disease e.g. renal artery disease or due to some endocrinal disorders e.g. pheochromocytoma, Cushing's syndrome and primary aldosteronism.

Systemic arterial blood pressure is determined by cardiac output and total peripheral resistance. In most of the cases, rise in BP is due to increase in total peripheral resistance.

Clinically, hypertension can be divided into three stages e.g. mild, moderate and severe hypertension. The diastolic blood pressure between 90-104 mmHg is graded as mild, 105-114 mmHg is graded as moderate and above 115 mmHg is graded as severe hypertension. The person having systolic blood pressure more than 160 mmHg with low diastolic blood pressure is termed as 'isolated systolic hypertension' commonly seen in elderly person.

The blood pressure is mainly controlled by two systems. Firstly through the baro-receptors and the adrenergic nervous system. The baroreceptor reflexes protect the circulation against stresses which shows the changes in the arterial blood pressure. Secondly through **renin angiotensin system**, which is involved in the pathogenesis of some forms of secondary hypertension. **Renin** is a proteolytic enzyme released from the juxtaglomerular cells of kidneys. The reaction between renin and plasma protein, serum globulin (angiotensinogen) forms an inactive compound 'angiotensin I' (decapeptide), which further changed into '**angiotensin II**' (octapeptide) by the action of angiotensin converting enzyme (ACE) and is the most powerful vasoconstrictor agent. Angiotensin II also stimulates the synthesis and release of aldosterone from adrenal cortex of adrenal gland.

The drugs used in the treatment of hypertension can be classified as in table 4.2.1.

Table 4.2.1: *Classification of antihypertensive agents.*

I.	**Centrally acting sympathetic inhibitors**	
	Clonidine (ARKAMIN)	75-225 μg/day
	Methyldopa (ALPHADOPA)	0.5-2 g/day
II.	**Adrenergic neurone blocking agents**	
	Reserpine (ADELPHANE)	0.25-0.5 mg OD
	Guanethidine (ISMELIN)	10-50 mg OD
III.	**Adrenergic receptor antagonists**	
i.	**Alpha blockers**	
	Prazosin (PRAZOPRESS)	0.5 mg BD, maintained at 3-20 mg BD
	Terazosin (OLYSTER)	2-10 mg/day
	Doxazosin (DOXACARD)	2-8 mg/day
	Phentolamine (FENTANOR)	2-5 mg IV
	Phenoxybenzamine (FENOXENE)	20-60 mg/day oral, 1 mg/kg IV
ii.	**Beta blockers**	
	Propranolol (CIPLAR)	10-80 mg TDS, 2-8 mg IV
	Metoprolol (BETALOC)	100-450 mg/day
	Atenolol (BETACARD)	50-100 mg/day
	Sotalol (SOTAGARD)	80-480 mg/day
	Pindolol (PINADOL)	10-30 mg/day
	Celiprolol (CELIPRESS)	100-200 mg/BD-TDS
iii.	**Alpha & beta blockers**	
	Carvedilol (CARDIVAS)	12.5-50 mg OD
	Labetalol (NORMADATE)	100-200 mg TDS, 50 mg IV
IV.	**Angiotensin converting enzyme (ACE) inhibitors**	
	Captopril (CAPOTRIL)	25-100 mg TDS
	Enalapril (ENCARDIL)	10-20 mg OD-BD
	Lisinopril (BIDPRIL)	5-20 mg/day
	Ramipril (RAMIPRESS)	2.5-10 mg OD
	Perindopril (PERIGARD)	4-8 mg OD
	Benzapril (BENACE)	10-40 mg OD-BD
	Also available omapatrilat, Quinapril, Trandolapril	
V.	**Angiotensin II receptor (type AT_1) antagonist**	
	Losartan potassium (LOSACAR)	25-100 mg OD
	Irbesartan (IROVEL)	150-300 mg OD
VI.	**Calcium channel blockers**	
	Verapamil (VASOPTEN)	40-160 mg TDS
	Diltiazem (DILZEM)	30-60 mg TDS-QID
	Nifedipine (CALCIGARD)	5-20 mg TDS, oral/SL
	Amlodipine (AMLODAC)	5-10 mg OD
	Also available Felodipine, Lacidipine, Benidipine, Nilmodipine	
VII.	**Direct vasodilators**	
	Hydralazine (NEPRESOL)	2-50 mg BD
	Sodium nitroprusside (NIPRESS)	0.1-0.3 mg/min IV infusion
	Nicorandil (ZYMCOR)	5-20 mg BD
VIII.	**Diuretics**	
	(For details see chapter 'Diuretics')	

Centrally Acting Drugs

CLONIDINE

It is an imidazoline derivative with a partial agonist action. It **stimulates presynaptic, α_2 receptors** in vasomotor centre of brain causing decreased sympathetic outflow which results in fall of blood pressure and bradycardia.

After oral administration the absorption is almost complete and rapid. It penetrates easily into CNS. Half to two third of oral dose is excreted unchanged in urine.

Adverse effects include drowsiness, dry mouth, sedation, restlessness, anxiety, nightmares, dizziness, sleep disturbances, skin rash, urticaria, nausea, constipation, indigestion and impotence.

Abrupt withdrawal may result in severe rebound hypertension, hepatic dysfunction and renal dysfunction.

It is **indicated** in hypertension of all grades except pheochromocytoma, glaucoma and migraine. It is also useful in opiate, alcohol and nicotine withdrawal. It also attenuates vasomotor symptoms of menopausal syndrome.

METHYLDOPA

It is α-methyl analogue of DOPA, the precursor of dopamine and noradrenaline.

It is converted to alpha methyl noradrenaline which stimulates central alpha$_2$ adrenergic receptors in brain thereby decreasing sympathetic outflow. It decreases peripheral resistance more than heart rate or cardiac output.

After oral administration bioavailability is low because of extensive metabolism. It is partly metabolized and partly excreted unchanged in urine.

Adverse effects include dizziness, postural hypotension, sedation, dry mouth, headache, sleep disturbances, depression, anxiety, impotence, blurred vision, constipation, skin rash, arthralgia, fatigue, anorexia, haemolytic anemia, parkinsonian signs, drug fever and hepatitis.

It is **indicated** in mild to moderate hypertension.

Adrenergic Neurone Blockers

RESERPINE

It is an alkaloid obtained from the roots of '*Rauwolfia serpentina*.' It is known to **deplete the catecholamines – adrenaline, noradrenaline and dopamine** from the various sites in the body. It also depletes 5-hydroxytryptamine (serotonin).

Hypotension develops gradually and is due to depletion of noradrenaline from peripheral adrenergic nerve endings.

Adverse effects include nasal congestion, flushing, bradycardia, postural hypotension, water and salt retention and CHF may be precipitated.

It also causes miosis, salivation, increased gastric acid secretion. CNS side effects include lethargy, apathy, psychic depression which may result in suicidal tendencies and weight gain.

Endocrinal disturbances include gynecomastia and impotence.

Because of its serious side effects and limited efficacy, it is not much used now clinically.

Guanethidine is another agent which inhibits release of noradrenaline. Causes sodium and water retention and may precipitate CHF. Endocrinal side effects are more common e.g. impotence and inhibition of ejaculation. It is also not used now clinically.

ADRENERGIC RECEPTOR ANTAGONISTS

The detailed pharmacology of alpha and beta blockers is already discussed in chapter 'Adrenergic blocking agents'. Only adrenergic blockers used in hypertension are discussed here.

PRAZOSIN

It selectively blocks post synaptic α_1 adrenergic receptors due to which vasodilatation occurs. The haemodynamic effects are decreased arterial pressure and reduction in venous and arterial tone.

It shows first pass metabolism in liver and it is highly bound to plasma proteins.

Adverse effects include postural hypotension, dizziness, tachycardia, palpitation, headache, weight gain, dry mouth, nausea, diarrhoea, constipation, nasal stuffiness, priapism and skin rash.

TERAZOSIN

It is an **α_1 adrenoceptor antagonist** and is a close structural analog of prazosin. It has a long duration of action.

It selectively blocks α_1 adrenoceptors due to which vasodilatation occurs and the blood pressure is reduced.

After oral administration it is almost completely absorbed. It is highly bound to plasma proteins and is metabolised in liver. About 10% terazosin is excreted unchanged in urine. It crosses the placenta.

Adverse effects include marked hypotension with first dose of terazosin, drowsiness, dizziness, nausea, blurred vision, nasal congestion, peripheral ederna, syncopal episodes and headache. In patients with BPH postural hypotension has been reported more than in those with hypertension.

It is **indicated** in mild to moderate hypertension, symptomatic relief of urinary obstruction in patients of benign prostatic hypertrophy.

DOXAZOSIN

It effectively controls blood pressure over 24 hours suppressing early morning BP rise. It increases insulin sensitivity, improves lipid profile.

It is extensively metabolised in the liver mainly by O-demethylation or hydroxylation. Approximately 4.8% is excreted in the faeces as unchanged drug.

Adverse effects include postural hypotension (rarely associated with fainting), dizziness, headache, fatigue/malaise, vertigo, edema, asthenia, somnolence, nausea and rhinitis.

It is **indicated** in mild to moderate, hypertension, treatment of both urinary outflow obstruction, obstructive and irritative symptoms associated with BPH.

PROPRANOLOL

It is **β_1, β_2 adrenergic receptor blocker** with membrane stabilising activity.

It selectively and competitively antagonises the action of catecholamines mediated through adrenergic receptors. It decreases heart rate, force of cardiac contraction. During longterm therapy, the blood pressure falls in patients of hypertension. The renin secretion is inhibited.

After oral administration it is absorbed almost completely but a large portion of the dose is metabolised in liver before reaching systemic circulation as a result the bioavailability of propranolol is reduced. It is highly bound to plasma proteins.

Adverse effects include fatigue, tiredness, skin rash, fever, depression, nightmares, sexual dysfunction, nausea, epigastric distress, cold extremities and hypoglycaemia.

It is **indicated** in hypertension, cardiac arrhythmias, longterm management of MI, hypertrophic subaortic stenosis, pheochromocytoma, migraine prophylaxis, angina pectoris, essential tremors.

The detailed pharmacology of propranolol is discussed in chapter 'Adrenergic blocking agents.'

METOPROLOL

It is a relatively **selective β_1 adrenergic antagonist with no agonist activity**. It reduces plasma renin activity in hypertensive patients.

After oral administration its absorption is good and rapid. It is metabolised extensively in body and shows first pass metabolism in liver (less than propranolol).

Adverse effects include headache, dizziness, nausea, vomiting, skin rash, diarrhoea, nightmares, hypotension and bradycardia.

It is **indicated** in hypertension, angina pectoris, cardiac arrhythmia, post MI patients, adjunctive management of thyrotoxicosis and prophylaxis of migraine.

ATENOLOL

It is a **cardioselective β_1 blocker with insignificant intrinsic sympathomimetic activity**.

After oral administration it is incompletely absorbed, excreted largely in urine as unchanged drug.

Adverse effects include bradycardia, nausea, vomiting, epigastric discomfort, dizziness, fatigue, tiredness, skin rash, leg pain, cold extremities because of peripheral arterial insufficiency.

It is **indicated** in hypertension, angina pectoris and acute MI.

PINDOLOL

It is a **non-selective β adrenergic blocker with partial agonist activity**.

It is absorbed efficiently after oral administration and is metabolised in liver.

Adverse effects include dizziness, nausea, vomiting, headache and sleep disturbances.

CARVEDILOL

It **competitively blocks β_1, β_2 and α_1 adreno-receptors**. It lacks sympathomimetic activity and has vasodilating properties which are exerted mainly through β_1 blockade. It reduces both systolic and diastolic blood pressure without reflex tachycardia.

After oral administration it is rapidly and extensively absorbed. Metabolism is primarily hepatic.

Adverse effects include postural hypotension, dizziness, headache, fatigue, Gl disturbances and dry eyes.

LABETALOL

It is a **mixed antagonist (α_1 and non-selective β-receptor antagonist)**. It has intrinsic sympathomimetic activity which is largely confined to β_2 adrenergic receptors. It is more potent in blocking β than a receptors. It is a potent hypotensive agent especially useful in pheochro-mocytoma.

After oral administration it is well absorbed and extensively metabolised in liver.

ACE Inhibitors

These drugs act primarily by suppressing renin-angiotensin-aldosterone system.

The main action of all ACE inhibitors is to **inhibit conversion of angiotensin I** (inactive) **to angiotensin II** (active). They **inhibit the angiotensin converting enzyme** (ACE). Hence, angiotensin II production is inhibited. Decrease in angiotensin II results in dilatation of peripheral vessels leading to a reduction in systemic vascular resistance and a decreased aldosterone secretion. They can be administered safely in patients of hypertension with diabetes mellitus or bronchial asthma. ACE inhibitors are efficacious drugs, are well tolerated and are useful antihypertensive drugs. ACE inhibitors are also used in coronary artery diseases. They reduce cardiovascular morbidity and mortality by improving coronary perfusion, reducing ventricular hypertrophy and remodeling and preventing progression of coronary atherosclerosis. However, the cellular mechanisms underlying the beneficial effects of ACE inhibitor are not fully understood.

They are now first line drug in all grades of hypertension. They can be safely combined with diuretics and β blockers.

CAPTOPRIL

After oral administration it is absorbed rapidly, the drug is partly metabolised and partly excreted unchanged in urine. The excretion is impaired in renal dysfunction.

Adverse effects include dry cough, skin rash, loss of taste, hyperkalemia, vertigo, headache, nausea, vomiting, hypotension, fatigue, neutropenia (rare), proteinuria and anaemia.

It is **indicated** in all grades of hypertension, CHF and scleroderma crisis.

ENALAPRIL

Enalapril maleate is an orally active angiotensin converting enzyme (ACE) inhibitor, it **lowers peripheral vascular resistance without causing an increase in heart rate**. The maleate salt (enalapril) allows better absorption after oral administration. It is an ideal drug for hypertensive patients who are intolerant to beta-blocker therapy. It also shows promise in the treatment of congestive heart failure. Following oral administration, enalapril is rapidly absorbed and hydrolysed to

enalaprilat – a highly specific, long acting, non-sulphydryl angiotensin converting enzyme (ACE) inhibitor.

It is **indicated** in all grades of essential hypertension and renovascular hypertension where standard therapy is ineffective or inappropriate because of adverse effects and in congestive heart failure. It should be used as an adjunctive therapy with digitalis and/or diuretics.

Enalapril is well tolerated in most patients. The most common **side effects** include dizziness, headache, nausea, diarrhoea, fatigue, muscle cramps, rash and cough. Other side effects are angioneurotic edema, hypotension, urticaria which are rare.

LISINOPRIL

It is lysine derivative of enalaprilat. Mechanism of action is same as other ACE inhibitors. After oral administration it is absorbed incompletely and slowly.

Adverse effects include dizziness, cough, hyperkalemia, headache, hypotension and angioedema.

RAMIPRIL

Ramipril is a long acting ACE inhibitor and is converted to active metabolite – ramiprilat.

Ramipril in patients with mild to moderate hypertension results in a reduction of both supine and standing blood pressure. In patients of acute myocardial infarction with CHF, ramipril reduced total mortality, progression of heart failure and CHF-related hospitalizations.

ANGIOTENSIN ANTAGONISTS

LOSARTAN

Angiotensin II is a potent vasoconstrictor, stimulant of aldosterone secretion and an important component in the pathophysiology of hypertension. Both losartan and its principal active carboxylic acid metabolite. (10-40 times more potent than losartan) **block the vasoconstrictor and aldosterone secreting effects of angiotensin II by selectively blocking the binding of angiotensin II to the AT_1 receptor** found in many tissues (e.g. vascular smooth muscle, adrenals). Losartan does not inhibit ACE (kininase II), the enzyme that converts angiotensin I to angiotensin II and degrades bradykinin.

Losartan potassium is well tolerated. Bioavailability is 33% due to hepatic first pass metabolism. It is 98% plasma protein bound. It is activated in liver. Both parent compound and active compound are excreted in urine.

Adverse effects seen most often are dizziness or light-headedness and rash. Angioedema (involving swelling of face, lips and/or tongue) have been rarely reported. There is also headache, asthenia, fatigue and dizziness.

IRBESARTAN

It is a **specific antagonist of AT_1 receptors** with a much greater affinity (more that 8,500 fold) for the AT_1 receptor than for the AT_2 receptor and no agonist activity.

Irbesartan is an orally active agent that does not require biotransformation into an active form. It is rapidly absorbed from the

GIT and undergoes metabolism in liver to inactive metabolites. It is about 90% bound to plasma proteins. It is excreted as unchanged drug and metabolites in the bile and urine.

Adverse effects are headache, sinus abnormality, cough, pharyngitis, diarrhoea, rhinitis, urinary tract infection, rash, anxiety/ nervousness, and muscle cramp. However, most side effects have been mild and transient in nature. Rare cases of hypersensitivity reaction, occasionally severe (e.g. anaphylaxis), have been reported.

It is **indicated** in mild to moderate hypertension, either alone or in combination with other antihypertensive agents.

Calcium Channel Blockers

Calcium channel blockers interfere with the calcium entry into the myocardial and vascular smooth muscles and thereby decreasing the availability of the intracellular calcium.

Calcium channel blockers depress the contractility of the myocardium and decrease the cardiac work and the requirement of oxygen. This effect proves to be beneficial in the treatment of angina pectoris.

VERAPAMIL

It **increases coronary blood flow and causes vasodilatation**. It has antiarrhythmic action also and it decreases peripheral vascular resistance.

After oral administration it is bound to plasma proteins and it is metabolised to biologically active metabolite.

Adverse effects include nausea, constipation, hypotension, flushing, dizziness, vertigo, pedal edema, nervousness and paraesthesias.

It is **indicated** in tachycardias, such as paroxysmal supraventricular tachycardia, atrial fibrillation/flutter with tachyarrhythmia, extra systoles, hypertensive crisis, acute coronary insufficiency (spasm), angina pectoris, vasospastic angina, myocardial infarction and hypertension.

DILTIAZEM

Diltiazem is a calcium ion influx inhibitor which **inhibits the transmembrane influx of calcium ions into cardiac muscle and smooth muscle** without changing serum calcium concentration.

Diltiazem is well absorbed from gastrointestinal tract and is subject to extensive first pass metabolism. It is 70% bound to plasma proteins. It is excreted as metabolites in bile and urine.

Adverse effects include headache ankle edema, hypotension, dizziness, flushing, weight gain, nausea, GI disturbances including anorexia, nausea, vomiting, constipation diarrhoea and taste disturbances. Occasionally there is gingival hyperplasia, skin rash and transient elevation in liver enzyme values.

It is **indicated** in the treatment of mild to moderate essential hypertension and in the management of chronic stable angina and angina due to coronary artery spasm.

NIFEDIPINE

It causes coronary vasodilatation and increases coronary blood flow. It reduces the total peripheral vascular resistance and systolic and diastolic blood pressure is reduced. It causes reflex tachycardia.

Adverse effects include headache, flushing, palpitation, nausea, vomiting and edema.

It is **indicated** in vasospastic angina, chronic stable angina, hypertension, hypertensive emergency, hypertrophic cardiomyopathy, peripheral vascular disorders, congestive heart failure, acute myocardial infarction, myocardial preservation during surgery, migraine, oesophageal spasm and exercise induced bronchial asthma.

AMLODIPINE

Amlodipine is a long-acting calcium channel blocker that **inhibits the transmembrane influx of calcium ions into vascular smooth muscle and cardiac muscle**. By inhibiting calcium ion influx it directly dilates vascular smooth muscle.

After oral administration of S-amlodipine besylate, bioavailability is 65-80%. Approximately 93% drug is bound to plasma proteins. It is extensively converted to inactive metabolites via hepatic metabolism. It is excreted in urine as 10% parent drug and 60% of the metabolites.

Amlodipine is generally well tolerated. The most commonly observed **side effects** are headache, edema, fatigue, flushing and dizziness.

Other side effects include nausea, abdominal pain, somnolence, palpitations, muscle cramps, frequency of micturition or nocturia, cough, breathlessness, epistaxis, impotence, nervousness and conjunctivitis.

It is **indicated** in the treatment of essential hypertension and angina pectoris.

DIRECT VASODILATORS

HYDRALAZINE

It **acts directly on arteriolar smooth muscle** to **cause relaxation**. It decreases diastolic pressure more than systolic blood pressure by lowering peripheral vascular resistance. Due to preferential arteriolar dilatation, postural hypotension is uncommon. It increases heart rate and cardiac output.

After oral administration its absorption is almost complete and rapid. It is subject to significant first pass metabolism in liver.

Adverse effects include nausea, vomiting, tachycardia, dizziness, fatigue, weakness, palpitations, headache, paresthesia, tremor, constipation, anxiety, nasal congestion, lupus like syndrome and sleep disturbances.

It is **indicated** in hypertension (moderate or severe) and hypertension with renal involvement.

SODIUM NITROPRUSSIDE

It has a brief duration of action. It relaxes directly arteriolar and venous smooth muscle. It decreases both preload and afterload thus both cardiac output and peripheral resistance are reduced.

It is given parenterally and onset of action occurs quickly (within 1 minute). On stopping IV infusion, the effect dissipates rapidly. It is converted to NO by endothelial cells and RBCs which relaxes vascular smooth muscle. It is converted to thiocyanate in liver which is excreted slowly.

Adverse effects include nausea, vomiting, nervousness, palpitation, sweating, headache, disorientation, methaemoglobinaemia.

It is **indicated** in hypertensive crisis, congestive heart failure and acute mitral regurgitation.

❑❑❑

CHAPTER 4.3 Antianginal Agents

Angina pectoris is a symptom of ischaemic heart disease. It develops as a result of an imbalance between the oxygen supply and oxygen demand of the myocardium. There is a paroxysmal chest pain which occurs when coronary blood flow is inadequate to supply required amount of oxygen to myocardium. There is a characteristic radiating pain in distribution in left arm, chest, jaw and neck region. This pain is mainly brought about by exertion/excitement when oxygen demand of heart increases and myocardial perfusion is decreased. Decrease in myocardial perfusion is due to deposition of atherosclerotic plaques in blood vessels. These plaques are due to accumulation of cholesterol and other lipid compounds which develop as patches on inner side of tunica intima of blood vessels i.e. subintimal layer.

The drugs used in the treatment of angina pectoris are classified as in table 4.3.1.

GLYCERYL TRINITRATE

Glyceryl trinitrate (GTN) releases nitrite ion (NO_2^-) which is further metabolised to NO by enzymatic step involving reaction with tissue sulphydryl (–SH) groups in vascular smooth muscles.

NO released by GTN activates soluble, cytosolic form of guanylyl cyclase in vascular smooth muscles by interacting with haem group in the enzyme. This converts GTP to cGMP. cGMP dephosphorylates myosin light chain kinase and prevent myosin interaction with actin leading to relaxation.

Pharmacodynamics

Action is almost exclusively on smooth muscle cells.

Effect on vascular smooth muscles: Both large arteries and veins relax in response to GTN. But in small doses, marked venorelaxation is seen leading to reduced preload. This causes decrease in stroke volume which is compensated with reflex tachycardia.

Arterioles relax less than venules because GTN evokes reflexes by baroreceptors which respond to decreased arterial pressure leading to reflex sympathetic discharge causing tachycardia and increased cardiac contractility.

Table 4.3.1: *Classification of antianginal agents.*

I. **Nitrates**	
Glyceryl trinitrate (Nitroglycerine; ANGISED)	2.5-15 mg BD-TDS, 0.5 mg SL, 2.5-6.5 mg SR
Amyl nitrate (VAPOROLE)	0.3 ml capsule inhalation
Isosorbide dinitrate (SORBITRATE)	5-10 mg TDS-QID SL, 40-80 mg SR BD
Isosorbide 5-mononitrate (MONOTRATE)	10-20 mg/day, 40 mg SR
Erythrityl tetranitrate (CARDILATE)	(30-60 mg/day oral, 5-10 mg SL)
Pentaerythritol tetranitrate (PERITRATE)	30 mg/day
II. **Beta blockers**	
Propranolol, atenolol etc. (For details see chapter on 'Antihypertensive drugs').	
III. **Calcium channel blockers**	
Verapamil, nifedipine etc. (For details see chapter on 'Antihypertensive drugs').	
IV. **Potassium channel openers**	
Nicorandil, diazoxide etc. (For details see chapter on 'Antihypertensive drugs').	
V. **Miscellaneous**	
Dipyridamole (PERSANTIN)	25-100 mg TDS
Nicotinyl xanthinate (COMPLAMINA)	300-600 mg TDS

Effect on coronary blood of flow: Myocardial oxygen extraction is nearly maximum at rest, so, there is little reserve to meet increased demands. So, increased myocardial demand for O_2 can only be met by increased coronary blood flow which depends on diastolic pressure and duration of diastole because coronary blood flow is negligible during systole.

Pharmacokinetics

They are administered through buccal, sublingual and parenteral routes. Skin ointments are also available. GTN is rapidly inactivated by hepatic first pass metabolism. So, oral tablets which are swallowed are ineffective.

Excretion is primarily as glucuronide derivatives of the denitrated metabolite via kidney. IV infusion has rapid onset of action but effects are quickly reversed on stopping the infusion. So, it is used only in treatment of severe, recurrent angina at rest.

Adverse Effects

1. **Throbbing headache:** It is due to arteriolar dilatation of meningeal arteries. It usually decreases over a few days if treatment is continued and can be controlled by decreasing the dose.
2. **Weakness and dizziness:** It may arise due to postural hypotension especially if patient is standing in a single position for a while. This is because, venodilatation results in 'venous pooling' i.e. accumulation of blood in peripheral vessels leads to postural hypotension.
3. **Flushing:** It is due to arteriolar dilatation in face and neck region.
4. **Sweating:** Arteriolar dilatation in arteries beneath the skin tends to warm up and sweating is the body's mechanism to dispel heat.
5. **Tachycardia and palpitation:** In small doses of GTN, arteriolar dilatation results in decreased arterial pressure. This leads to reflex sympathetic dis-

charge causing tachycardia and increased cardiac contractility. So, palpitation are felt.

6. **Methaemoglobinemia:** Its a rare adverse effect.

   Methaemoglobin has very low affinity for oxygen, so large doses of nitrites can result in pseudocyanosis (reduced O_2 carrying capacity), tissue hypoxia and death.

   Usually, even large doses of GTN and other organic nitrates do not raise plasma levels of nitrite dangerously high.

7. **Fainting:** Venodilatation leads to increased capacity (venous pooling) leading to marked hypotension. This can cause syncope/temporary loss of consciousness.

Indications

Sublingual tablet: Angina pectoris.

Intravenous: Unstable angina, coronary vaso-spasm, left ventricular failure accompanying MI, hypertension and during cardiac surgery.

Ointment/transdermal patch: Prevention of angina pectoris.

ISOSORBIDE DINITRATE

It can be given sublingually and orally for treatment of angina. Mechanism of action is same as nitrates.

Adverse effects include throbbing headache, sweating, skin rash, palpitation, flushing, weakness and dizziness.

It is **indicated** in acute attacks (sublingually) and chronic prophylaxis (orally) of angina pectoris and coronary insufficiency. In acute myocardial infarction, CHF and acute LVF.

ISOSORBIDE-5-MONONITRATE

It has a longer duration of action and mechanism of action is same as nitrates.

After oral administration hepatic first pass metabolism is less than isosorbide dinitrate, hence, systemic bioavailability is more.

It is **indicated** in pulmonary hypertension, prophylaxis of angina pectoris, post myocardial infarction therapy, CHF and acute LVF. It is not recommended for acute attacks of angina.

ERYTHRITYL TETRANITRATE

It is used for chronic prophylaxis of angina pectoris. Tolerance may develop to pharmacological actions.

Adverse effects include flushing, headache, dizziness, methaemoglobinaemia and drug rash.

It is **indicated** in treatment and prophylaxis of exertional and vasospastic angina.

PENTAERYTHRITOL TETRANITRATE

It is used for chronic prophylaxis of angina pectoris. Tolerance may develop to pharmacological actions.

Beta blockers, calcium channel blockers and potassium channel openers detailed pharmacology is given in chapter 'Antihypertensive drugs'.

OTHER ANTIANGINAL DRUGS

DIPYRIDAMOLE

It is a **coronary dilator** and claimed to dilate coronary resistance vessels. It probably

act by inhibiting the uptake and degradation of adenosine (a local mediator involved in auto regulation of coronary flow in response to ischemia). It has also weak platelet inhibiting action. It reversibly inhibits platelet phosphodiesterase hence cAMP concentration is increased and there is reduction of platelet reactivity.

Adverse effects include nausea, dizziness, skin rash and headache. Though it is not useful as an antianginal drug, but it has been employed for prophylaxis of coronary and cerebral thrombosis in post MI and post stroke patients, as well as to prevent thrombosis in patients with prosthetic heart valves.

❑❑❑

CHAPTER 4.4 Antiarrhythmic Agents

CARDIAC ARRHYTHMIAS

Cardiac arrhythmias is a group of disorder characterized by an abnormal cardiac rhythm and arise as a result of disorders of impulse formation or conduction or both.

Tachyarrhythmias (sinus rate more than 100 per minute) are produced by a disturbances of impulse generation or of impulse conduction in the heart. Tachyarrhythmias due to disturbed impulse formation are associated with irregular and rhythmic discharge from ectopic pacemaker activity in areas of the heart other than the SA node. The characteristic of myocardial cells, which enables them to generate spontaneous depolarization, is called **automaticity**.

Bradycardia can be due to depressed sinus automaticity and AV block. Bradyarrhythmias manifest as slow heart rate (less than 50 to 60 beats per minute in sleep). Depressed SA nodal automaticity lead to missing beats and bradycardia. AV block can be due to high vagal activity and side effect of certain drugs e.g. digitalis and β-blockers.

Antiarrhythmic drugs can be classified as in table 4.4.1.

SODIUM CHANNEL BLOCKERS

By limiting the conductance of Na^+ (and K^+) across cell membrane, they interfere with depolarization and decrease responsiveness to excitation thereby reducing rate of phase of phase 4 depolarisation in automatic cells.

QUINIDINE

It is an alkaloid obtained from the bark of cinchona and is a dextro isomer of anti-malarial drug 'quinine'. Its sodium channel blocking property results in an increased threshold for excitability and decreased automaticity. As a consequence of its potassium channel blocking properties, it prolongs action potential in most cardiac cells.

Pharmacological Actions

Cardiac actions:

a. **Excitability:** Quinidine depresses the excitability of cardiac tissues.

Table 4.4.1: *Classification of antiarrhythmic agents.*

I. **Class I: Sodium channel blockers**	
Quinidine (NATCARDINE)	200-400 mg TDS-QID
Procainamide (PRONESTYL)	50 mg/kg/day oral, 50 mg/min slow IV
Disopyramide (NORPACE)	100-200 mg TDS-QID, 2 mg/kg slow IV
Lignocaine (XYLOCARD)	1 mg/kg slow IV (bolus) then 1-3 mg/min IV infusion
Phenytoin sodium (DILANTIN)	100-400 mg/day oral, 100 mg IV (max 600 mg/day)
II. **Class II: Beta adrenergic blockers**	
Propranolol, etc. (Detailed pharmacology is discussed in chapter 'Antihypertensive agents' and Adrenergic blocking agents').	
III. **Class III: Drugs that prolong effective refractory period by prolonging action potential**	
Amiodarone (ALDARONE)	200 mg TDS
Bretylium	5-10 mg/kg bolus IV then 0.5-2 mg/min IV infusion
IV. **Class IV: Calcium channel blockers**	
Verapamil, diltiazem etc. (Detailed pharmacology is discussed in chapter 'Antihypertensive agents').	
V. **Miscellaneous**	
Adenosine (ADENOCOR)	6-12 mg IV bolus.
Atropine	0.6-2 mg IM (Used for AV block)
Sympathomimetics (e.g. adrenaline, isoprenaline and orciprenaline are also used for AV block).	
Digitalis (DIGOXIN)	0.25-0.5 mg IV for paroxysmal supraventricular tachycardia (PSVT), atrial flutter and atrial fibrillation

b. **Automaticity:** Quinidine decreases the slope of slow diastolic depolarisation (phase 4 of action potential) and thus decreases the spontaneous rate of firing of pacemakers. By depressing the entry of sodium into the cell during depolarization, quinidine depresses diastolic depolarization and ultimately automaticity.

c. **Conductivity:** Quinidine depresses interventricular and atrioventricular conductivity. PR and QRS intervals are also prolonged. Also decreases the rate of rise of action potential.

d. **Effective refractory period:** Quinidine depresses the potassium efflux during repolarization and prolongs repolarization. The refractory period increases due to its antivagal action. Its antivagal action prolongs the refractory period of atrium and shortens that of AV node. The antivagal action on the AV node causes paradoxical tachycardia in a patient of atrium fibrillation.

e. **Contractility:** Quinidine produces a negative inotropic action on the heart and contractility is depressed with toxic doses.

f. **AV conduction:** Quinidine depresses the conduction in atrium and Purkinje system.

g. **Electrophysiological effect (effect on ECG):**

1. It reduces the rate of rise of action potential i.e. phase zero of action potential which is due to depolarisation.

2. Increase in the duration of ventricular systole (QT interval).
3. Decrease in amplitude of T waves.
4. Depression of ST segment.
5. Reduction in conduction velocity (widening of QRS complex).

Extracardiac actions:

a. Quinidine in normal individuals produce a **decrease in blood pressure** after oral and IV administration.
b. Quinidine has got **antimalarial**, **antipyretic**, **oxytocic** and **skeletal muscle relaxant activity** also.

It is well absorbed orally, undergoes extensive hepatic oxidative metabolism. 90% quinidine is bound to plasma protein. The drug is distributed to most tissues except brain. About 20% is excreted unchanged by the kidney.

Adverse effects include SA block or arrest, high grade AV block, ventricular tachycardia, arrhythmia or ventricular asystole, polymorphic ventricular tachyarrhythmia, hypotension (particularly when given IV), cinchonism, tinnitus, loss of hearing, gastrointestinal upset, severe headache, diplopia, photophobia, etc.

It is **indicated** in prevention of atrial arrhythmia, atrial fibrillation or flutter, paroxysmal supraventricular tachycardia, ventricular premature beats and ventricular tachycardia.

PROCAINAMIDE

It has got quinidine like cardiac property. It **depresses the excitability of both atria and ventricles**. Contractility and conductivity are also depressed. It has got minimal vagolytic action.

It decreases the rate of rise of action potential and prolongs the effective refractory period.

After oral administration it is absorbed quickly, about 20% is bound to plasma protein up to and 70% of a dose is excreted in urine in unchanged form.

Adverse effects include renal failure, hypotension (when given IV), anorexia, nausea, vomiting, Q-T prolongation. Rarely there is diarrhoea, giddiness, psychosis, hallucination, mental depression, hypersensitivity, agranulocytosis, myalgia, angioedema, skin rash, digital vasculitis. Procainamide can cause syndrome that resembles SLE, which is reversible on discontinuation of procainamide; leukopenia and thrombocytopenia.

It is **indicated** in ventricular arrhythmia, ventricular premature depolarization and paroxysmal ventricular tachycardia, supra-ventricular tachycardia and atrial arrhythmia.

DISOPYRAMIDE

It has got **anticholinergic and membrane depressant properties** and like quinidine, it is effective against most of the atrial and ventricular arrhythmias. It has no effect on sinus rate.

Adverse effects include dry mouth, constipation, blurred vision, urinary urgency and occasional urinary retention, nausea, vomiting, diarrhoea, abdominal pain, hypoglycaemia, jaundice, coronary heart failure and hypotension.

It is **indicated** in atrial and ventricular arrhythmias in digitalised and non-digitalised patients, arrhythmias associated with Wolff-Parkinson-White (WPW) syndrome.

LIGNOCAINE

It is an amide local anaesthetic and has rapid onset of action. It **depresses diastolic depolarization and automaticity in ectopic foci in ventricular tissue**. Phase 4 depolarization in partially depressed Purkinje fibres and after depolarizations are antagonised. It does not depress AV conduction and decreases action potential duration, effective refractory period. It has no effect on BP.

Adverse effects include ventricular fibrillation, hypotension or massive cardiac arrest due to overdose, dizziness, paraesthesia, drowsiness, seizures, disorientation, respiratory arrest, nausea, vomiting, circulatory collapse and blurred vision.

It is **indicated** in prophylaxis or treatment of ventricular arrhythmias associated with MI, digitalis intoxication, ventricular tachyarrhythmia, in patients predisposed to ventricular arrhythmias during general anaesthesia.

PHENYTOIN SODIUM

It is a anticonvulsant drug and **depresses the ventricular automaticity and accelerates the AV conduction**. It also reduces the duration of action potential like quinidine. It also shortens the QT interval. It mainly blocks inactivated Na^+ channels. It is **used** for the suppression of ectopic beats and for prophylaxis of recurrent paroxysmal tachycardia and also for the treatment of rapid supraventricular or ventricular tachycardia.

It is also used in digitalis induced ventricular arrhythmia as it reverse the conduction block while accentuating the depression of automaticity (The detailed pharmacology is discussed in chapter 'Antiepileptic agents').

BETA-ADRENEGIC BLOCKERS

The detailed pharmacology of beta blockers is discussed in chapter 'Adrenergic blocking agents' and 'Antihypertensive agents'.

The antiarrhythmic action is due to cardiac adrenergic blockade. It decreases the slope of phase 4 depolarization and automaticity in SA node, Purkinje fibres and other ectopic foci. It also prolongs the effective refractory period of AV node and impedes AV conduction. ECG shows prolonged PR interval. It is **useful** in sinus tachycardia, atrial and nodal extrasystoles. It is also useful in sympathetically mediated arrhythmias in pheochromocytoma and halothane anaesthesia.

DRUGS PROLONGING ACTION POTENTIAL

By prolonging repolarization, AP is widened and ERP is increased, so the tissues remain refractory even after full repolarization.

AMIODARONE

It is a long acting antiarrhythmic drug. It contains iodine and may cause disorders of thyroid function.

It blocks inactivated sodium channels. It also decreases calcium current and transient outward, delayed rectifier and inward rectifier potassium currents. It is a potent inhibitor of abnormal automaticity. It prolongs duration of action potential, refractoriness in Purkinje and ventricular muscle fibers.

Amiodarone is slowly and poorly absorbed after oral administration. It is metabolised slowly in liver to active metabolite.

Adverse effects include hypotension due to vasodilatation and depression of myocardial performance is frequent with the IV route. Heart block, bradycardia, corneal microdeposits, photosensitivity, hepatitis, gastrointestinal upset may occur.

It is **indicated** in tachyarrhythmias associated with WPW syndrome, atrial flutter and fibrillation, paroxysmal tachyarrhythmias not responding to other agents. Ventricular tachycardia and ventricular arrhythmia refractory to other treatment.

BRETYLIUM

It has **direct action on myocardium and interferes with the neuronal release of catecholamines** and has direct antiarrhythmic property. Bretylium may reverse the shortening of action potential duration caused by ischemia. It acts due to K^+ channel blockade.

It is **used** in the treatment of ventricular tachycardia and ventricular fibrillation.

CALCIUM CHANNEL BLOCKERS

The detailed pharmacology is discussed in chapter 'Antihypertensive agents'.

These drugs inhibit Ca^{2+} mediated slow channel inward current, thus inhibiting Ca^{2+} mediated depolarization. Phase 4 depolarization in SA node and Purkinje fibres is reduced. They also prolong AV nodal effective refractory period thus AV conduction is slowed. There is also negative inotropic action.

It is **indicated** in PSVT, to control ventricular rate in atrial flutter or atrial fibrillation.

❑❑❑

CHAPTER 4.5 Antihyperlipidemic Agents

These drugs are used for treatment of hyperlipidemia. They lower the levels of lipoproteins and lipids in blood. The plasma lipids are present in lipoproteins after combining with apoproteins. They are high density lipoproteins (HDL), low density lipoproteins (LDL), very low density lipoproteins (VLDL) and intermediate density lipoproteins (IDL).

Atherosclerosis is main cause of cardiovascular deaths. It is characterized by a localised plaque in the intima and is composed of cholesterol esters, deposition of fibrous proteins and calcification. These plaques may narrow the arterial lumen and can cause distalischemia. The coronary and cerebral circulation are main sites of atherosclerosis. Raised levels of VLDL, LDL

Table 4.5.1: *Classification for antihyperlipidemic agents.*

I.	**HMG CoA reductase inhibitors**	
	Lovastatin (LOVASTROL)	10-40 mg/day
	Simvastatin (SIMCARD)	5-20 mg/day
	Atorvastatin (ATOCOR)	10-80 mg/day
	Pravastatin (PRASTATIN)	40 mg/day
II.	**Fibric acid derivatives**	
	Clofibrate (ATROMID)	0.5-1 g BD
	Gemfibrozil (GEMPAR)	600 mg before meals
III.	**Agents inhibiting production of VLDL and lipolysis in adipose tissue**	
	Nicotinic acid	100 mg TDS, increased to 2-6 g/day
IV.	**Interferes with intestinal absorption of cholesterol**	
	Cholestyramine	4 g TDS
	Colestipol	5-10 g TDS
V.	**Inhibit synthesis of LDL**	
	Probucol	500 mg BD after meals
VI.	**Miscellaneous**	
	Gugulipid (GUGLIP)	25 mg TDS

and IDL are atherogenic, while HDL is protective because it facilitates removal of cholesterol from tissues.

The drugs used in the treatment of hyperlipidemia are classified as in table 4.5.1.

HMG CoA Reductase Inhibitors

Also known as statins. HMG CoA reductase (Hydroxymethyl-Glutaryl Coenzyme A Reductase) inhibitors block the synthesis of cholesterol in liver by competitively inhibiting HMG CoA reductase activity, also cause depletion of critical intracellular pools of sterols and increased transcription of LDL receptors leading to enhanced removal from plasma of LDL cholesterol and LDL precursors. They also reduce hepatic synthesis of VLDL, increase plasma HDL. Reduction of LDL occurs over 4-6 weeks.

LOVASTATIN

It is a **potent HMG CoA reductase inhibitor.** This enzyme catalyzes the conversion of HMG CoA to mevalonate in liver which is an important early and rate limiting step in the cholesterol synthesis. It **causes marked reduction in LDL cholesterol** and also raise HDL level and may lower the triglyceride level. After oral administration it is extensively metabolised in liver and metabolites are excreted in bile.

Adverse reactions include arthralgia, myopathy, vertigo, tremor, memory loss, alteration of taste, peripheral neuropathy, anxiety, insomnia, depression, hepatitis cholestatic jaundice, abdominal pain, alopecia, blurred vision etc.

It is **indicated in** primary hypercholesterolemia and hyperglyceridemia.

SIMVASTATIN

Simvastatin, is twice as potent as lovastatin.

Simvastatin has been shown to **reduce both normal and elevated low-density lipoprotein (LDL)** cholesterol concentrations. Apolipoprotein B, VLDL cholesterol and plasma triglycerides also reduce and can produce increase in HDL cholesterol.

Simvastatin reduces total cholesterol, LDL cholesterol and triglycerides by 25%, 35%, and 10% respectively. The increase in HDL is upto 12%.

Adverse effects are flatulence, diarrhoea, constipation, nausea, abdominal pain, cramps, heart burn and dysgeusia. Rarely myopathy, rhabdomyolysis with acute renal failure may also occur.

Other adverse effects include headache, dizziness, rashes/pruritus, impotence insomnia, blurring of vision and lens opacities.

Simvastatin is **indicated** in patients with coronary heart disease and hypercholesteremia, for the reduction of elevated total and LDL cholesterol in patients with primary hypercholesterolemia (type IIa and IIb hyperlipoproteinemia), combined hypercholesterolemia and hypertriglyceridemia.

Simvastatin is also used in combination with nicotinic acid. It is found to be the most useful drug combination for the treatment of dyslipidemias associated with coronary artery disease. It is particularly effective in normalizing the lipid profiles of patients with familial combined dyslipidemia.

ATORVASTATIN

Atorvastatin **reduces total cholesterol, LDL-cholesterol and apolipoprotein B**

hypercholesterolemia and mixed dyslipidemias. Atorvastatin also reduces VLDL-cholesterol and TG and produces variable increases in HDL-cholesterol and apolipoprotein A1. Atorvastatin reduces LDL-cholesterol in patients with familial hyper-cholesterolemia (FH).

Atorvastatin is generally well tolerated. **Adverse effects** include constipation, flatulence, dyspepsia, abdominal pain, headache, nausea, myalgia, diarrhoea, asthenia and insomnia.

Dose related and reversible elevated serum ALT levels have also been reported.

Elevated serum CPK levels have been reported in some patients but only rarely patients have concurrent muscle pain, tenderness or weakness.

It is **indicated** as an adjunct to diet to reduce elevated total cholesterol, LDL-cholesterol and TG levels in patients with primary hypercholesterolemia, diabetic dyslipidaemia or mixed hyperlipidemia, hypertriglyceridemia, dysbetalipoproteinemia and familial hypercholesterolemia.

PRAVASTATIN

Pravastatin sodium besides increasing LDL cholesterol catabolism, also **inhibits LDL-cholesterol production by inhibiting hepatic synthesis** of VLDL-cholesterol, the LDL-cholesterol precursor. These effects result in a reduction of total cholesterol, LDL-cholesterol, VLDL-cholesterol, apolipoprotein B and trigly-cerides, whilst increasing (HDL-cholesterol) and apolipoprotein A. It has little effect on cholesterol synthesis in other tissues.

Pravastatin is administered orally in the active form and is rapidly absorbed, with peak plasma levels occurring 1 to 1.5 hours after dosing. Pravastatin undergoes extensive first-pass extraction in the liver, which is its primary site of action. It is 50% bound to plasma proteins.

Adverse effects include rash, myalgia, headache, non-cardiac chest pain; rarely nausea/vomiting, diarrhoea and fatigue may occur.

Pravastatin is indicated as an adjunct to diet in patients with primary hypercholesterolemia, mixed dyslipidemia, elevated serum triglyceride levels and primary dysbetalipoproteinemia who do not respond adequately to diet.

FIBRIC ACID DERIVATIVES

These **activate lipoprotein lipase** which is a key enzyme in degradation of VLDL resulting in lower circulating triglycerides. These drugs lower triglyceride levels by 20-50% with 10-15% decrease in LDL cholesterol and a 10-15% increase in HDL cholesterol.

CLOFIBRATE

It has a specific action on type III hyperlipo-proteinemia and also reduces VLDL and LDL but because of its association with a small increase in risk of gastrointestinal and hepatobiliary neoplasia, it is seldom used.

GEMFIBROZIL

Gemfibrozil reduces plasma triglycerides by 40 to 55% by decreasing the concentration of VLDL. Its effectiveness is less in lowering LDL.

It also decrease hepatic synthesis and secretion of VLDL. The lowering of triglyceride plasma levels may be due to reduction in hepatic synthesis of VLDL and increase in VLDL clearance.

It is completely absorbed from gastrointestinal tract and is excreted in urine.

Adverse effects include nausea, diarrhoea, abdominal pain, dyspepsia, fatigue, skin rash, weight gain, leucopenia, alopecia, blurred vision etc.

NICOTINIC ACID

Nicotinic acid and nicotinamide together represent the essential vitamin niacin in the diet. Of these two, only nicotinic acid is active as a lipid modifying drug. Nicotinic acid is preferred in patients with triglyceride levels exceeding 200 mg/dl because bile acid sequestrants tend to raise triglyceride levels. Nicotinic acid **reduces production of VLDL by liver, thus its degradation products IDL and LDL are subsequently reduced. It inhibits lipolysis in adipose tissue** and increases activity of lipoprotein lipase. It has no effect on cholesterol and bile acid metabolism. Combination drug therapy has been shown to decrease cholesterol levels in hyperlipidemic patients.

Adverse effects include, flushing, itching, vomiting, diarrhoea and dyspepsia. It may also lead to hyperpigmentation of skin, liver dysfunction, hyperglycaemia and hyperuricaemia.

It is **indicated** in type III, IV & V hypertriglyceridemia. It lowers VLDL and raise HDL level and it is administered with HMG CoA reductase inhibitors e.g. simvastatin.

CHOLESTYRAMINE AND COLESTIPOL

They are useful only in hyperlipoproteinemias involving elevated levels of LDL i.e. type IIa, IIb and V. They are basic ion exchange resins. They are neither digested nor absorbed in the gut. **They bind bile acids in intestine and interrupt their enterohepatic circulation, leading to increased faecal excretion of bile salts and cholesterol**. There is increased hepatic conversion of choles-terol to bile acids. More LDL receptors are expressed on liver cells leading to increased clearance of IDL, LDL and indirectly of VLDL.

Adverse effects include nausea, heart burn, constipation and acidosis etc.

PROBUCOL

It is **cholesterol lowering agent with antioxidant property**. It is only **1/10** absorbed when given orally. It reduces the serum cholesterol levels without reduction in serum triglycerides level and also reduces the HDL levels. It has no effect on VLDL and triglyceride levels.

Adverse effects include headache, dizziness, diarrhoea and eosinophilia.

GUGULIPID

Is an indigenous drug obtained from gum guggul used for treatment of hyperlipidemia, hypercholesterolemia and hypertriglyceridemia.

❑❑❑

CHAPTER 4.6 Plasma Expanders

Plasma substitutes/expanders are high molecular weight substances when infused intravenously into blood stream retain fluid in the vascular compartment and exert oncotic pressure. But before infusing into the blood stream, the following requirement may be present.

- Should have same oncotic pressure with plasma.
- Should remain in blood stream for adequate period.
- Should not be disposed rapidly by metabolic degradation or by excretion.
- Should remain stable on storage.
- Should not interfere with blood grouping and cross matching.
- Should be compatible with other IV fluid and other drugs.
- Should be easily sterilized.
- Should be pharmacologically inert and have a viscosity suitable for infusion into blood stream.

They are used in conditions where blood plasma has been lost e.g. shock, burn cases, severe trauma and extensive tissue damage as a temporary measure till the blood can be arranged. These do not have O_2 carrying capacity.

The clinically used plasma expanders are classified as in table 4.6.1.

HUMAN ALBUMIN

It is obtained from heat treated pooled human plasma. 100 ml of 20% human albumin solution is osmotic equivalent of 800 ml of whole blood. It draws and holds additional fluid from tissues. It can used irrespective of patient's blood group. For optimum benefit it should be used with electrolyte solutions. It does not interfere with coagulation and there is no risk of sensitization.

Table 4.6.1: *Classification of plasma substitutes/ expanders.*

I.	Human albumin (20% solution; ALBUSAFE)
II.	**Dextran**
	Dextran 70 (Mol. wt. 70,000; 6% solution; LOMODEX-70)
	Dextran 40 (Mol. wt. 40,000; 10% solution; LOMODEX-40)
III.	Degraded gelatin polymer – polygeline (3.5% in electrolyte solution; HAEMACCEL)
IV.	Hydroxyethyl starch (HES; Hetastarch; 6% solution; HESTAR)
V.	Polyvinylpyrrolidone (PVP; 3.5% solution in buffered normal saline; OSMOPLASMA)

It is **used** in burns, shock, in patients of acute liver failure and on dialysis.

DEXTRAN

They are most commonly used plasma expanders. It is polysaccharide isolated from beet sugar which is formed by the action of *Leuconstec mesenteroides*. It is available in mainly two forms depending upon the molecular weight. Dextran 70 (mol. wt. 70,000) available in 6% solution and Dextran 40 (mol. wt. 40,000) available in 10% solution. They are infused intravenously in the treatment of shock. Dextran 40 acts more rapidly than dextran 70. It decreases the blood viscosity and prevents the sludging of RBC's. Dextran 70 remains in circulation for longer period (upto 24 hrs) and is slowly excreted by glomerular filtration.

It is commonly used cheap plasma expander and can be stored for a longer period of time but it may interfere with blood grouping and cross matching. It may trigger anaphylactic reaction characterized by urticaria, bronchospasm and decrease in blood pressure etc. It can also prolong bleeding time by interfering in coagulation of blood.

DEGRADED GELATIN POLYMER – POLYGELINE

It is a polypeptide and exerts oncotic pressure similar to albumin. It remains in circulation for 12 hours and is slowly excreted by the kidney. It does not interfere with blood grouping and cross matching.

It is a plasma substitute which corrects circulatory insufficiency due to plasma/ blood volume deficiency, absolute (e.g., resulting from bleeding) or relative (e.g., resulting from a shift in the blood volume between the circulatory compartments).

Side effects include transient skin reactions (urticaria, wheals), hypotension, tachycardia, bradycardia, nausea/vomiting, dyspnoea, a rise in temperature and/or chills may occasionally occur. In rare cases of severe hypersensitivity reactions leading to shock.

If side effects occur, the infusion should be discontinued at once. Anaphylactic reactions associated with polygeline are due to histamine release.

It is **indicated** in hypovolaemic shock, loss of blood and plasma (e.g., trauma, burns, preoperative autologous blood or plasma donation), and for priming the heart-lung machine. In addition, it can be used as a vehicle for various drugs.

HYDROXYETHYL STARCH

It is similar to glycogen, the starch molecule is substituted to a selected degree to achieve a distinct plasma retention and volume effect. It improves haemodynamics, macrocirculation, microcirculation, organ function, oxygen supply.

After IV administration it is enzymatically metabolised by endogenous amylase. The smaller fragments undergo rapid glomerular filtration. The 6% iso-oncotic infusion solution allows precise blood volume control and leads to an effective stabilisation of blood volume, whereas 10% hyperoncotic infusion solution has a greater expansive volume effect. It improves plasma volume for 24 hours or more.

Adverse effects include anaphylactoid reactions, manifesting as itching, chills, urticaria, shock and bronchospasm. In rising doses it can influence coagulation mechanism without triggering clinical haemorrhage.

POLYVINYLPYRROLIDONE (PVP)

It is a synthetic, water soluble polymer of molecular weight approximately 40,000. It is 3-5% solution in buffered physiological saline administered intravenously. It produce agglutination of RBC's and therefore interferes with blood grouping and cross matching and also releases histamine. It also binds certain drugs i.e. insulin, penicillin etc. Because of these drawbacks, it is less commonly used.

Plasma expanders are not used in severe anaemia, cardiac failure, pulmonary edema and renal failure.

Apart from colloidal plasma expanders crystalloid (electrolyte) fluids are used in certain clinical conditions.

DEXTROSE (5%) SOLUTION

1. It is used in prevention of:
   - Dehydration of all types.
   - Excessive tissue protein catabolism.
   - Depletion of liver glycogen.
   - As vehicle for IV administration of numerous drugs.
2. When oral intake of food and water is limited as in pre and postoperative patients or in the patients with severe hepatic or cardiac or GIT disease.
3. Correction of deficit of water as in case of inadequate intake and excessive losses in urine and perspiration.
4. In the treatment of ketosis in starvation, diarrhoea, vomiting or high fever.
5. In promotion of sodium excretion when there is excess sodium in the body due to excessive use of electrolyte solutions.
6. To provide adequate calories to the body.

NORMAL SALINE

It is **indicated** in:

1. When alkalosis is present alongwith fluid loss.
2. In case of severe salt depletion when rapid electrolyte restoration is essential.
3. In the treatment of low salt syndrome which may occur in presence of heart failure, renal impairment, during surgery, etc. In these cases chloride loss frequently exceeds sodium loss.
4. In severe salt depletion resulting from excessive fluid loss due to sweating, vomiting, diarrhoea, etc.

RINGER LACTATE

Ringer lactate (contain calcium chloride, potassium chloride, sodium chloride and sodium lactate) is **indicated** in:

1. For replacing the deficit of ECF due to decreased water intake or increased secretion of water even in absence of marked acid base disturbance.
2. In case of burns, infections, fractures, peritoneal irrigation etc. For the restoration of normal ECF balance during surgery.
3. In moderate metabolic acidosis which occurs in cases of mild renal insufficiency, infant diarrhoea, diabetic ketosis etc.
4. In diabetes mellitus to provide potassium to ECF.
5. During or after giving anaesthesia, to correct metabolic acidosis which results from disturbed respiration.

❑❑❑

CHAPTER 4.7 Diuretics and Antidiuretics

Diuretics are the agents which increase the rate of urine formation by the kidneys, or which cause a net loss of sodium and water in urine, i.e. the diuretics increase the urine output of ions and fluids from the kidneys.

Clinically, diuretics are among the most widely prescribed drugs used in the management of hypertension and various edematous states like congestive heart failure, nephrotic edema and in some cases of edema in pregnancy.

Almost all diuretics exert their action at the luminal surface of the renal tubule cells. Their mechanism of action includes interaction with specific membrane transport proteins like thiazides, furosemide etc., osmotic effects which prevent the water permeable segments of the nephron from absorbing water like mannitol, and specific interaction with enzyme like carbonic anhydrase inhibitors i.e. acetazolamide, and hormone receptors in renal epithelial cells like spironolactone.

They are classified as in table 4.7.1.

BENZOTHIAZIDES

The main action of thiazides is exerted on the early segment of distal tubule or cortical diluting segment. They **inhibit reabsorption of sodium and chloride**. The thiazides enter the tubule partly by glomerular filtration and partly by active secretion into the proximal tubule. At usual therapeutic doses, the major portion of the diuresis is due to an inhibition of reabsorption in the more distal parts of the nephron.

Pharmacodynamics

In maximal doses, chlorothiazide will markedly increase excretion of water, Na^+, K^+, Cl^- and HCO_3^-. Chlorothiazide due to its weak carbonic anhydrase activity, can cause some loss of bicarbonate in therapeutic dose.

Because of the marked inhibitory action on sodium reabsorption, a large amount of sodium is made available to the distal tubule where exchange of potassium with sodium takes place, this causes potassium loss.

Thiazides, due to their direct action on blood vessels and on sodium metabolism produce a mild hypotension. They also tend

Table 4.7.1: *Classification of diuretics.*

Drug	Dose
I. Benzothiazides and related compounds	
a. Thiazides	
Chlorothiazide (DIURIL)	0.5-2 g/day
Polythiazide (NEPHRIL)	1-3 mg/day
Cyclopenthiazide (NAVIDREX)	0.5-1.5 mg/day
Benzthiazide (FOVANE)	25-100 mg/day
b. Thiazide like compounds	
Chlorthalidone (HYTHALTON)	50-200 mg/day
Xipamide (XIPAMID)	20-60 mg/day
Indapamide (LORVAS)	2.5 mg/day
II. High ceiling or loop diuretics	
a. Sulphamoyl derivatives	
Furosemide (Frusemide; LASIX)	20-80 mg/day
Bumetanide (BURINEX)	1-5 mg/day
b. Phenoxyacetic acid derivatives	
Ethacrynic acid (EDECRIN)	50-150 mg/day
III. Carbonic anhydrase inhibitors	
Acetazolamide (DIAMOX)	250-500 mg/day
IV. Potassium - sparing diuretics	
a. Directly acting	
Triamterene (DYTIDE)	50-100 mg/day
Amiloride (MIDAMOR)	5-10 mg/day
b. Aldosterone antagonist	
Spironolactone (ALDACTONE)	25-200 mg/day
V. Osmotic diuretic	
Mannitol (OSMITROL)	1-2 g/kg as 10 to 20% solution IV
Isosorbide (ISMOTIC)	1.5 g/kg as oral solution
Urea (sterile; UREAPHIL)	40-120 g IV in 4% or 30% solution
VI. Organic mercurials	
Mersalyl sodium (SALYRGAN)	1-2 ml of 100 mg/ml solution IM twice weekly
Meralluride (MERCUHYDRIN)	1-2 ml IM twice weekly
VII. Miscellaneous or minor diuretics	
a. Acidifying or alkalinizing salts	
Ammonium chloride	2-4 g/day
Potassium citrate	0.3-1 g TDS
b. Xanthines	
Aminophylline	250-500 mg IV

to reduce glomerular filtration rate by their action to reduce blood volume, also decrease positive free water formation. Although this response is less than that seen with ADH-deficient diabetes insipidus patients treated with ADH, it is sufficient to reduce significantly urinary frequency and water consumption.

Pharmacokinetics

All thiazides and related compounds are well absorbed from the GIT and begin to produce diuresis within one hour after oral administration, but the duration is variable, which are due to variation in rates of renal tubular secretion and clearance, metabolism, and enterohepatic circulation. Approximately 50 percent of an oral dose is excreted in urine within 6 hours. Most of the agents undergo little hepatic metabolism and excreted as such. However indapamide is extensively metabolized.

Adverse Reactions

In the presence of severe renal and hepatic disease, these drugs may precipitate renal failure or hepatic coma. The most important toxic effect associated with thiazide therapy is hypokalemia and hypochloremic alkalosis.

The thiazides may induce hyperglycemia and aggravate pre-existing diabetes mellitus, the pharmacological effect of oral hypoglycemic agents may also be reduced.

Occasionally, they can cause allergic reactions like rashes, photosensitivity, thrombocytopenic purpura, dermatitis etc.

Therapeutic Uses

1. ***Edema:*** Thiazides are useful adjunctive therapy in controlling the edema associated with CHF and cirrhosis.
2. ***Hypertension:*** They are widely used in the treatment of hypertension with or without edema and often serve as the first drug of choice.
3. ***Diabetes insipidus:*** They reduce urine volume in both pituitary and renal diabetes insipidus. They are especially valuable for the latter in which ADH is ineffective.

HIGH-CEILING OR LOOP DIURETICS

These are the most efficacious agents available for inducing marked water and electrolyte excretion. The peak diuresis is far greater than that observed maximally with other diuretics. The drugs in this group include furosemide, bumetanide and ethacrynic acid and the main site of action is the thick ascending limb of loop of Henle, thus they are often called 'loop diuretics.'

The high-ceiling diuretics act primarily by inhibiting electrolyte reabsorption in the thick ascending limb of the loop of Henle. As much as 20% of the filtered Na^+ may be reabsorbed in the loop of Henle.

These agents bind to Cl^- binding site of Na^+-K^+-$2Cl^-$ cotransporter glycoprotein and inhibit its transport function in ascending limb of loop of Henle.

These agents tend to increase renal blood flow without increasing filtration rate, which reduces fluid and electrolyte reabsorption in the proximal tubule and may augment the initial diuretic response.

Pharmacodynamics

After oral administration, the intense

diuretic action starts within one hour and lasts up to 4 to 6 hours. Furosemide produces more loss of chloride than sodium, potassium loss also occurs, which is probably an indirect effect due to the large Na^+ load reaching to the distal tubules. In low doses, these drugs do not appreciably effect HCO_3^- or H^+ excretion.

Pharmacokinetics

All the loop diuretics are rapidly absorbed from the GIT, usually within 30 minutes after oral, and 5 minutes after IV administration. The bio-availability of furosemide is about 60% while that of bumetanide is nearly 100%. They are extensively bound to plasma proteins, but they are rapidly secreted by the organic acid transport system of the proximal tubule. They produce a peak diuresis in about 2 hours with a total duration of diuretic action of 6 to 8 hours.

Furosemide is mainly excreted unchanged by glomerular filtration as well as tubular secretion.

Adverse Reactions

Abnormalities of fluid and electrolyte imbalance are the most common forms of clinical toxicity, overdose may result in rapid reduction of blood volume, dizziness, orthostatic hypotension, headache, hypokalemia.

Gastrointestinal symptoms of nausea, vomiting, diarrhoea are common with ethacrynic acid.

Ototoxicity has been reported with all the three loop diuretics, which is seen more commonly in patients with renal insufficiency.

Therapeutic Uses

Edema: The high ceiling diuretics are effective for the treatment of edema of cardiac, hepatic or renal origin. They are the drug of choice in case of congestive heart failure. These are preferred initially in all cases for rapid mobilization of edema fluid.

IV administration of furosemide produces prompt relief in acute pulmonary edema (acute left ventricular failure, following myocardial infarction). This is due to the vasodilator action that precedes the saluretic action.

In the management of refractory edema, the high ceiling diuretics may be used in conjunction with other types of diuretics. They are also useful for forced diuresis in hypnotic or other poisonings.

BUMETANIDE

Bumetanide is chemically similar to furosemide. It induces very rapid diuresis. The site and mechanism of action is similar to furosemide but it is 40 times more potent than furosemide.

It is highly effective in pulmonary edema. **Adverse effects** such as hyperuricaemia, potassium loss and ototoxicity are less than furosemide.

ETHACRYNIC ACID

Ethacrynic acid is chemically distinct from the thiazides and furosemide but ceiling effect is similar. It is a phenoxyacetic acid derivative that also contains an adjacent ketone and methylene group.

It does not inhibit carbonic anhydrase. Loss of potassium is less marked but chance of hypochloremic alkalosis are greater. It is an irritant and upon oral administration it produces diarrhoea, gastrointestinal bleeding may occur at higher dose. Chances of hearing loss are greater. So, due to their uniform toxicity, they are no longer used.

CARBONIC ANHYDRASE INHIBITORS

ACETAZOLAMIDE

It is a potent, noncompetitive reversible carbonic anhydrase inhibitor. Carbonic anhydrase is an enzyme which catalyses the reversible reaction

$$H_2O + CO_2 \rightleftharpoons H_2CO_3$$

Carbonic anhydrase influences the tubular reabsorption of sodium in proximal tubule where biocarbonate absorption occurs and in the distal tubule where sodium is exchanged for potassium or hydrogen ion and bicarbonate is formed as the accompanying anion. The hydration of carbon dioxide takes place under the influence of enzyme carbonic anhydrase which forms carbonic acid which dissociates and breaks into hydrogen and carbonate ions.

Acetazolamide **inhibits the enzyme carbonic anhydrase, and interferes with the ability of the renal tubules to produce and secrete hydrogen ions**. And, the diuretic action is due to the decreased sodium biocarbonate absorption in proximal tubules and diminished hydrogensodium exchange in the distal tubules.

Pharmacokinetics

All the carbonic anhydrase inhibitors are well absorbed after oral administration. Peak concentrations in plasma occur with in 2 hours and persists for 12 hours after a single dose. Acetazolamide is excreted unchanged in urine. **Ethoxzolamide** is similar to acetazolamide but more potent.

Adverse Reactions

Serious toxic reactions include acidosis, hypokalemia, drowsiness and paresthesia are common with larger doses.

Hypersensitivity reactions are rare, they consists of fever, skin reactions, bonemarrow depression and sulfonamide like renal lesions.

Drug induced osteomalacia has been reported with the simultaneous use of phenytoin.

Therapeutic Uses

Carbonic anhydrase inhibitors are rarely used as primary diuretics, because of self-limiting action, production of acidosis, and hypokalemia. They are used in:

i. Glaucoma, as adjuvant to miotics.
ii. In urinary tract infections or to alkalinise urine to promote the excretion of acidic drugs.
iii. In petit mal epilepsy as adjuvant.
iv. In the management of periodic paralysis.
v. Effective in ameliorating the symptoms of acute mountain sickness.

DIRECTLY ACTING DIURETICS

TRIAMTERENE AND AMILORIDE

Triamterene and amiloride are non-steroidal potassium sparing diuretics, which **interfere**

with transport in the late segments of the nephron by blocking the luminal Na^+ channels thus indirectly inhibiting K^+ excretion. They slightly increase sodium excretion and decrease potassium excretion, particularly when it is high due to high potassium intake or use of diuretics that enhances potassium loss.

In addition to these effects, all the potassium sparing diuretics are capable of inhibiting urinary H^+ secretion in the distal tubule and cortical collecting duct.

Pharmacokinetics

About 50% of an oral dose of each agent is absorbed. Triamterene is about 60 percent bound to plasma proteins, while amiloride is bound to a lesser extent. Both drugs are secreted in the proximal tubule, presumably by the organic cation secretory mechanism.

Adverse Reactions

The serious toxic effect is hyperkalemia. Triamterene produces relatively few other side effects which includes nausea, vomiting, dizziness etc. Megaloblastic anaemia has been reported in patients with alcoholic cirrhosis, which is probably due to inhibition of dihydrofolate reductase in patients with reduced folic acid intake.

Therapeutic Uses

Both drugs are used in conjunction with other diuretics like thiazide or loop diuretics to augment natriuresis and reduce loss of potassium. Triamterene may be used in the treatment of congestive heart failure, cirrhosis and the edema caused by secondary hyperaldosteronism. Amiloride is also useful in lithium induced diabetes insipidus.

POTASSIUM SPARING DIURETICS

SPIRONOLACTONE

It is a **steroid** and **aldosterone antagonist**. Aldosterone acts on the late distal tubules and collecting tubule cells by combining with an intracellular receptor which induces the formation of aldosterone induced protein, which promotes Na^+ reabsorption and K^+ secretion.

Spironolactone also increases Ca^{2+} excretion through a direct effect on tubular transport. In relatively high concentrations, it can inhibit the biosynthesis of aldosterone.

Pharmacokinetics

The oral bioavailability of spironolactone is about 70%. It is extensively bound to plasma proteins and is completely metabolized in liver. **Canrenone is a major active metabolite of spironolactone**, which can be converted enzymatically into canrenoate (hydrolytic product). Canrenoate has no intrinsic activity, but it can exert their effects by virtue of its interconversion with canrenone.

Adverse Reactions

In patients with renal insufficiency, spironolactone may induce hyperkalemia.

Minor side effects include drowsiness confusion, gastrointestinal upset, gynaecomastia and menstrual irregularities.

Therapeutic Uses

Spironolactone is generally used in combination with other, more efficacious diuretics.

i. It is widely used in the treatment of hypertension and in the management of refractory edema.
ii. Hypokalemia: Potassium sparing diuretics have been used in patients with low serum K^+ resulting from other diuretics, like thiazide and loop diuretics.
iii. Edema: It has been used in cirrhotic and nephrotic edema.

OSMOTIC DIURETICS

Osmotic diuretics are non-electrolytes, freely filterable at the glomerulus, undergo limited reabsorption by the renal tubules. The amount of diuresis produced is proportional to the quantity of osmotic diuretic, therefore for more diuresis, a large quantity of osmotic diuretic should be given. The primary effect of osmotic diuretics involves an increased fluid loss caused by osmotically active diuretic molecule. This results in reduced reabsorption of sodium and water in proximal tubule and since the tubule is permeable to water, there is a passive back diffusion of water, such a process keeps the tubular fluid isotonic.

They also tend to increase glomerular filtration rate.

MANNITOL

Mannitol is not absorbed from the GIT and must be given IV and is osmotically more active than urea.

Mannitol is useful in clinical conditions which are characterized by hypotension and decreased glomerular filtration. It is useful in maintaining kidney function under these conditions, even at low rates of filtration a sufficient amount of mannitol may enter the tubular fluid to exert an osmotic effect and thus continue urine formation.

It is also used to reduce intraocular pressure prior to eye surgery for glaucoma. Mannitol has been used to reduce cerebral edema.

The adverse reactions associated with mannitol administration are nausea, vomiting, headache and hypernatremia.

UREA

Urea is administered intravenously and useful for reducing a raised cerebrospinal fluid pressure during neurosurgery and cerebral edema after head injury.

Urea is contraindicated in patients with severe impairment of renal, hepatic or cardiac function due to their potential effect on expansion of the extracellular fluid volume.

ISOSORBIDE

Isosorbide is an orally active diuretic, most commonly used in the emergency treatment of acute angle-closure glaucoma.

ORGANIC MERCURIALS

In earlier twenties, these agents were diuretics of choice, but after the introduction of thiazides and loop diuretics, the organomercurials have been almost replaced.

Mercurials **depress the tubular reabsorption of sodium at several sites** including loop of Henle and some portions of proximal and distal tubules. They **inhibit the reabsorption of Cl^- and Na^+.**

The mercury ion is capable of causing local or systemic toxicity. For local irritation, they are combined with theophylline in an attempt to diminish the irritative toxicity at the site of injection. IV administration may lead to ventricular arrhythmias. They cause hepatocellular damage and even precipitate hepatic failure. They can also lead to low salt syndrome, hypochloraemic alkalosis and potassium depletion.

Miscellaneous Compounds

Ammonium Chloride

Ammonium chloride was used earlier along with mercurials, as they act best in acidosis, but now-a-days, it is not used as diuretic.

It is converted to urea in liver and free hydrogen ion are liberated in the body which tilt the buffer system towards acidosis.

Potassium Citrate

Potassium citrate alkalinises the urine and increases its volume. They are used to change the pH of urine.

ANTIDIURETICS

Antidiuretic agents reduce urine volume and are used in the treatment of diabetes insipidus. They are classified as in table 4.7.2.

VASOPRESSIN

The antidiuretic hormone is an octapeptide released from the posterior lobe of pituitary gland. It is used in the treatment of diabetes insipidus. ADH reduces the total urine volume and absence of this hormone cause diabetes insipidus. ADH **acts on collecting duct cells to increase their water permeability. It acts on V2 receptors** in collecting duct and regulate their water permeability through cAMP production.

ADH in larger dose increases the blood pressure by direct stimulation of vascular smooth muscle. It also stimulates the smooth muscle of gastrointestinal tract and increase the peristalsis. It is inactive orally because it is destroyed by trypsin. It can be administered by any parenteral route or by nasal spray. Vasopressin is **indicated** in diabetes insipidus and in treatment of postoperative abdominal varices.

Table 4.7.2: *Classification of antidiuretics.*

I.	**Antidiuretic hormone (vasopressin)**	
	Vasopressin (VASOPIN)	5-20 U SC/IM
	Desmopressin (MINIRIN):	0.2-0.4 mg/day HS
II.	**Thiazide diuretics**	
	Hydrochlorothiazide (Details are given in section on 'Diuretics')	25-50 mg TDS
III.	**Miscellaneous agents**	
	Carbamazepine (Antiepileptic drug, MAZETOL)	200-600 mg BD
	Chlorpropamide (Oral hypoglycemic agent, DIABINESE)	100-50 mg OD

Adverse effects include nausea, belching, abdominal cramps, hypersensitivity reactions etc.

DESMOPRESSIN

Desmopressin is a synthetic analogue of vasopressin. Two chemical changes have been made to natural hormone, namely dissemination of cysteine and substitution of 8-L-arginine by 8-D-arginine. These structural changes result in a compound with significantly increased antidiuretic potency, very little activity on the smooth muscles, hence the avoidance of undesirable pressor effects. Desmopressin proved to be a highly selective diuretic agent with a ratio between antidiuretic and vasopressor activity in excess of 2,000 : 1. Desmopressin is more stable than vasopressin and this is reflected in its prolonged duration of action.

Desmopressin is a pure **V2 receptor** agonist. When bound to V2 receptors in the kidney, **it increases the permeability of the collecting ducts and tubules thereby enhancing water reabsorption and reducing the volume of urine** produced without any pressor effects.

Oral administration of 0.1-0.2 mg desmopressin provides an antidiuretic effect lasting for 8-12 hours. Desmopressin does not cross blood brain barrier and maximal plasma concentrations are reached within 2 hours. After oral administration, t½ varies between 2.0 hours and 3.2 hours. 65% of oral desmopressin absorbed is excreted unchanged in the urine. It is also used as a nasal spray.

Adverse effects include headache, nausea and stomach pain and in very rare cases epistaxis. Treatment without concomitant restriction of water intake may lead to water retention with accompanying signs and symptoms (reduced serum sodium, weight gain and in serious cases, convulsions).

Therapeutic Uses

- Nocturia in adults.
- Primary nocturnal enuresis.
- Central diabetes insipidus: Desmopressin is preparation of choice.

❑❑❑

Section 5

Autacoids

CHAPTER 5.1

Histamine and Antihistaminic Agents

The term 'autacoid' is derived from Greek, *autos* – self and *akos* – remedy. These are formed in various tissues of the body and generally act locally at the site of synthesis and release in the body. They have also been called **'local hormones'** and differ from hormones which are secreted from endocrine glands. The hormones are produced by specific cells (endocrine glands), and are transported through circulation to the distant target organs while autacoids are produced in tissues rather than in glands.

The important autacoids include:

- Histamine,
- Hydroxytryptamine (5-HT, serotonin),
- Prostaglandins,
- Leukotrienes, and
- Kinins.

HISTAMINE

Histamine is a potent biogenic amine, occurs in tissues in almost all forms of life and released in a free state in response to injury or to any antigenantibody reaction. Histamine is an imidazole compound, formed by decarboxylation of the amino acid L-histidine, a reaction catalyzed by the enzyme histidine decarboxylase.

Histamine is found in most of the tissues, present in various biological fluids. In most tissues, histamine exists in bound form in granules, in mast cells or basophils. These mast cells are especially rich at sites of potential tissue injury i.e. skin, lungs, liver, GIT etc. and is unevenly distributed. It is also present in many venoms (of bees & wasps), bacteria and plant tissues.

Histamine Receptors

The present evidence indicates that histamine act on **three types of receptors namely H_1, H_2 & H_3**.

The contraction of smooth muscle, increase in vascular permeability and mucus secretion are mediated by H_1 receptors and is associated with increase in intracellular cyclic GMP. These type of effects are competitively blocked by H_1 receptor antagonists (antihistaminics) like mepyramine.

Table 5.1.1: *Classification of antihistaminic agents.*

I. **Ethanolamines**	
Diphenhydramine (BENADRYL)	25-50 mg/day
Dimenhydrinate (DRAMAMINE)	25-50 mg/day, IM
II. **Ethylenediamines**	
Pyrilamine maleate (DORANTAMIN)	25-50 mg/day
Tripelennamine	25-50 mg/day
III. **Alkylamines**	
Pheniramine maleate (AVIL)	25-50 mg/day, IM
Chlorpheniramine maleate (PIRITON)	2-4 mg/day, IM
Triprolidine (ACTIDIL)	2.5-5 mg/day
IV. **Phenothiazines**	
Promethazine (PHENERGAN)	25-50 mg/day, IM
Promethazine chlorotheophyllinate (AVOMINE)	25-75 mg/day
V. **Piperazines**	
Cyclizine hydrochloride (MAREZINE)	50 mg/day
Meclizine hydrochloride (ANCOLAN)	25-50 mg/day
Buclizine (LONGIFENE)	25-50 mg/day
VI. **Piperidines:**	
Loratidine (LORMEG)	10 mg OD
Fexofenadine (ALLEGRA)	60-180 mg OD
Astemizole (STEMIZ)	10 mg/day
VII. **Miscellaneous compounds**	
Cetirizine (CETZINE)	10 mg/day
Levocetirizine (TECZINE)	5 mg/day
Cyproheptadine (Antihistaminic/antiserotonin; PERIACTIN)	4 mg/day
Cinnarizine (Antivertigo; STUGERON)	25-50 mg/day

ANTIHISTAMINICS

Antihistaminics are classified in table 5.1.1.

Pharmacological Actions

Most of the antihistaminics (H_1-receptor antagonists) have similar pharmacological actions and conventionally can be discussed together.

1. **Antihistaminic action:** The antihistaminics blocks histamine effects at a variety of sites. They inhibit most responses of smooth muscles to histamine. They antagonize the stimulant actions of histamine on various smooth muscles of the respiratory system, gastrointestinal tract, the uterus and the blood vessels. They inhibit the hypertensive effect (in rabbits & guinea pigs) and hypotensive effect (in cat & dog) produced by histamine. They also reduced the triple response induced by histamine injection.

Histamine induced bronchospasm in many animal species, especially in guinea pigs can easily be antagonized by antihistaminics.

2. **Action on central nervous system:** Majority of antihistaminic drugs produce variable degree of CNS depression i.e. sedation, drowsiness and sleep. Drugs like diphenhydramine, promethazine are potent sedatives and is often accompanied by inability to concentrate.

The newer H_1-antagonists such as terfenadine and astemizole are claimed to have little or no sedative action. Astemizole is also claimed to be free of autonomic blocking effects. Loratidine is claimed to have little autonomic and CNS blocking effects.

3. **Antimotion sickness effect:** Several H_1-antagonists have significant property in preventing motion sickness. This effect was first observed with drug, dimenhydrinate and subsequently with other drugs like diphenhydramine, promethazine and other piperazine derivatives.
4. **Anticholinergic effects:** Many of the H_1-antagonists also tend to inhibit responses to acetylcholine that are mediated by muscarinic receptors. The newer agents, terfenadine and astemizole have no effect on muscarinic receptors.
5. **Adrenergic blocking effect:** H_1-antagonists, specially of phenothiazine subgroups have weak alpha-receptor blocking effect.
6. **Antiparkinsonism effects:** Because of anticholinergic property, some H_1-antagonists have significant suppressant effect on the parkinsonism like symptoms.
7. **Local anaesthesia:** Most of the H_1 antagonists block sodium channels in excitable membranes in the same way as procaine and lignocaine. The drugs like diphenhydramine and promethazine are occassionally used to produce local anaesthesia in patients allergic to local anaesthetic drugs.
8. **Antiserotonin effect:** Drugs, like cyproheptadine is promoted as an antiserotonin agent.

Pharmacokinetics

H_1-antagonists are well absorbed from the gastrointestinal tract. Following oral administration, antihistaminic effect is manifested within 30 minutes, peak plasma concentration is achieved in 2 to 3 hours and effects usually last 4 to 6 hours. However, drugs in piperazine subgroups especially chlorcyclizine and meclizine, the actions persists for 8 to 12 and 12 to 24 hours respectively.

The drugs are mainly metabolized in the liver by hydroxylation and glucuronide conjugation, widely distributed throughout the body and excreted in the urine.

Adverse Reactions

The most common side effect, common to all H_1 antagonists other than terfenadine and astemizole is **sedation**. Other untoward reactions include fatigue, dizziness, tinnitus, lassitude, blurred vision, diplopia, euphoria, nervousness, tremor and insomnia.

Side effects include loss of appetite, nausea, vomiting, epigastric distress, constipation or diarrhoea. Side effects due to antimuscarinic actions of H_1-antagonists include dryness of mouth, bladder disturbances.

Therapeutic Uses

H_1 antagonists have a widespread value in the symptomatic treatment of various disorders.

1. **Hypersensitivity reactions:** To prevent allergic reactions or to treat their symptoms, in which histamine is the primary mediator, the H_1-antagonists are the drugs of choice and are often quite effective. They are used primarily to treat allergic reactions produced by the release of histamine e.g., edematous states, pruritus, allergic rhinitis and urticaria. They are generally more effective in acute conditions and are used only for symptomatic relief.
2. **Motion sickness:** Drugs like promethazine, promethazine chlorotheophyllinate, diphenhydramine, dimenhydrinate, cyclizine and meclizine have value in prophylaxis of motion sickness.
3. **Antivertigo:** Drugs line cyclizine, cinnarizine, dimenhydrinate, diphenhydramine are used in the treatment of vertigo.
4. **Antiparkinsonism:** Based on anticholinergic property, some H_1-antagonists such as diphenhydramine can be used in the early stages of treatment of parkinsonism.
5. **Local anaesthetics:** In patients allergic to procaine H_1-antagonists, such as diphenhydramine and tripelennamine have been used successfully as local anaesthetic.

NEWER ANTIHISTAMINICS

CETIRIZINE

Cetirizine is a potent antihistaminic with a low potential for drowsiness at pharmacologically active doses and with additional antiallergic properties. It is a selective H_1 antagonist with negligible effects on other receptors and is, therefore, virtually free from anti-cholinergic and anti-serotonin effects. Cetirizine inhibits the histaminemediated 'early' phase of the allergic reaction and also reduces the migration of inflammatory cells such as eosinophils and the release of mediators associated with 'late' allergic response.

Cetirizine is **indicated** for the symptomatic treatment of perennial allergic rhinitis, seasonal allergic rhinitis, chronic idiopathic urticaria, conjunctivitis and pruritus in adults and children above two years of age.

Side effects include headache, dizziness, drowsiness, dry mouth and gastrointestinal discomfort.

LEVOCETIRIZINE

The second generation H_1-receptor antagonist cetirizine is a reacemate consisting of equal quantities of 2 enantiomers, levocetirizine [(R)-enantiomer] and dextrocetirizine [(S)-enantiomer]. *In vitro* and human pharmacodynamic studies have provided evidence that levocetirizine is the more active enantiomer, accounting for most or all clinical antihistaminic activity of racemic cetirizine; this activity of levocetirizine is seen at half the dose of cetirizine.

Levocetirizine exhibit a 2-fold higher affinity for human H_1-receptors than cetirizine, and is about 10 fold more potent than the (S)-enantiomer. Levocetirizine dissociates more slowly from the H_1-receptor than the (S)-enantiomer.

It is well absorbed with an oral bioavailability of 85%. Onset of action occurs within one hour.

Indications for levocetirizine remain the same as those of cetirizine.

Adverse reactions include headache, fatigue etc.

FEXOFENADINE

It is a pharmacologically active metabolite of terfenadine, is a non sedating antihistaminic with selective peripheral H_1 receptor antagonist activity.

Fexofenadine inhibited antigen-induced bronchospasm and histamine release from mast cells. No anticholinergic or alpha adrenergic-receptor blocking effects were observed. Moreover, no sedative or other CNS effects were observed. Fexofenadine does not cross the blood-brain barrier. It inhibits skin wheal and flare responses produced by histamine injection. Following single and twice daily oral administration, antihistaminic effects occurred within 1 hour, achieved a maximum at 2-3 hours, and lasted a minimum of 12 hours.

Fexofenadine hydrochloride is rapidly absorbed into the body following oral administration, with Tmax occurring at approximately 1-3 hours post dose. It is 60-70% plasma protein bound.

Side effects include headache, fatigue, drowsiness, nausea, tachycardia, palpitations, dry mouth, GIT disturbances, taste disturbances, photosensitivity, dysmenorrhoea and menstrual disorders.

The newer antihistaminics agents e.g. **Azelastine** inhibits histamine release and also inflammatory reactions evoked by leukotrienes and plasma activating factor (PAF). It is used for seasonal and perennial allergic rhinitis in the form of nasal spray. **Mizolastine**, a non-sedating antihistaminic is used in allergic rhinitis and urticaria. **Ebastine**, another non-sedating antihistaminic is used in nasal and skin allergies.

H_2-RECEPTOR ANTAGONISTS

As discussed earlier, H_2 receptors are responsible for histamine induced gastric acid secretion. H_2-receptors antagonists such as cimetidine, ranitidine, famotidine etc. are used in the treatment of peptic ulcer and are discussed in chapter 'Antiulcer agents'.

❑❑❑

CHAPTER 5.2 Serotonin and its Antagonists

5-HYDROXYTRYPTAMINE (5-HT, SEROTONIN)

5-Hydroxytryptamine is widely distributed in plant and animal tissues, mast cells, platelets, the enterochromaffin cells located throughout the gastrointestinal tract, and in certain regions of the brain. It is also present in the venoms and stings. Some fruits such as bananas, pineapples, tomatoes and plums contain considerable amount of 5-HT.

It is an indole ethylamine formed in biological systems from the amino acid L-tryptophan by hydroxylation with tryptophan hydroxylase enzyme, followed by the decarboxylation by the nonspecific aromatic L-amino acid decarboxylase. 5-HT is then taken up into secretory granules and stored.

Pharmacological Actions

Cardiovascular system: 5-HT can directly stimulate or relax smooth muscles via 5-HT_1 & 5-HT_2 receptors and can influence the release of noradrenaline from adrenergic nerves and stimulate endothelial cells to release EDRF and prostaglandins. It acts directly to constrict the arteries and increases the peripheral vascular resistance. The released adrenaline from adrenal medulla, affects ganglionic transmission and evokes cardiovascular reflexes.

On heart, 5-HT has weakly direct positive inotropic and chronotropic effects, that are mediated by 5-HT_1 receptors. 5-HT_3 receptors are also present on vagal nerve endings in the coronary bed, which evoke bradycardia and hypotension.

A characteristic 'triphasic response' is observed after intravenous injection. The early transient fall in blood pressure is due to stimulation of chemoreceptors. The second phase, pressor effect is due to vasoconstriction. The final depressor phase is due to vasodilator action on the skeletal muscle.

Smooth muscle: 5-HT stimulates smooth muscles, it increases the motility of the small intestine, stomach and also large intestine by which peristalsis is increased & diarrhoea can occur.

It also constricts bronchial smooth muscles, but is less potent than histamine. It

Table 5.2.1: *Classification of 5-HT antagonists.*

I.	**Ergot alkaloids and derivatives**	
	Ergotamine	1-3 mg/day, 0.25-0.5 mg SC/IM
	Lysergic acid diethylamide (LSD)	
	2-Bromolysergic acid amide (BOL)	
	Methysergide (Congener of LSD; SANSERT)	2 mg BD-TDS
	Metergoline	
II.	**Antihistaminics**	
	Cyproheptadine (PERIACTIN)	4 mg/day
	Cinnarizine (STUGERON)	25-50 mg/day
III.	**Phenothiazines**	
	Chlorpromazine (LARGECTIL)	25-100 mg/day, IM
IV.	**Selective 5-HT blockers**	
	Ketanserin (SUFREXAL)	10-30 mg/day
	Pizotifen (PIZOTYLINE)	0.5-1 mg/day

can also stimulate the smooth muscles of uterus.

Nerve endings: 5-HT is less potent than histamine in releasing catecholamines from adrenal medulla. 5-HT_3 receptors located on various sensory neurons mediate a depolarising response, which may cause pain & itching.

5-HT Antagonists

5-HT antagonists are classified in table 5.2.1.

Many of the drugs are partial agonists or antagonise certain action of 5-HT but stimulate others. The two drugs that are usually classified as 5-HT antagonist namely methysergide and cyproheptadine is used as a potent 5-HT_1 antagonist, while another drug, ketanserin is highly selective for blocking $5HT_2$ receptors.

METHYSERGIDE

Chemically, methysergide is 1-methyl-d-lysergic acid butanolamide, congener of methylergonovine and of LSD.

It antagonises the vasoconstrictor and pressor effect of 5-HT as well as the action of the amine on a variety of extravascular smooth muscles.

It has been **used** for migraine prophylaxis, vascular headaches, postgastrectomy dumping syndrome and also used to combat diarrhoea and malabsorption in carcinoid patients.

Common **side effects** include nausea, vomiting, heartburn, diarrhoea. Central effects include drowsiness, weakness, nervousness, insomnia, confusion, excitement and hallucinations.

CYPROHEPTADINE

Chemically, it is a phenothiazine derivative and has equal potency at both H_1-histamine and 5-HT receptors as an antagonist. As H_1-histamine antagonist it has been used in various allergic conditions. It increases the appetite and promotes weight gain.

As 5-HT antagonist it is **used** in controlling intestinal manifestations of carcinoid and postgastrectomy dumping syndrome. In addition, it has weak anticholinergic and sedative properties also.

Side effects include drowsiness, dry mouth, weight gain and confusion.

KETANSERIN

Ketanserin is a highly selective 5-HT_2 antagonist and has no significant action on 5-HT_1 & 5-HT_3 receptors. It blocks 5-HT induced vasoconstriction, platelet aggregation and contraction of airway smooth muscle.

In addition, it has adrenergic, H_1 and dopaminergic blocking activity also. Ketanserin is an effective antihypertensive, but the mechanism of action is not clear.

Side effects include dry mouth, sedation, nausea, dizziness etc.

❑❑❑

CHAPTER 5.3 Prostaglandins and Leukotrienes

Eicosanoids – Prostaglandins and Leukotrienes

In 1935, von Eular demonstrated a substance present in the extracts of human seminal fluid, which caused contraction of the isolated intestine and uterine muscle. This substance was named as 'prostaglandin' (PG) because of its probable origin from the prostate gland. In 1962, the structure of two prostaglandins namely PGE_1 & PGF_{2a} were elucidated and in 1964, PGE_2 was biosynthesized.

Biosynthesis and Metabolism

Prostaglandins (PG's) and leukotrienes (LT's) are biologically active derivatives of 20 carbon atom polyunsaturated essential fatty acids, which contains 3, 4 or 5 double bonds (e.g. 5, 8, 11, 14-eicosatetraenoic acid i.e., arachidonic acid).

In human being, arachidonic acid is the most important precursor for the biosynthesis of eicosanoids. Arachidonic acid is formed from linoleic acid in most mammalians by desaturation and carbon elongation to dihomog-linolenic acid and subsequent desaturation.

Inhibitors of Eicosanoid Biosynthesis

Salicylates and related non-steroidal anti-inflammatory drugs inhibit cyclooxygenase, thus all the PG's formed by this pathway i.e. PGG_2, PGE_2, PGD_2, PGF_{2a}, TXA_2 and prostacyclin can not be synthesized.

Pharmacological Actions

Uterus: Uterine smooth muscle from pregnant women are uniformly contracted by PGF's. PGI_2 and high concentrations of PGE_2 produce relaxation. While, nonpregnant human uterus are contracted by PGF's but relaxed by PGE's.

Bronchial muscle: Bronchial and tracheal muscle are contracted by PGF's & PGD_2 and relaxed by PGE's. Asthmatic patients are sensitive to PGF_{2a} and PGE_1 & PGE_2 causes bronchodilatation. LTC_4 & LTD_4 are bronchoconstrictors.

Gastrointestinal tract: Longitudinal muscle is contracted by PGE_2 & PGF_{2a}, while circular muscle is contracted by PGI_2 & PGF_{2a} and relaxed by PGE_2.

PGE's & PGI_2 also inhibit gastric acid secretion stimulated by gastrin or histamine.

Cardiovascular system: PGE's are potent vasodilators. However, PGF's constricts arterioles and veins. PGI_2 inhibits the aggregation of human platelets *in vitro.* TXA_2 is a very powerful inducer of platelet aggregation. LTB_4 stimulates the aggregation of polymorphonuclear leukocytes.

Endocrine system: Systemic administration of PGE_2 increases circulating concentration of ACTH, GH, prolactin & gonadotrophins.

It has also been observed in experimental animal that PG's cause regression of corpus luteum and reduction in secretion of progesterone.

Central & peripheral nervous system: PGE_1 & PGE_2 increase body temperature. They also contribute importantly to the genesis of the signs and symptoms of inflammation. When injected intracerebroventrically, PGE_2 produces sedation, rigidity and increased body temperature.

Kidney: PGE_2 and PGI_2 increases water, Na^+ and K^+ excretion and have a diuretic effect. Prostaglandins probably modulate renal blood flow and may serve to regulate urine formation. It also plays a role in the regulation of the secretion of renin (PGI_2, PGE_2 & PGD_2 evoke release of renin). PGE_2 and PGI_2 cause renal vasodilatation while TXA_2 causes renal vasoconstriction.

Uses of Prostaglandins

1. **Abortifacient:** Intra-amniotic administration of PGF_{2a} produced abortion with less severe adverse effects. It is used to induce second trimester abortion & usually administered as a single 40 mg intraamniotic injection.
   Synthetic PGE_2 analogues are also used as suppositories for abortion. It directly affects the collagenase of the cervix and also stimulates the contraction of the uterus.

2. **Induction of labour:** PG's do not have any advantage over oxytocin for the induction of labour. The adverse effects of the prostaglandins are slightly higher than that produced by oxytocin. PGF_{2a} has more gastrointestinal toxicity than PGE_2 and is a bronchoconstrictor also. Oral PGE_2 is superior to oral oxytocin. PGE_2 & PGF_{2a} is used in place of oxytocin in renal failure patients.

Table 5.3.1: *Classification of prostaglandin analogues.*

PGE_1	Misoprostol (CYTOTEC) 200 µg/day oral Rioprostil
PGE_2	Enprostil Arbaprostil Trimoprostil Dinoprostone (PROSTIN E_2)
PGI_2	Carbacyclin Iloprost
$PGF_{2\alpha}$	Dinoprost (PROSTIN F_2 ALPHA)

15-methyl-PGF_{2a} is used to control postpartum haemorrhage when oxytocin and ergot alkaloids fail to control the bleeding.

3. **Peripheral vascular diseases:** Infusion or intraarterial injection of prostacyclin (PGI_2) improves potency of blood vessels in certain peripheral vascular diseases. Infusion of PGI_2 can also reduce the infarct size in immediate postmyocardial infarction period.
4. **Respiratory system:** PGE_2 is a powerful bronchodilator when given in aerosol form, but due to its irritant action on bronchial mucosa its clinical utility is limited.
5. **Renal system:** PGE_1, PGE_2 & PGI_2 increase glomerular filtration through their vasodilatory effects and increase water & sodium excretion.
6. **Gastric ulcer:** PGE_2 & PGI_2 has been found to promote healing in gastric ulcer. PGE's are cytoprotective at low doses and inhibit gastric acid secretion at higher doses.
7. PGE_1 (Alprostadil) is being used as IV infusion in infants with congenital heart defects, to maintain the patency of ductus arteriosus.

LEUKOTRIENES

The leukotrienes play a major role in the inflammatory response to injury and are implicated in the pathogenesis of many inflammatory diseases, most notably asthma, allergic rhinitis, cystic fibrosis, glomerulonephritis, rheumatoid arthritis, psoriasis, and inflammatory bowel disease. Several highly effective cysteinyl leukotriene receptor antagonists and synthesis inhibitors are now in late stage clinical development and are coming in to the market for the treatment of asthma. There are indications that these new compounds are steroid sparing in their actions. The development of leukotriene receptor antagonists and synthesis inhibitors for the treatment of other inflammatory conditions is currently a highly active area of research.

❑❑❑

CHAPTER 5.4 Drugs Used in Cough and Asthma

Cough is a protective reflex which helps in expulsion of respiratory secretion or foreign particles which are irritant to respiratory tract. Irritation to any part of respiratory tract starting from pharynx to lungs carried impulses by afferent fibres in vagus and sympathetic nerve to the cough centre in the medulla oblongata. Cough may be **dry** (without sputum or unproductive) or **productive** (with sputum production). There are certain factors which are responsible for production of cough e.g.

i. *Environmental factors:* Certain irritant pollutants, dust, smoking, automobile smoke.
ii. Upper respiratory tract infection.
iii. Acute lung infections, asthma and certain pleural diseases e.g. pleural effusion.
iv. Chronic pulmonary ailments e.g. tuberculosis, chronic bronchitis & lung cancer etc.
v. Drug induced cough.

The various drugs and their combination used in cough are clasified as in table 5.1.1.

PHARYNGEAL DEMULCENTS

These are the agents which are generally administered in the form of lozenges, cough drops and cough linctus. They produce the soothing action on throat directly and by increasing the flow of saliva and provide symptomatic relief from dry cough.

EXPECTORANT

Expectorants are the drugs which **increase the production of bronchial secretion** and **reduce its viscosity to facilitate its removal by coughing**. Expectorants can stimulate the expulsion of respiratory secretion either directly or reflexly. Certain volatile oils of plant origin such as oil of lemon, anise, eucalyptus by steam inhalation route increase the respiratory secretion by its **direct action**. Another compound, guaiacol, which is obtained from wood creosote or synthetically prepared, directly increase bronchial secretion and syrup tolu (Tolu balsum) act in same way.

The second type is **reflex expectorant**, which acts by stimulating the gastric reflexes which help to increase the respiratory

Table 5.4.1: *Classification for drugs used in cough.*

	Drug	Dose
I.	**Pharyngeal demulcents**	
	Certain lozenges, linctus and cough drops containing glycerine, liquorice and syrups.	
II.	**Expectorants**	
	Sodium and potassium citrate Sodium and potassium acetate Potassium iodide Ammonium chloride & carbonate	0.3-1 g TDS. Used in various preparations as expectorant
	Acetylcysteine	3-5 ml of 10-20% (as aerosol)
	Bromhexine	8 mg TDS (used with ambroxol and cetirizine also)
	Guaiphenesin	100-300 mg TDS
	Syrup of Vasaka	2-4 ml TDS
	Syrup of Tolu	0.3-0.6 g TDS
III.	**Antitussive**	
i.	**Opioids**	
	Codeine (as linctus)	10-30 mg/day
	Pholcodeine	10-15 mg/day
ii.	**Non-opioids**	
	Noscapine	15-30 mg/day
	Dextromethorphan	10-20 mg/day
	Pipazethate	40-80 mg/day
iii.	**Antihistaminics**	
	Chlorpheniramine (PIRITON)	2-5 mg/day
	Diphenhydramine (BENADRYL)	15-25 mg/day
	Promethazine (PHENARGAN)	15-25 mg/day

secretions. Certain salts which are used as emetics, when used in subemetic dose, increase the bronchial secretion and expel it out, they are known as **saline expectorants**.

Ammonium salts (as chloride and carbonate) are gastric irritant in nature and reflexly increase bronchial secretion.

Potassium salts (as iodide) act by both direct action and reflexly to increase the respiratory secretions and decrease its viscosity thus they are easy to expel out. Potassium iodide is generally used for cough associated with chronic bronchitis and asthma but it interferes with thyroid function tests, so it is dangerous in patients sensitive to iodine and chronic use can induce hypothyroidism and goitre.

Sodium and **potassium citrate** and **acetate** act by increasing bronchial secretion by their salt actions.

Certain alkaloids such as **vasicine** obtained from plant *Adhatoda vasica* act as potent expectorant and mucolytic agent. **Bromhexine**, a derivative of vasicine depolymerises mucopolysaccharides directly and by liberating lysosomal enzymes. Another compound **acetylcysteine** opens disulfide bonds in mucoproteins present in sputum and decrease its viscosity. **Carbocisteine** acts in same manner.

Erdosteine is recently introduced mucolytic with unique protective functions for the respiratory tract. It is **indicated** in the treatment of acute and chronic airway diseases such as bronchitis, rhinitis, sinusitis, laryngopharyngitis and exacerbations of chronic bronchitis.

ANTITUSSIVES

They are central cough suppressants and **act centrally to raise the threshold of cough centre and inhibit the cough reflex** by suppressing the coordinating cough centre in the medulla oblongata. They are mainly used in dry (unproductive) cough and are ineffective in cough due to pleural disease.

Codeine, which is an opium alkaloid is most commonly opiate used as antitussive and more selective for cough centre. Like morphine, it depresses cough centre but is less constipating and abuse liability is low. It is relatively safe drug used in cough along with analgesic property and it's only important adverse effect is constipation.

Pholcodeine is similar to codeine in efficacy and is longer acting. It has no analgesic or addicting property.

Noscapine is another opium alkaloid of benzylisoquinoline group. It is used as antitussive with no analgesic and drug abuse or drug dependence property. It is contraindicated in asthmatic patients as it releases histamine which can cause bronchoconstriction.

Dextromethorphan is a synthetic compound and its dextroisomer is used as antitussive and is as effective as codeine without any addiction liability.

Pipazethate is another synthetic compound of phenothiazine category used as antitussive with little analgesic and sedative properties.

ANTIHISTAMINICS

Many H_1 antihistaminics have been added to antitussive/expectorant formulations. They do not act on cough centre but provide relief due to their sedative and anticholinergic action.

BRONCHODILATORS

Bronchodilators are helpful in individuals with cough and bronchoconstriction due to bronchial hyperreactivity. They help by improving the effectiveness of cough in clearing secretions.

ANTIASTHMATIC AGENTS

BRONCHIAL ASTHMA

Asthma is a disease characterized by an increased responsiveness of the trachea and bronchi to a variety of stimuli and manifests as narrowing of the airways that changes in severity either spontaneously or as a result of therapy. The impairment of air flow in asthma is caused by three abnormalities:

a. Constriction of bronchial smooth muscle (bronchoconstriction).
b. Swelling of bronchiolar mucosa (bronchial edema).
c. Excessive bronchial secretions.

The drugs used in management of bronchial asthma can be classified as in table 5.4.1.

SYMPATHOMIMETICS

β_2-agonists are invariably used in the symptomatic treatment of asthma. Epinephrine and ephedrine are structurally related to the catecholamine norepinephrine, a neu-

Table 5.4.2: *Classification for antiasthmatic drugs.*

I. Bronchodilators	
i. Sympathomimetics (adrenergic receptor agonists)	
Adrenaline, ephedrine, isoprenaline, orciprenaline, salbutamol, terbutaline, salmeterol, bambuterol etc.	
ii. Methylxanthines (theophylline and its derivatives)	
Theophylline (THEOLONG)	200-400 mg TDS
Hydroxyethyl theophylline (DERIPHYLLIN)	250-500 mg/day oral/IM/IV
Theophylline ethanolate of piperazine (CADIPHYLLATE)	250-500 mg/day oral/IV
iii. Anticholinergics	
Atropine methonitrate (BROVON INHALANT)	2.5-10 mg/day oral/IM, 1-2 mg (aerosol)
Ipratropium bromide (IPRATOP)	40-80 µg day (aerosol)
II. Mast cell stabilizer	
Sodium cromoglycate (CHROMOTOP)	2 mg by aerosol TDS-QID, 2% nasal spray (FINTAL)
Ketotifen (AIRYFEN)	1-2 mg/day
III. Corticosteroids	
Beclomethasone dipropionate (BACLATE INHALER)	100-200 µg TDS-QID
Beclomethasone (200 µg) with salbutamol (AEROCORT ROTACAPS)	2 rotacaps TDS-QID
IV. Leukotriene pathway inhibitors (newer compounds)	
Montelukast (MONTAIR)	10 mg HS
Zafirlukast (ACCOLATE)	20 mg/day

rotransmitter of the adrenergic nervous system. They also protect effectively against the challenge with various bronchoconstrictor agents and may inhibit microvascular leakage into the airway. β_2-agonists are the drug of choice to relieve acute exacerbation of asthma and prevent bronchoconstriction following exercise or other stimuli. After inhalation the β_2 agonists have rapid onset of action (within minutes), but are active only for 4 to 6 hours.

Their **adverse effects** are dose-related and are more common after oral than aerosol administration because of the manifold higher dose required for oral drugs. Some of the important β_2-agonists like salmeterol, terbutaline and salbutamol are invariably used as bronchodilators both oral as well as aerosol inhalants. Salmeterol is long-acting analogue of salbutamol in which the amine substituent is a long lipophilic chain, but found to be slower in achieving the peak bronchodilatation effect. The detailed pharmacology is discussed in chapter 'Adrenergic Agents'.

Specific agents used in bronchial asthma are discussed here.

SALBUTAMOL

It is highly selective β_2-adrenergic stimulant having a prominent bronchodilator action. It has poor cardiac action compared to isoprenaline. It is given by oral as well as inhalation route by nebulizer. Palpitation, restlessness, nervousness are the common side effects with salbutamol.

TERBUTALINE

It is highly selective β_2 agonist similar to salbutamol, useful by oral as well as inhalational route.

SALMETEROL

It is newer long acting selective β_2 adrenergic agonist with slow onset of action, **used** for maintenance therapy in asthma, nocturnal asthma and asthma induced by exercise.

The β_2 selective adrenergic agonists are most widely used drugs for the treatment of asthma. They are effective after oral and inhaled administration and have a longer duration of action. Albuterol (salbutamol), salmeterol, bitolterol, pirbuterol are available as aerosol pack in metered dose.

BAMBUTEROL

It is a latest selective adrenergic β_2 agonist with long plasma half life and given once daily in a dose of 10-20 mg orally.

Methylxanthines (Theophylline and Its Derivatives)

Among the methylxanthines, aminophylline is most commonly used drug in the treatment of bronchial asthma. It is a stable mixture of theophylline and ethylenediamine. These drugs inhibit the enzyme phosphodiesterase, this inhibition results in higher concentration of intracellular cyclic AMP. Increased cAMP leads to bronchodilatation, cardiac stimulation and vasodilatation.

Pharmacological Actions

CNS: The caffeine and theophylline are pharmacologically CNS stimulants and produce alertness and cortical arousal, but in higher doses causes restlessness, nervousness and insomnia.

CVS: Methylxanthines stimulate the heart and increase the force of myocardial contraction. Tachycardia is more common with theophylline. Cardiac output is increased in CHF patients.

Smooth muscles: Methylxanthines relax smooth muscles especially bronchi in asthmatic patients. Theophylline produces sustained bronchodilator action.

Kidney: Methylxanthines exert mild diuretic action by inhibiting tubular reabsorption of sodium and water, In addition, it increases renal blood flow and glomerular filtration rate.

Skeletal muscles: Methylxanthines facilitate neuromuscular transmission by increasing acetylcholine release.

Mast cells: Methylxanthines inhibit the release of histamine and other mediators from mast cells which indirectly help in the management of bronchial asthma.

THEOPHYLLINE

Theophylline has two distinct action: smooth muscle relaxation (i.e. bronchodilatation) and suppression of the response of the airways to stimuli (i.e. non-bronchodilator prophylactic effects). Bronchodilatation is mediated by inhibition of two isozymes of phosphodiesterase (PDE III and to a lesser extent, PDE IV) while non-bronchodilator prophylactic actions are mediated through one or more different molecular mechanisms, that do not involve inhibition of PDE III or antagonism of adenosine receptors. Theophylline increases the force of contraction of diaphragmatic muscles.

It is well absorbed orally. It is distributed to all tissues and is 50% plasma protein bound. It is extensively metabolized in liver by demethylation and oxidation. Only 10% is excreted unchanged in urine.

Adverse Effects

Side effects are usually associated with the increasing serum concentration of theophylline and includes nausea, vomiting, headache, insomnia, tachypnea, epigastric pain, palpitation, hypotension, irritability. Higher doses can cause persistent vomiting, cardiac arrhythmias, intractable seizures, tachycardia. Other side effects include alopecia, hyperglycemia, inappropriate ADH syndrome, rash.

ANTICHOLINERGICS

Anticholinergics, like atropine and its derivative ipratropium bromide **block cholinergic pathways that cause airway constriction**. They may provide added bronchodilator effect in patients who are receiving $beta_2$-adrenergic agents for asthma.

The detailed pharmacology is discussed in chapter 'Cholinergic blocking agents.'

MAST CELL STABILIZERS

SODIUM CROMOGLYCATE

It is a synthetic chromone derivative, highly effective in preventing asthma attacks. **It inhibits degranulation of mast cells by trigger stimuli.** It **also inhibits the release of various asthma provoking mediators** e.g. histamine, leukotrienes, platelet activating factor (PAF) and interleukins (IL's) from mast cells. It prevents the late response and subsequent bronchial hyperresponsiveness by acting on inflammatory cells such as macrophages or eosinophils. It does not produce bronchodilatation and also does not antagonize the constrictor effect of histamine etc. therefore not found beneficial in acute attack of asthma and **used for prophylaxis only**.

Sodium cromoglycate is not absorbed orally and is to be administered by aerosol. Only a small fraction of inhaled drug is absorbed systemically and it is rapidly excreted unchanged in urine and bile.

Adverse reactions reported are bronchospasm, throat irritation and rarely headache, dizziness, rashes and nasal congestion.

Therapeutic Uses

1. **Bronchial asthma:** It is used for prophylactic treatment of bronchial asthma.
2. **Allergic rhinitis:** Two percent aqueous nasal spray (FINTAL nasal spray) is used for nasal decongestion although it is not a nasal decongestant.
3. **Allergic conjunctivitis:** Two percent aqueous eye solution (FINTAL eye

drop) is used in allergic conjunctivitis in chronic cases.

KETOTIFEN

It is a cromolyn analogue. It is an antihistaminic (H_1 antagonist) and probably inhibits airway inflammation induced by platelet activating factor (PAF) in primate. It is not a bronchodilator. It is **used** in asthma and symptomatic relief in atopic dermatitis, rhinitis, conjunctivitis and urticaria. It is absorbed orally and well tolerated. Bioavailability is 50% due to first pass metabolism and is primarily metabolized. The common **side effects** include dry mouth, sedation, dizziness and nausea.

CORTICOSTEROIDS

Like mast cell stabilizer, corticosteroids do not relax airway smooth muscle directly but **reduce bronchial reactivity, increase airway caliber, suppress inflammatory response to antigen antibody reaction or trigger stimuli and reduce the frequency of asthma exacerbations**. They produce more sustained symptomatic relief than any bronchodilator and mast cell stabilizer.

Systemic steroids are used in both severe chronic asthma and in acute emergency of asthma (*status asthmaticus*).

Among the **inhaled steroids**, beclomethasone is a halogenated corticosteroid ester used in aerosol form. It suppresses asthma by a topical antiinflammatory action without causing any systemic side effects. They reduce the bronchial hyperreactivity and increase the peak expiratory flow rate in asthmatic patients. They are not effective during an acute attack or in status asthmaticus. **Side effects** are sore throat, hoarseness of voice, dysphonia, oropharyngeal candidiasis.

LEUKOTRIENE PATHWAY INHIBITORS

Apart from histamine, leukotrienes liberated during inflammation are more powerful bronchoconstrictor and longer acting. Leukotrienes also increase bronchial mucus secretion and increase vascular permeability. All the leukotrienes are derived from 5-lipoxygenase pathway of arachidonic acid and are synthesized by a variety of inflammatory cells in the airways e.g. eosinophils, mast cells, basophils and macrophages. The LTB_4, C_4 & D_4 exert many effects known to occur in bronchial asthma, including bronchoconstriction and increased bronchial reactivity. The drug, **montelukast** (LTB_4 antagonist) and **zafirlukast** (LTD_4 antagonist) have the advantage of being used when taken orally in asthmatic patients.

MONTELUKAST

It is a **cysteinyl leukotriene receptor antagonist** indicated for the management of persistent asthma. It has been shown to have substantial blockade of airway leukotriene receptors 24 hours after oral dosing. Montelukast appears to be a useful alternative or adjunct to inhaled corticosteroid therapy in adults and an alternative to sodium cromoglycate in children.

❑❑❑

Section 6

Drugs Acting On Blood

CHAPTER 6.1 Coagulants and Anticoagulants

Thrombogenesis is an abnormal state of haemostasis leading to the formation of arterial and venous thrombus, also known as white and red thrombus respectively. **Haemostasis** is the spontaneous arrest of bleeding from the damaged blood vessels. The immediate haemostatic response to a damaged blood vessel is vasospasm and, after few seconds, platelets stick to the exposed collagen of the damaged endothelium (platelet adhesion) and to each other (platelet aggregation). Certain agents e.g. thromboxane A_2 (from arachidonic acid metabolic pathway) is synthesized within platelets and induces thrombogenesis and vasoconstriction and prostacyclin I_2 (PGI_2) inhibits thrombogenesis.

Coagulation of blood comprises the formation of fibrin. There are thirteen factors (synthesized in liver) which are involved in the coagulation of blood.

Review of Clotting Mechanism

Haemostasis: Haemostasis refers to the arrest of blood loss from a damaged blood vessel i.e. stoppage of bleeding. The mechanism is essential to maintain life. In case of any damage to a blood vessel, the haemostatic response must be:

- Quick.
- Controlled & localised to region of damage.

Three basic measures taken by the body to reduce and stop blood loss are:

i. Vascular spasm.
ii. Platelet plug formation.
iii. Clotting or coagulation.

Clotting: Normally, blood remains liquid as long as it is flowing within intact smooth blood vessels. But on damage to the blood vessel and/or if blood is extracted from the blood vessel, there is conversion of liquid to gel state. This gel, on solidification gives a clot. The process of conversion of liquid to gel is termed as **coagulation**.

Clotting involves several factors called **clotting factors**. These include calcium, several inactive enzymes synthesized by hepatocytes and various molecules associated with platelets and/or released by the damaged tissue. The clotting factors are denoted by Roman numeral, denoting the order of their discovery (Table 6.1.1).

Table 6.1.1: *Clotting factors.*

I.	Fibrinogen.
II.	Prothrombin.
III.	Thromboplastin.
IV.	Calcium.
V.	Proaccelerin.
VI.	Accelerin.
VII.	Serum prothrombin conversion accelerator.
VIII.	Antihaemophilic factor.
IX.	Plasma thomboplastin component.
X.	Stuart Prower factor.
XI.	Plasma thromboplastin antecedent.
XII.	Hageman factor.
XIII.	Fibrin stabilizing factor.

Stages of Clotting

Formation of prothrombinase: It can be formed by extrinsic pathway and intrinsic pathway.

Extrinsic pathway: This pathway has fewer steps than the intrinsic pathway and occurs rapidly, within a matter of seconds if the trauma is severe. It is called the extrinsic pathway because a protein tissue factor, also called thromboplastin or coagulation factor III, takes into the blood stream from outside and initiates the formation of prothrombinase. Tissue factor is released from the surface of the damaged cells. It activates factor VII. Factor VII combines with factor X, activating it. Factor X in the presence of Ca^{++} combines with factor V to give active enzyme prothrombinase.

Intrinsic pathway: This pathway is more complex and is much slower. It is so named as the activators are in direct contact with the blood in the intact blood vessels. No outside tissue damage is required. Rough vessels with exposed collagen is sufficient. Contact with collagen activates factor XII. This in turn activates factor IX. Factor IX joins factor VIII and this gives active factor X. Factor X joins with calcium to bring about the formation of prothrombinase.

Once prothrombinase has been formed, the **common pathway** is followed. In stage 2, prothrombinase and calcium catalyze the conversion of prothrombin to thrombin. In stage 3, thrombin, in the presence of calcium converts soluble fibrinogen to insoluble fibrin threads.

COAGULANTS

These are the agents which promote coagulation and are mainly used in any haemorrhagic condition. They are classified as in table 6.1.2.

VITAMIN K

Vitamin K is a fat soluble vitamin found primarily in leafy green vegetables. There are two normal forms exist, K_1 found in food (called phytonadione), K_2 found in human tissue (synthesized by intestinal bacteria) known as menaquinone. The synthetic compound is known as K_3. Synthetic analogues of natural vitamin also show biological activity. Most of the vitamin K is synthesized by intestinal microorganisms and there is a risk of vitamin K deficiency in new born infants.

Vitamin K is necessary for final stage of

Table 6.1.2: *Classification of coagulants.*

I. **Vitamin K** (along with other vitamins available)	0.66 mg OD-BD
Vitamin K analogues	
Menapthone (KAPLIN)	5-20 mg/day
Menadione (STYPINDON)	10-30 mg TDS
Phytomenadione	10 mg/ml IM/day
Botropase	1 ml BD-TDS IM
Ethamsylate (ALSTAT)	250-500 mg TDS
Adenochrome monosemicarbazone (STYPTOCID)	10-30 mg BD-TDS
Feracrylum (HEMOLOK)	Applied locally on affected surface
Aprotinin (APROTIN)	Upto 2 million KIU IV injection
II. **Other**	
Tranexamic acid (TEXID)	15-25 mg/kg BD-QID oral, 10-15 mg/kg slow IV TDS
Polidocanol (SCLEROL)	Local application
Sodium tetradecyl (SETROL)	1-3% solution

synthesis of coagulation factors (mainly factor II, VII, IX and X) in liver. In synthesis of coagulant proteins vitamins K is converted to an epoxide which is subsequently reduced to vitamin K. Vitamin K is metabolised in liver and metabolites are excreted in bile and urine.

The **deficiency** of vitamin K occur due to liver disease, jaundice, malabsorption syndromes and chronic use of antimicrobial agents.

Adverse effects include haemolysis especially in infants and person with G-6-PD deficiency. Menadione can cause jaundice, and haemolysis in infants.

Therapeutically, vitamin K is **used** in prophylaxis and treatment of deficiency of clotting factor due to dietary deficiency of vitamin K, chronic antimicrobial therapy, malabsorption syndrome, obstructive jaundice, liver diseases such as cirrhosis and hepatitis, in neonates to prevent or treat haemorrhagic disease of new born; to counteract the overdosing of oral anticoagulants (phytomenadione is most effective as it acts most rapidly).

BOTROPASE

It is a aqueous solution of haemocoagulase isolated from venom of *Bothrops jararaca* and *B. atorox* containing normal saline. It is **indicated** in primary and secondary post-operative internal and external haemorrhage.

ETHAMSYLATE

It **inhibits prostacyclin synthetase enzyme** resulting in the prevention of prostacyclin induced vasodilatation and corrects abnormal platelet function. It is mainly **used** to control haemorrhage in epistaxis, haemoptysis, haematemesis, menorrhagia and postsurgical conditions.

ADENOCHROME MONOSEMICARBAZONE

It exerts its haemostatic action by **reducing capillary fragility**, and is **indicated** in epistaxis, haematuria, retinal haemorrhage and secondary haemorrhage from wounds.

FERACRYLUM

It is a **local haemostatic** and antiseptic agent. The haemostatic effect of feracrylum is based on the formation of synthetic complex consisting of its adduct with plasma proteins principally albumin. Like other biodegradable polymers, the feracrylum-albumin complex formed gets broken down over a period of time.

Adverse effects include burning sensation.

It is **indicated** as adjunct to conventional haemostatic procedures in capillary and venule oozing in various surgical and diagnostic procedures, dental extraction and oral surgeries.

APROTININ

It is a naturally occurring proteolytic enzyme inhibitor acting on plasmin and kallikrein.

It **inhibits plasmin and kallikrein, thus directly affecting fibrinolysis**. It also inhibits the contact phase activation of coagulation which both initiates coagulation and promotes fibrinolysis.

After IV injection rapid distribution of aprotinin occurs into the total extracellular space leading to a rapid initial decrease in plasma concentration. It has a plasma half-life of 2.5 hours. After a single IV dose 25-40% is excreted in the urine over 48 hours. It is accumulated primarily in the kidney (it is actively absorbed by the proximal tubules).

Adverse effects include local thrombophlebitis, hypersensitivity reactions (skin eruptions, tachycardia, pallor/cyanosis, dyspnoea, nausea or anaphylactic shock) may occur.

It is **indicated** in patients at high risk of blood loss following open heart surgery with extracorporeal circulation, life threatening haemorrhage due to hyperplasminaemia, hyperfibrinolytic haemorrhage occurring post-traumatically and postoperatively e.g. in obstetrics and gynaecology.

TRANEXAMIC ACID

Tranexamic acid produces an antifibrinolytic effect by **blocking the lysine binding site on plasminogen** which is essential for binding to fibrin and thereby prevents the activation of plasminogen on the surface of fibrin.

Tranexamic acid is absorbed from the GIT with peak plasma concentration at about three hours. Bioavailability is about 30 to 50 percent. It is widely distributed throughout the body and has very low protein binding. It diffuses across the placenta and is distributed into breast milk. It has a plasma half life of about two hours. It is excreted in the urine mainly as unchanged drug.

Adverse effects include dose related gastrointestinal disturbances, hypotension particularly after rapid IV administration and transient disturbance in colour vision rarely.

It is **used** for prophylaxis and control of bleeding in gynaecological and obstetric surgery, haemorrhage associated with IUCD insertion, conisation of the cervix, intra- and postoperative haemorrhage (cardiac surgery with cardiopulmonary bypass, coronary artery bypass grafting), total knee replacement, gastrointestinal bleeding, local and general fibrinolysis, epistaxis, prosta tectomy, haemoptysis and haemorrhage after dental extraction.

POLIDOCANOL

It is a sclerosing agent for bleeding oesophageal varices, varicose veins, bleeding gastroduodenal ulcers etc.

SODIUM TETRADECYL

IV injection causes intimal inflammation and thrombus formation occluding the injected vein. Subsequent formation of fibrous tissue results in partial or complete vein obliteration.

It is **indicated** in the treatment of small, uncomplicated varicose veins of the lower extremities, haemangioma, ganglionoma, oesophageal varices.

ANTICOAGULANTS

These are the drugs used to reduce the coagulability of blood. They can be classified as in table 6.1.3.

HEPARIN

Heparin is a heterogenous mixture of sulfated mucopolysaccharides and quick acting anticoagulant which shows efficacy both *in vitro* and *in vivo* and having a molecular weight from 4,000 to 40,000 depending upon the type of preparations. Its biological activity is dependent upon the plasma protease inhibitor antithrombin III, which inhibits clotting factor proteases by forming equimolar stable complexes with them.

It **acts by activating plasma antithrombin III** which rapidly inhibits activated coagulation factors IXa, Xa, XIa and XIIa, plasmin, kallikrein and thrombin, thus inhibiting conversion of fibrinogen to fibrin.

Heparin is well absorbed after subcutaneous administration and is not effective orally, and metabolized mainly in liver. It is not secreted in milk and does not cross placental barrier.

Adverse effects include bleeding, alopecia (reversible), bleeding from gums, unexplained bruising, osteoporosis and rarely hypersensitivity, thrombocytopenia and hyperkalemia.

It is **indicated** in the prophylaxis and treatment of deep vein thrombosis in major surgery and pulmonary embolism, treatment of atrial fibrillation with embolisation, prophylaxis and treatment of peripheral arterial embolism.

LOW MOLECULAR WEIGHT HEPARINS (LMWH)

These are prepared by enzymatic or chemical hydrolysis of conventional heparin, their molecular weight varies from 3,000 to 7,000. They are absorbed more completely than the conventional heparin preparation and having longer duration of action.

It is obtained as fragments of commercial grade heparin which is produced by chemical or enzymatic depolymerisation. It contains less pentasaccharide sequences with a high affinity for antithrombin III.

LMWH exerts its **action mostly by antithrombin mediated inhibition of factor Xa.** But some thrombin inhibition by LMWH is

Table 6.1.3: *Classification of anticoagulants.*

I.	**Parenteral anticoagulants**	
•	Heparin (INHEP)	5,000-10,000 U IV stat and maintained at 5,000 U 4-6 hourly
•	***Low molecular weight heparin (LMWH)***	
	Nadroparin (FRAXIPARINE)	3075-4100 IU OD SC
	Enoxaparin (CLEXANE)	20-40 mg OD SC
	Reviparin (CLIVARINE)	13.8 mg OD SC
	Dalteparin (FRAGMIN)	100-200 U/kg OD
	Pamparin (FLUXUM)	6400 IU OD SC
	Ardeparin (INDEPARIN)	2500-5000 IU OD SC
•	***Semisynthetic heparinoids***	
	Ancrod	2 U/kg IV infusion
	Heparan sulfate	
	Danaparoid	
	Lepirudin	
II.	**Oral anticoagulants**	
	Warfarin (WARF)	30 mg (loading) & maintained on 2.5-10 mg/day (usual dose is 10-15 mg/day)
	Bishydroxycoumarin (DICUMAROL)	200 mg × 2 days (loading), maintained on 50-100 mg/day
	Acenocoumarol (ACITROM)	8-28 mg/day (loading), maintained on 2-10 mg/day
	Phenindione (DINDEVAN)	200 mg/day (loading), maintained on 50-150 mg/day
III.	**Fibrinolytics**	
	Streptokinase (PROKINASE)	7,50,000-1.5 million IU in 1 hr IV infusion
	Urokinase (URIDAN)	50,000-2.5 lac IV infusion
	Alteplase (ACTILYSE)	10 mg IV (bolus) upto 100 mg in 3 hrs

retained and is of importance for the antithrombotic effect.

LMWH have higher bioavailability after subcutaneous injection than standard, heparin. LMWH binds less than heparin to plasma proteins. The clearance of LMWH is mainly renal, independent of dose and slower than metabolic clearance of heparin.

Adverse effects include thrombocytopenia, haemorrhage, injection site ecchymoses, osteoporosis, sensitivity phenomenon.

It is **indicated** in prevention and treatment of deep vein thrombosis and pulmonary embolism in surgical patients, prevention of extracorporeal thrombosis during haemodialysis.

The clinically used low molecular weight heparins are **enoxaparin, reviparin, dalteparin, nadroparin, ardeparin** and **tinzaparin** etc.

HEPARINOIDS

Ancrod is an enzyme obtained from Malayan pit viper venom. It produces heparin like effect by degrading fibrinogen into an unstable form of fibrin.

Danaparoid containing mainly heparan sulfate isolated from porcine intestinal mucosa and is used in heparin induced thrombocytopenia and deep venous thrombosis.

Lepirudin is a recombinant derivative of hirudin (direct thrombin inhibitor secreted by salivary glands of leech). It inhibits thrombin directly and is mainly used in heparin induced thrombocytopenia.

HEPARIN ANTAGONISTS

The agents like **protamine sulfate** react with the strongly acidic groups of heparin and can abolish its anticoagulant activity. Approximately 1 mg of protamine sulfate neutralizes 80 to 100 units of heparin. It is **used** only in severe bleeding or when heparin action needs to be terminated rapidly e.g. after cardiac or vascular surgery.

ORAL ANTICOAGULANTS

They act by interfering with synthesis of vitamin K dependent clotting factors in liver. They act as competitive antagonists of vitamin K and reduce plasma levels of clotting factors in a dose dependent manner. They act by interfering with regeneration of active form of vitamin K. Factor VII levels are reduced first followed by factor IX, X and II.

ACENOCOUMAROL

It takes at least 48 to 72 hours for the anticoagulant effect to develop fully.

Acenocoumarol is absorbed nearly completely after oral administration. It is highly bound to plasma proteins and it crosses the placental barrier.

Adverse effects include haemorrhage, rash, alopecia, diarrhoea, hepatic dysfunction, nausea, vomiting and pancreatitis.

It is **used** in venous thromboembolism, pulmonary embolism, atrial fibrillation and for prophylaxis after insertion of prosthetic heart valves.

WARFARIN

It is most commonly used oral anticoagulants employed for long term anticoagulant therapy and having less toxic effects including alopecia and dermatitis. It is rapidly and completely absorbed from intestines and is 99% plasma protein bound. It crosses the placental barrier and is secreted in milk. The other properties are same as acenocoumarol.

PHENINDIONE

The mechanism of action and adverse effects are same as acenocoumarol. It produces more serious nonhaemorrhagic toxic effects, their use is now very limited.

FIBRINOLYTICS

These are agents used to lyse clot to recanalise occluded blood vessels, mainly used in coronary arteries.

STREPTOKINASE

It is a purified preparation of bacterial protein obtained from β hemolytic streptococci.

It acts by forming a complex with circulating plasminogen that binds loosely to fibrin and it converts plasminogen to plasmin. It has no intrinsic activity. It is given by parenteral route and has a short plasma half life.

Adverse effects include fever, allergic reactions, bleeding from different sites, rarely anaphylaxis, arrhythmias, bronchospasm.

It is **indicated** in acute myocardial infarction, pulmonary embolism, deep vein thrombosis, arterial thrombosis, acute thrombosis of central retinal vessels, extensive coronary emboli and severe iliofemoral thrombophlebitis.

UROKINASE

It is obtained from cultures of human renal cells in tissue culture and it is a proteolytic enzyme. It activates plasminogen directly. Plasmin acts on fibrin and fibrinolysis occurs. It is non antigenic.

Adverse effects include drug fever and haemorrhage.

It is **used** for myocardial infarction, for venous thrombosis and pulmonary embolism.

ALTEPLASE

Also known as recombinant tissue Plasminogen Activator (rt-PA). It is produced by recombinant DNA technology from human tissue culture. It specifically activates plasminogen bound to the fibrin clot. This minimises the risk of systemic bleeding.

It is non antigenic and has a plasma t½ of 4-8 min.

Adverse effects are nausea, fever, mild hypotension, rash, pruritus and localised bleeding.

It is **used** in lysis of suspected occlusive coronary artery thrombi associated with evolving MI in adults.

PLATELET INHIBITING DRUGS

These drugs interfere with platelet function and may be useful in prophylaxis of thromboembolic disorders. Thromboxane A_2 (TXA_2) from platelets promote and prostacyclin (PGI_2) from vessel wall inhibit platelet aggregation.

ABCIXIMAB

It binds to the intact glycoprotein IIb/IIIa receptor of human platelets, which is a member of the integrin family of adhesion receptors and the major platelet surface receptor involved in platelet aggregation. The drug **inhibits platelet aggregation by preventing the binding of fibrinogen, von Willebrand factor** and other adhesive molecules to GP IIb/IIIa receptor sites on activated platelets.

Adverse effects include bleeding, thrombocytopenia, human antichimeric antibody development, atrial fibrillation/flutter, complete AV block, palpitation, SVT, constipation, ileus, abnormal thinking, dizziness.

It is **indicated** for platelet aggregation inhibition as adjunct to percutaneous transluminal coronary angioplasty or atherectomy (PTCA).

ASPIRIN

In small doses aspirin **inactivates irreversibly platelet enzyme cyclooxygenase**, hence **thromboxane A_2 is not synthesised**. The effect of enzyme inactivation lasts till the life of platelet.

It is **indicated** in prophylaxis in cases of increased risk of blood clotting, myocardial infarction, coronary bypass, transluminal angioplasty, stroke, transient ischaemic attack and unstable angina.

❑❑❑

CHAPTER 6.2

Haematinics

(Drugs Used in Anaemia)

Anaemia is the decrease in number of red blood cells or hemoglobin content caused by blood loss, deficient erythropoiesis, excessive hemolysis, or combination of these changes. Iron deficiency anaemia is probably the most common nutritional deficiency in the world. It is estimated that at least 500 million people are affected. Iron deficiency anaemia is much more common in developing countries, as people are consuming too little food or a limited variety of food.

Infants and young children have higher iron requirement. For the first six months of life, these requirements are met by iron store in the infant's body alone with supplementation from breast or formula milk. Iron requirement increases during adolescence because of growth, muscle development and, for girls, at the start of menstruation. Adult women have higher iron requirement because of menstrual losses. During pregnancy it is not necessary to have extra iron in the diet because absorption increases and menstruation stops. The fetus is likely to get enough iron even if its mother has low stores, but mother becomes anaemic.

Anaemia may be classified into different groups according to the pathophysiology.

1. Dietary deficiency anaemia, which is due to deficient supply of various factors e.g. iron, folic acid, vitamin B_{12}, vitamin C and pyridoxine which are essential for normal blood formation.
2. Anaemia due to blood loss e.g. in severe gastric blood loss (ulcers), protozoal or worm infestation.
3. Anaemia due to excessive destruction, of blood e.g. sickle cell anaemia and haemolytic anaemia.
4. Anaemia due bone narrow depression e.g. aplastic and hypoplastic anaemia.

IRON

The body iron is distributed mainly in two forms, one as haem in haemoglobin and cytochrome oxidase enzyme and other as iron bound to protein as storage compounds ferritin and hemosiderin, and as transport iron bound to transferrin. The total body iron in human adult is approximately 3.5 g out of which 66% is in haemoglobin and 25% is stored as ferritin and hemosiderin and rest is in muscles and enzyme.

Iron absorption occurs predominantly in the duodenum and upper jejunum. The physical state of iron entering the duodenum greatly influences its absorption. At physiological pH, ferrous iron is rapidly oxidized to the insoluble ferric form. Gastric acid lowers the pH in the proximal duodenum, enhancing the solubility and uptake of ferric iron. When gastric acid production is impaired, iron absorption is reduced substantially. Ascorbic acid enhances iron absorption. Ascorbic acid mobilizes iron from iron-binding proteins *in vivo,* which in turn could catalyze lipid peroxidation. Iron absorption is inhibited by antacids, phytates, phosphates and tetracyclines.

The iron is transferred by the mucosal epithelium to the body and is bound to plasma transferrin in the ferric state. In the plasma, iron takes part in a dynamic transferrin-iron equilibrium and is distributed into vascular and interstitial extravascular compartment. 50 to 60% of transferrin is extravascular. The plasma iron pool in adults is about 3 mg and has an estimated turnover of 20 to 30 mg per 24 hours. Daily and obligatory **losses** of iron in healthy men are about 1 mg; in healthy menstruating women these average 2 mg and in either case are compensated by a net absorption of 1 to 2 mg from the intestine, which enters the mobile pool of transferrin iron.

Pharmacokinetics

After oral administration iron is absorbed in ferrous form. The conversion of ferric iron to ferrous iron is aided by hydrochloric acid. Iron is transported via **transferrin**. When body stores of iron are high, ferric iron combines with apoferritin to form **ferritin**. Ferritin is the protein of iron storage. About 80 percent iron in plasma goes to erythroid marrow. The excretion of iron is minimal. Only little amount of iron is lost by exfoliation of intestinal mucosal cells and trace amount is excreted in urine, sweat and bile.

After confirmation of iron deficiency iron therapy can be given by oral or parenteral route. Generally oral iron therapy is given unless the patient is suffering from severe anaemia, malabsorption syndrome, gastrectomy or patient is showing adverse effects to oral iron therapy.

Uses

Nutritional iron deficiency anaemia; other causes in which iron deficiency can occur are pregnancy, lactation, infants, children. In patients with malabsorption syndrome, patients who are taking NSAIDs for long period, patients with chronic inflammatory disease and in patients of gastrectomy.

Preparations of iron alone or in combination with vitamin B_{12}, folic acid or other vitamins are available (see table 6.2.1).

Most of the oral formulations contain one of the iron compound with many vitamins, amino acids, liver extract, minerals, folic acid, appetite stimulants (cyproheptadine like compound).

Adverse Effects

Oral administration can cause nausea, vomiting, epigastric pain, metallic taste, staining of teeth, constipation and diarrhoea both can occur, but constipation is more common.

Table 6.2.1: *Classification for iron preparations.*

Preparation	Dose
Ferrous sulphate (Hydrated salt 20% iron, exsiccated salt 30% iron; FERSOLATE).	200-600 mg/day
Ferrous gluconate (12% iron; FERRONICUM).	300-1200 mg/day
Ferrous fumarate (33% iron; AUTRIN).	100-300 mg/day
Colloidal ferric hydroxide (50% iron; NEOFERUM).	200-800 mg/day

Other forms of iron which are present in different pharmaceutical preparations are ferric ammonium citrate, ferrous succinate, iron choline citrate, ferrous amionate, iron calcium complex, carbonyl iron, ferric glycerophosphate, haemoglobin, elemental iron, ferrous glycine sulphate, glycerinated haemoglobin, and iron (III) hydroxide polymaltose complex (equivalent to elemental iron).

Parenteral preparations: Iron dextran (IMFERON) & Iron-sorbitol citric acid complex (JECTOFER).

The parenteral administration can cause local pain at the site of injection. The other adverse effects include headache, fever, flushing, palpitation, dyspnoea, chest pain, metallic taste and even disorientation and temporary loss of taste.

IV administration can cause anaphylactic reaction characterized by circulatory collapse and even deaths have been reported.

Treatment of Acute Iron Poisoning

1. Gastric lavage with 1% sodium bicarbonate solution to remove any undissolved iron tablets.
2. Administration of milk or egg yolk to complex iron.
3. Specific iron binding chelating agent like desferrioxamine mesylate (5-10 g in 100 ml isotonic saline) or calcium diethylene triamine pentaacetate (DTPA) 35-40 mg/kg or calcium disodium acetate (35-40 mg/kg).
4. Electrolytes and other fluids to correct metabolic acidosis and hypotension.
5. Supportive administration of various agents e.g. anticonvulsants drugs to control convulsions.

ERYTHROPOIETIN

It is produced primarily by peritubular cells in the proximal tubule of the kidney. In anaemia renal secretion of erythropoietin increases rapidly manifold. Erythropoietin levels are always detectable in plasma.

It exerts its action by binding to receptor on surface of erythroid precursor cells. There is increase in intracellular concentration of calcium and arachidonate and changes in intracellular phosphorylation. It stimulates proliferation, maturation and haemoglobin formation by committed erythroid progenitors.

Recombinant human erythropoietin is available. It is given by parenteral route (IV or SC).

It is **used** in the treatment of anaemia of chronic renal failure, in anaemia of patients with AIDS who are being treated with zidovudine and anaemia associated with cancer chemotherapy.

Adverse effects include exacerbation of or new onset of hypertension and seizures in patients with renal disease.

❑❑❑

Section 7

Drugs Acting On GIT

CHAPTER 7.1

Laxatives and Antidiarrhoeal Agents

LAXATIVES

These are the drugs which promote the evacuation of bowels and used in constipation.

They are classified as in table 7.1.1.

Bulk Forming Agents

These contain natural or semisynthetic hydrophilic colloidal derivatives of cellulose.

These drugs act to increase the volume of stool by absorbing water and as a result softening of faeces occurs. These are safe drugs (except in patient with strictures when intestinal obstruction may be precipitated). Adequate hydration of the patient is to be maintained. The onset of action occurs in 12-24 hours after oral intake.

Osmotic Laxatives

These solutes are not absorbed in intestine. They retain water osmotically in bowel lumen and distend the bowel thereby increasing peristalsis indirectly. These agents should be administered with plenty of water. The administration of sodium salts is to be avoided in patients of cardiac failure, renal failure and hepatic failure.

LACTULOSE

It is a semisynthetic disaccharide of fructose and lactose. It is not digested or absorbed in small intestine thereby withdrawing water into bowel lumen. It breaks down in colon to form more osmotically active products. It also causes reduction in ammonia in hepatic coma.

Table 7.1.1: *Classification of laxatives.*

I. Bulk forming agents	Ispaghula, methylcellulose, psyllium
II. Osmotic laxatives	Magnesium salts, (sulphate, hydroxide), sodium salts (sulphate, phosphate), lactulose, glycerol suppositories
III. Stool softener	Liquid paraffin, docusate sodium
IV. Stimulant laxatives	Bisacodyl, senna, phenolphthalein, danthron, sodium picosulphate, castor oil

Stool Softener

Docusate acts by its detergent action which reduces the surface tension.

LIQUID PARAFFIN

It is a petroleum hydrocarbon, an inert viscous liquid. It is a faecal softener and causes lubrication of hard scybali by coating them. Paraffin lubricates the passage of faeces. It is not absorbed and is safe.

It is **indicated** in postoperative constipation. **Dose:** CREMAFFIN 10-15 ml/day.

Adverse effects include aspiration pneumonia, perianal pruritus, healing in perianal region may be delayed, unpleasant taste, the absorption of fat soluble vitamins may be affected. Long-term administration is not recommended.

DOCUSATES

It is an anionic detergent which softens the stool by water accumulation in intestinal lumen and emulsifies the colon contents. It is **indicated** in obstetric, habitual, geriatric, paediatric constipation or when straining is to be avoided (recent myocardial infarction, severe hypertension, post-operative cases, abdominal hernia), fissures, haemorrhoids and bed ridden patients. **Dose:** 100-200 mg/day.

Side effects include nausea, cramps and abdominal pain.

Stimulant Laxatives

These drugs exert their laxative action by increasing motility of colon. They mainly alter absorptive and secretory activity by inhibiting $Na^+ K^+$ ATPase in mucosal cells, leading to water and electrolyte accumulation in lumen. Colicky pain may occur and on the long term use may lead to hypokalemia. These drugs are to be avoided in pregnancy and children. The onset of action occurs in 6-12 hours after oral administration.

BISACODYL

It is stimulant laxative, when administered orally or as a rectal suppository it produces increased peristalsis by direct action on the mucosa of the colon, usually resulting in a soft, formed stool.

It is **indicated** in all forms of constipation, e.g. in bedridden patients, due to change of food or environment, illness or digestive disorders; relief of evacuation in painful conditions such as haemorrhoids; pre and postoperatively; pre-paration for barium enema; preparation of colon for proctosigmoidoscopy. **Dose:** DULCOLAX 5-15 mg HS oral and suppository (5-10 mg).

SODIUM PICOSULPHATE

In the colon, sodium picosulphate is converted in to the active comound bis-(p-hydroxy diphenyl) pyridyl methane (BHPM) which stimulates propulsive activity of the colon, prevents absorption of water in the colonic lumen and promotes accumulation of water.

Following oral administration sodium picosulphate is not absorbed. In colon it is converted to the active metabolite BHPM, by the action of arylsulphatases secreted by the colonic bacteria.

Prolonged use or overdosage can precipitate the onset of an atonic non-functioning colon and hypokalemia.

It is **indicated** in constipation e.g. in patients with cardiovascular disease, hernia and anorectal disorders, the elderly and postoperatively; bowel clearance before radiography, endoscopy, labour or surgery.

It is **contraindicated** in intestinal obstruction, undiagnosed abdominal symptoms.
Dose: CREMALAX 5-10 mg HS.

SENNA

It is an anthraquinone laxative. It is not active as such but after oral intake when it reaches colon the bacteria liberate anthrones, which is the active form. Active form acts on myenteric plexus to increase peristalsis. It also inhibits salt and water absorption in colon.

It is **indicated** in intestinal evacuation for radiological examination and atonic constipation.

Adverse effects include vomiting, nausea, fixed drug eruptions, skin rash. It is **contraindicated** in spastic constipation, electrolyte imbalance, intestinal obstruction, lactation.

Dose: As powder 0.6-10 gm. HS

ANTIDIARRHOEAL AGENTS

Diarrhoea is defined as frequent passage of liquid faeces with or without blood and mucus. It occurs due to various causes, infective or non infective.

The antidiarrhoeal agents can be classified as in table 7.1.2.

Antidiarrhoeals are given for symptomatic relief of diarrhoea. The first step in treatment of acute diarrhoea is replacement of fluid and electrolytes. If due to diarrhoea there is severe dehydration, it requires immediate hospitalization for IV fluid and electrolyte replacement. Antidiarrhoeal drugs are administered for obtaining symptomatic relief in acute diarrhoea but have untoward effects. Alongwith antidiarrhoeal drugs, antispasmodics are administered in those patients who have diarrhoea with abdominal pain.

Table 7.1.2: *Classification of antidiarrhoeal agents.*

I. **Rehydrating solutions:** Containing NaCl, KCl, $NaHCO_3$ (for parenteral administration) and sodium chloride, potassium chloride, sodium citrate and glucose as oral formula (ORS).	
II. **Absorbents & bulk forming agents**	
Kaolin	2-4 g/day
Pectin	100-300 mg/day
Psyllium	8-16 g/day
Ispaghula	8-16 g/day
Methyl cellulose	4-6 g/day
III. **Antimotility & antisecretory drugs**	
Codeine	30-60 mg TDS
Loperamide (LOPAMIDE)	4-16 mg/day
Diphenoxylate with atropine (LOMOFEN)	5 mg QID
Sulfasalazine (SALAZOPYRIN)	1-3 g QID
Mesalazine (MESACOL)	2-4 g/day
IV. **Antimicrobial drugs**	
Details are given in chapter 'Chemotherapeutic agents'.	

Absorbents and Bulk Forming Drugs

They are colloidal bulk forming agents which swell by absorbing water. They modify the consistency and frequency of stools. They are used for functional bowel disease associated with diarrhoea. They are safe substances but their effect occurs slowly.

Antimotility and Antisecretory Drugs

Antimotility drugs are opioid drugs. They increase small bowel smooth muscle tone and segmentation activity. They also reduce propulsive movements and decrease intestinal secretions while increasing absorption. They mediate these actions through μ receptors.

LOPERAMIDE

It has a direct action on intestinal musculature and having a weak anticholinergic property. It is **used** to treat acute and chronic diarrhoea. **Adverse effects** include addominal cramps and skin rash.

DIPHENOXYLATE

Chemically it is an opioid, related to pethidine. It is **used** in acute and chronic diarrhoea but since it crosses the blood brain barrier it can cause CNS effect similar to opioids. Atropine is added with diphenoxylate (LOMOFEN) to discourage abuse.

Loperamide and codeine are preferred to diphenoxylate in chronic diarrhoea, because they have less tendency to produce drug dependence. Long-term use of these drugs may aggravate irritable bowel syndrome. These drugs are used cautiously in attacks of colitis because there is increased risk of toxic megacolon. Also all these drugs should be used with caution in elderly because faecal impaction may occur leading to abdominal obstruction. These are usually not prescribed for bacterial diarrhoea in children because by delaying the passage of liquid faeces there is proliferation of pathogens which is undesirable.

SULFASALAZINE

It is an antisecretory drug. It is 5-aminosalicylic acid with linked sulfapyridine through azo bond. The drug is poorly absorbed from the intestine and the azo linkage is broken down by the bacterial flora in the distal ileum and colon to release 5-aminosalicylic acid (5-ASA) and sulfapyridine. 5-ASA inhibits locally prostaglandin synthesis, decreases mucosal secretion. It is **used** in rheumatoid arthritis and ulcerative colitis. **Side effects** include fever, rashes, blood dyscrasias, nausea, vomiting and headache.

MESALAZINE

5-ASA is prepared as delayed release preparation by coating with acrylic polymer, which releases 5-ASA in distal ileum and colon. It is **used** in ulcerative colitis to prevent relapses.

Olsalazine and **balsalazine** are the newer compounds of 5-aminosalicylic acid linked with azo bonds.

Antimicrobial Therapy

Antimicrobials have a limited role in treatment of diarrhoea because only a small percentage of diarrhoeas are caused by bacterial infection. Majority of cases are due to non infective causes, Rota virus and food poisoning in which antimicrobial therapy has no role.

Specific antimicrobial drugs are discussed in chapter 'Chemotherapeutic agents.'

❑❑❑

CHAPTER 7.2 Emetics & Antiemetic Agents

EMETICS

Vomiting or emesis occurs due to stimulation of **vomiting/emetic centre** in medulla oblongata. The **chemoreceptor trigger zone** (CTZ) and nucleus tractus solitarius (NTS) are relays for the afferent impulses arising from GIT, throat and other viscera. There are different drugs e.g. morphine, digitalis glycosides, apomorphine etc. which stimulate the CTZ. While certain agents e.g. chlorpromazine and certain antihistaminics depress it. Vomiting due to irritants in the GIT especially upper region does not involve CTZ and is mediated directly by the vomiting centre. Histamine (H_1), serotonin (5-HT_3), dopamine (D_2) cholinergic (M) and opioid (μ) receptors on CTZ and NTS are involved in inducing vomiting. Impulses from vestibular centre also lead to stimulation of vomiting centre via H_1 and M receptors.

The drugs that produce or evoke vomiting are known as emetics. The most common compounds used are apomorphine and ipecacuanha.

APOMORPHINE

It is a semisynthetic opioid and act as dopami-nergic agonist on the CTZ. It is given by subcuta-neous/IM route in the dose of 6 mg and it produces vomiting within 15 minutes. Apomorphine induced vomiting can be antagonized by chlorpromazine.

Side effects include tremors, restlessness and in toxic doses it may cause convulsions and respiratory depression.

IPECACUANHA

It is used as tincture and syrup containing alkaloid emetine obtained from plant *Cephaelis ipeca-cuanha*. It act on both gastric mucosa and CTZ.

The emetics are **used** mainly in poisoning when gastric lavage facilities are not available. But in certain poisoning e.g. kerosene poisoning, corrosive acid or alkali poisoning, emetics are contraindicated. They are also not advisable in unconscious patients as they may aspirate vomitus.

ANTIEMETICS

These are the drugs which are used to prevent vomiting. They are classified in table 7.2.1.

The detailed pharmacology of phenothiazines e.g. chlorpromazine, triflupro-

Table 7.2.1: *Classification of antiemetics.*

I. **Anticholinergics**	
Dicyclomine, hyoscine etc.	Details are given in chapter 'Anticholinergic agents'
II. **Antihistaminics**	
Promethazine	
Promethazine theoclate (AVOMINE)	
Diphenhydrinate	
Diphenhydramine	
Doxylamine succinate etc.	Details are given in chapter 'Antihistaminic agents'.
III. **Dopamine antagonists**	
Chlorpromazine	10-25 mg/day oral/IM
Triflupromazine	10 mg/day oral/IM
Prochlorperazine (STEMETIL)	5-10 mg/day oral/IM
Domperidone (DOMSTAL)	10-40 mg TDS
Metoclopramide (PERINORM)	10 mg TDS oral/IM
IV. **5-HT$_3$ antagonists**	
Ondansetron (EMSETRON)	Dose depends upon the patient's requirement and stage.
Granisetron (GRANICIP)	
V. **Prokinetic agents**	
Cisapride (CIZA)	10-20 mg TDS
Mosapride (MOZA)	2.5-10 mg BD-TDS
Itopride (ITZA)	150 mg TDS

mazine and is discussed in chapter 'Psychopharmacological agents'. Only remaining compounds used as antiemetics are discussed here.

Dopamine Antagonists

PROCHLORPERAZINE

It blocks dopaminergic neurotransmission in brain and exerts its action **by blocking dopamine receptors in brain**. It is used in nausea and vomiting.

Side effects include drowsiness, dry mouth, skin rash, insomnia and other cholinergic effects.

DOMPERIDONE

It causes antiemetic action **by blocking dopamine (D$_2$) receptors** and it also increases gastric motility. It is absorbed orally but bioavailability is 15% due to first pass metabolism. It is completely biotransformed and metabolites are excreted in urine. It is **used** in nausea and vomiting in postoperative period, drug induced, radiation, uraemia, hepatitis, peptic ulcer. It is also useful in reflex oesophagitis.

Side effects include galactorrhoea, skin rash and gynaecomastia.

METOCLOPRAMIDE

It is a centrally acting dopamine antagonist and acts on CTZ by blocking D_2 receptors thereby preventing emesis. It also acts peripherally in GIT to enhance ACh release from muscarinic receptors, leading to increased gastric peristalsis and relaxing the pylorus and first part of duodenum. Thus it increases gastric emptying. It also increases tone of lower esophageal sphincter and prevents gastroesophageal reflux.

It is absorbed orally, partly conjugated in liver and excreted in urine.

It is **used** as antiemetic, for gastroesophageal reflux disease, dyspepsia and as gastrokinetic.

Adverse effects include drowsiness, diarrhoea, facial spasm, trismus, oculogyric crisis seen commonly in children and young adults.

On prolonged use leads to tardive dyskinesia in elderly, gynaecomastia, galactorrhoea and parkinsonism.

5-HT^3 ANTAGONISTS

ONDANSETRON

It causes antiemetic effect by **blocking 5-HT_3 receptor in brain and periphery.**

Absorbed orally and bioavailability is 60-70% due to first pass metabolism. Metabolised by hydroxylation and metabolites are excreted in urine and faeces.

It is **used** in nausea and vomiting induced by cytotoxic chemotherapy and radiotherapy and for the prevention of postoperative vomiting.

Side effects include headache, constipation, dizziness and allergic reactions.

GRANISETRON

It is newer compound. Mechanism of action is similar to ondansetron but can cause elevation of liver enzyme level e.g. SGOT, SGPT etc. It is mainly used in the management of nausea and vomiting induced by cytotoxic chemotherapy and radiotherapy.

Dolasetron is a new compound of the similar category acting by blocking 5-HT_3 receptor.

PROKINETIC AGENTS

CISAPRIDE

It is a selective 5-HT_4 agonist. It restores and increases motility throughout gastrointestinal tract. **It appears to increase the release of acetylcholine from myenteric plexus of the gut**.

It is absorbed orally (bioavailability 33%) and is metabolised in liver.

Adverse effects include abdominal cramps, diarrhoea, headache, convulsions and extrapyramidal effects. When used with imidazole antifungals/macrolide antibiotics, it may lead to Q-T prolongation and ventricular arrhythmias.

It is **indicated** in non-ulcer dyspepsia and gastroesophageal reflux disease and not mainly used as antiemetic.

MOSAPRIDE

Mosapride is a **selective 5-HT_4 receptor agonist** which is free from the extrapyramidal and proarrhythmic effects. It stimulates the 5-HT_4 receptor in the presynaptic nerve endings in the myenteric plexus **promoting the release of acetylcholine at the neuromuscular junction**, strengthening tone and contractions of the gut wall, in particular the tone of the lower oesophageal sphincter.

Adverse effects include nausea and diarrhoea.

It is **indicated** in gastroesophageal reflux disease and functional dyspepsia, diabetic gastropathy.

Renzapride is also a selective 5-HT_4 receptor agonist.

ITOPRIDE

It is a novel prokinetic agent, it **inhibits dopamine D_2 receptors at the parasympathetic nerve endings and thereby increases the release of acetylcholine.** It decreases the metabolism of acetylcholine by inhibiting the enzyme acetylcholinesterase.

It is highly protein bound (approx. 96%), metabolised in the liver by N-oxidation to inactive metabolites by the enzyme flavin-containing monooxygenase. It is excreted mainly by the kidneys in the form of metabolites and as unchanged drug.

Adverse effects include rash, itching sensation, tremor, increase in SGOT, SGPT levels, diarrhoea, abdominal pain, gynecomastia etc.

It is **indicated** in upper abdominal digestive symptoms associated with chronic gastritis.

❑❑❑

CHAPTER 7.3

Antacids and Antiulcer Agents

ANTACIDS

Antacids are basic compounds that neutralise acid in gastric lumen, have no effect on gastric acid secretion. They are quantitatively compared in terms of their acid neutralizing capacity (ANC), which is defined as the quantity of 1 N HCl (in MEq) that can be brought to pH 3.5 in 15 minutes by a unit dose of antacid preparation. An ideal antacid should be potent in neutralizing acid, inexpensive, not absorbed from GIT and contain negligible amounts of sodium, should be sufficiently palatable to be readily tolerated with repeated dosage and should be free of side effects. An ideal antacid is yet to be developed.

Role of antacids:

1. Is primarily in pain relief.
2. Higher dose given continuously can promote ulcer healing.
3. Are superior to H_2 blockers in bleeding peptic ulcer.

SYSTEMIC ANTACIDS

Systemic antacids e.g. sodium carbonate is water soluble and potent neutralizer, but is not suitable for the treatment of peptic ulcer because of risk of ulcer perforation due to production of carbon dioxide in the stomach. Systemic absorption lead to alkalosis, may worsen edema and CHF because of increased Na^+ load.

NON-SYSTEMIC ANTACIDS

They are insoluble and poorly absorbed compounds.

MAGNESIUM SALTS

Magnesium carbonate is most water soluble and reacts with hydrochloric acid at a slow rate. Magnesium hydroxide has low water solubility. It reacts with hydrochloric acid promptly. Magnesium trisilicate has low solubility and has the power to adsorb and inactivate pepsin and to protect the ulcer base.

ALUMINIUM HYDROXIDE

It is weak and slow reacting antacid. The aluminium ion relaxes smooth muscles, thus delays gastric emptying and causes constipation. It can also adsorb pepsin at pH > 3 but releases it at lower pH. It also prevents phosphate absorption.

MAGALDRATE

It is hydrated complex of hydroxy magnesium aluminate. It initially reacts with acid and releases $Al(OH)_3$ which then reacts more slowly. It is a good antacid, with prompt and sustained neutralizing action.

CALCIUM CARBONATE

It is a potent antacid with rapid acid neutralizing capacity, but on long term use, it can cause hypercalcemia, hypercalciuria and formation of calcium stones in the kidney.

Every single compound among the antacids have some serious side effects especially when used for longer period or used in elderly patients. To avoid these, the antacids combinations are used such as:

i. Magnesium salts produce laxative action while aluminium salts are constipating in nature, so combination of these two counteract their effect and are used commonly.
ii. Fast acting antacid e.g. magnesium hydroxide and slow acting antacid e.g. aluminium hydroxide are used together for sustained action.
iii. For reducing the systemic toxicity of individual compounds.

ANTIULCER AGENTS

PATHOGENESIS OF PEPTIC ULCERS

Peptic ulcers are chronic, most often solitary lesions that occur in any part of GIT exposed to the aggressive action of acid-peptic juices.

Duodenal ulcer patients have an increased capacity to secrete acid and pepsin, increased responsiveness to stimuli of acid secretion and more rapid gastric emptying.

Gastric ulcer patients have a low to normal levels of gastric acid, but never true achlorhydria. Some primary defect in gastric mucosal resistance is seen and also an increased tendency to back diffusion of H^+ ion. Other influences are thought to be decreased production of bicarbonate buffer, decreased blood flow which permits acid ions to accumulate.

The various drugs used in peptic ulcer are classified as in table 7.3.1.

H_2 RECEPTOR ANTAGONISTS

The H_2 antagonists in clinical use are analogs of histamine that competitively inhibit the interaction of histamine with H_2 receptors and are highly selective. They inhibit gastric acid secretion elicited by histamine and other H_2 agonists in a dose dependent manner. H_2 antagonists inhibit gastric acid secretion by food and fundic distension and also inhibit fasting and nocturnal acid secretion and they reduce both the volume and H^+ ion concentration of gastric juice.

Pharmacokinetics

The H_2 antagonists are well absorbed orally (60-80%) and its absorption is not affected with the presence of food in the stomach. They cross the placental barrier and secreted mostly in mother's milk. They are excreted in urine mostly in unchanged form.

Adverse Reactions

They produces headache, dizziness, dry mouth, rashes. CNS effects include restlessness, delirium, hallucinations, convulsion and coma. Intravenous bolus injection cause bradycardia, arrhythmia and

Table 7.3.1: *Classification of drugs used in peptic ulcer.*

I. **Drugs which reduce gastric acid secretion**	
i. ***H_2-receptor antagonists***	
Cimetidine (CIMETIN)	200-400 mg TDS-QID, 400 mg HS, 200-400 mg/day IM/IV
Ranitidine (HISTAC)	150 mg BD/HS, 50-100 mg/day IM/IV
Famotidine (FACID)	40 mg HS, 20 mg BD
Roxatidine (ZORPEX)	75-150 mg HS
Also available Nizatidine, Loxatidine.	
ii. ***Proton pump inhibitor***	
Omeprazole (OMIZAC)	20-60 mg OD
Pantoprazole (PANTOCID)	40 mg OD
Rabeprazole (VELOZ)	20 mg OD
Also available Esomeprazole, Lansoprazole	
iii. ***Prostaglandin analogues***	
Misoprostol (CYTOTEC)	200 μg QID
Enprostil	35-140 μg/day
Also available Rioprostil, Arbaprostil, Trimoprostil.	
II. **Ulcer healing agents**	
Carbenoxolone sodium (GASTRIULCER)	100 mg TDS
III. **Ulcer protective agents**	
Sucralfate (SUCRASE)	1 g one hr before each (3) meals and at bed time
IV. **Antacids (Neutralize gastric acid)**	
Systemic antacids	
Sodium bicarbonate	0.3-1.5 g TDS-QID
Nonsystemic antacids	
Magnesium carbonate	0.5-2 g/day
Magnesium hydroxide (MILK OF MAGNESIA)	0.3-1 g/day
Magnesium trisilicate	0.5-1 g/day
Aluminium hydroxide gel (ALUDROX)	0.5-1 g/day
Magaldrate (STACID)	400-800 mg/day
Calcium carbonate	0.5-1 g/day

cardiac arrest due to histamine release. The cimetidine has antiandrogenic action and can cause gynaecomastia, loss of libido and impotence, otherwise all other H_2 blockers are devoid of these side effects.

Therapeutic Uses

H_2 blockers are used in the treatment of:

- Duodenal ulcer.
- Gastric ulcer.
- Zollinger-Ellison syndrome (ZES).
- Gastroesophageal reflux.
- NSAID's induced ulcers.
- Prophylaxis of aspiration pneumonia.

CIMETIDINE

Low potency, short duration of action. Oral bioavailability is 60% and 2/3 is excreted unchanged in urine and bile. Incidence of adverse effects is 5%.

It has poor CNS entry but in elderly and in patients with impaired renal functions, CNS symptoms may occur. It displaces dihydrotestosterone from cytoplasmic receptors (antiandrogenic action) and inhibits estradiol degradation by liver. High doses given for longer periods produce gynaecomastia, decreased libido and impotence. It inhibits cytochrome P450 catalyzed hydroxylation of estradiol in men, also slowing metabolism of many drugs and concurrent administration of cimetidine will prolong the half life of many drugs (warfarin, phenytoin, theophylline, phenobarbital, benzodiazepines, propranolol, nifedipine, digitoxin, quinidine, mexiletine, tricyclic antidepressants).

RANITIDINE

5 to 8 times more potent than cimetidine. Produces higher suppression of gastric acid and action lasts longer than cimetidine. No clinically significant drug interaction and side effects are seen.

FAMOTIDINE

On a weight basis 20 times more potent than cimetidine and 7.5 times more potent than ranitidine in inhibiting basal and pentagastrin stimulated gastric acid secretion. It is a competitive-noncompetitive inhibitor of H_2 receptors. It has a longer duration of action. Oral bioavailability is 40-50% and is excreted unchanged (70%) in urine. Incidence of adverse effects is low.

It is more **useful** in ZE syndrome and prophylaxis of aspiration pneumonia.

ROXATIDINE

Roxatidine inhibit H_2 induced gastric secretion with a potency greater than cimetidine and in the same range as ranitidine. Its acetate salt is more than 95% absorbed after oral administration and rapidly converted to roxatidine by esterases in small intestine and liver. Plasma t½ is 6 hours. Peak plasma levels occur about 8 hours after dosing. Effects of the drug persist for about 12 hours.

It has **use** in prophylaxis of acid aspiration syndrome after induction of anaesthesia. In a dose of 150 mg HS as premedication affords reliable protection against the consequences of acid aspiration until 11 AM the next day and decreases the danger of aspiration by reducing the high volumes of gastric juice.

PROTON PUMP INHIBITOR

OMEPRAZOLE

Omeprazole is gastric proton pump inhibitor which reduces gastric acid secretion. It **inhibits the enzyme H^+K^+ATPase** in the parietal cells of gastric mucosa. It effectively inhibits both basal and stimulated acid secretion irrespective of the stimulus. It has quick onset of action and effective control of gastric acid secretion is achieved with once daily dosing. It has no effect on pepsin, intrinsic factor, juice volume and gastric motility. Proton pump inhibitors do not exhibit anticholinergic or H_2 receptor antagonistic properties.

Omeprazole distributes widely and is rapidly eliminated from plasma by metabolism in liver. The antisecretory effect persists for much longer as it strongly binds to $H^+ K^+$ ATPase. The disposition is not altered in patients with renal disease or in those undergoing haemodialysis. Increased age and liver disease delays plasma clearance of the drug but this does not necessitate dosage adjustment in these patients.

It is indicated in:

- Treatment of duodenal ulcer.
- Treatment of gastric ulcer.
- Treatment of reflux oesophagitis.
- For control of acid secretion in patients of Zollinger-Ellison syndrome.

It is well tolerated. Nausea, headache, diarrhoea, constipation and flatulence have been reported occasionally, Rarely skin rash has occurred in few patients.

RABEPRAZOLE

Rabeprazole belongs to substituted benzimidazole proton-pump inhibitors. In gastric parietal cells, **rabeprazole is protonated, accumulates and is transformed to an active sulfenamide**.

Following oral administration of 20 mg, rabeprazole is absorbed and can be detected in plasma by one hour. Rabeprazole is 96.3% bound to plasma proteins.

Rabeprazole is extensively metabolized. The thioether and sulfone are the primary inactive metabolites. 90% of the drug is eliminated in the urine, primarily as thioether carboxylic acid, its glucuronide and mercapturic acid metabolites.

It is **indicated** in erosive and ulcerative gastroesophageal reflux disease, healing of duodenal ulcers and Zollinger Ellison syndrome.

Adverse effects include nausea, diarrhoea, skin eruptions, headache and dizziness.

Other proton pump inhibitors e.g., **lansoprazole** is more potent than omeprazole and has higher bioavailability, rapid onset of action and longer duration of action. **Pantoprazole** is the new H^+K^+ATPase inhibitor with similar properties and action to omeprazole.

PROSTAGLANDIN ANALOGUES

PGE_2 and PGI_2 are the main prostaglandins synthesized by gastric mucosa. They decrease acid secretion and improve mucosal defense mechanism by:

- Stimulation of synthesis and release of mucus.
- Enhance bicarbonate production.
- Enhancement of tight junctions of cell membrane architecture.
- Inhibit gastrin production.
- Stimulation of a number of cellular transport processes.
- Stimulation of DNA content in damaged gastric mucosa by a process termed as cytoprotection.

The important use of prostaglandin analogues is in the arthritic patients who are on chronic use of NSAID's and are not responding to H_2 receptor antagonists.

MISOPROSTOL

200 μg QID was of similar efficacy to cimetidine 300 mg TDS in healing duodenal and gastric ulcer. Pain relief occurred more slowly than with cimetidine. Shown to heal erosions, ulcers due to NSAIDs.

ENPROSTIL

35-140 μg day heal duodenal and gastric ulcer but are less effective than H_2 receptor antagonists.

ULCER HEALING DRUGS

CARBENOXOLONE SODIUM

It is a steroid like triterpenoid synthetic derivative of glycyrrhizic acid (obtained from liquorice) and has been found to be effective in healing both gastric and duodenal ulcer without affecting volume or acidity of gastric juice.

It **acts by increasing mucus production, slowing turnover of gastric cells and increasing regeneration of cells around ulcer**. It also enhances pyloric tone preventing bile reflux. It retards PG's degradation in gastric mucosa. Its mineralocorticoid side effects lead to Na^+ and water retention and K^+ loss preclude its use on large scale.

ULCER PROTECTIVE AGENTS

SUCRALFATE

It is a basic aluminium salt of sucrose octasulfate. It polymerizes at pH < 4 to form a sticky, viscid yellow white gel which adheres to ulcer base. The gel **acts as a strong mechanical barrier** because of a strong electrostatic interaction of the drug with proteins at ulcer site. It also **binds to basic fibroblast growth factor preventing its degradation and thereby promotes healing**. It also protects from intracellular enzymes released from damaged cells. It also helps in formation of new blood vessels (angiogenesis) and helps in cell division (mitogenic). Sucralfate also **inhibits release of cytokines (immunomodulator)**. It also has antibacterial activity.

It precipitates surface proteins at ulcer base and act as a physical barrier, preventing acid, pepsin and bile from coming in contact with ulcer base. It also augments gastric mucosal PG synthesis thereby enhancing protective action. It has no acid neutralizing action.

It promotes healing of both gastric and duodenal ulcers and also prevents ulcer recurrence.

Topical sucralfate (4-10%) is also useful in management of decubitus ulcer, diabetic ulcers, chemical and thermal burns, radiation induced skin damage, vaginal ulceration, oral and genital ulceration.

Side effects include dry mouth, constipation, nausea, vomiting, rash, pruritus, dizziness. It adsorbs and interferes with absorption of tetracycline, cimetidine, digoxin and phenytoin.

❑❑❑

Section 8

Drugs Acting on Endocrine System

CHAPTER 8.1

Anterior Pituitary Hormones

The pituitary gland is situated in *sella turcica* or *hypophyseal fossa* of the sphenoid bone attached to the brain by a stalk which is continuous with the part of brain i.e. hypothalamus and there is a communication between the hypothalamus and the pituitary gland by means of nerve fibres and a complex of blood vessels. Pituitary gland consists of three parts – anterior lobe or *adenohypophysis*, posterior lobe or *neurohypophysis* and middle lobe or *pars intermedia*.

The anterior lobe secretes various trophic hormones, the posterior lobe is responsible for the secretion of oxytocin and antidiuretic hormone (vasopressin) and middle lobe secretes melanocyte-stimulating hormone (MSH) which may affect the synthesis of melanin.

ANTERIOR PITUITARY HORMONES

Anterior lobe of pituitary is the master gland of the endocrine system as a whole because it produces peptide trophic hormones which affect the other ductless/endocrine glands. The anterior lobe secretes the following hormones:

1. Growth hormone or somatotrophic hormone (GH & STH).
2. Thyroid stimulating hormone (TSH) or thyrotrophic hormone.
3. Adrenocorticotrophic hormone (ACTH).
4. Follicle stimulating hormone (FSH).
5. Luteinising hormone (LH) or interstitial cell stimulating hormone (ICSH).
6. Lactogenic hormone or prolactin.

GROWTH HORMONE

It is secreted by acidophil cells. Human growth hormone has a single straight chain polypeptide structure containing two intramolecular disulphide bridges and is composed of 188 amino acids.

It stimulates growth directly and in conjunction with other hormones. It stimulates the multiplication of the cells of epiphyseal cartilage and thus increases the length of the cartilage bone. After administration, there is an increased body growth due to its direct effect on the tissues. It stimulates the growth of muscles. It also increases the secretion of milk during lactation.

Growth hormone promotes protein metabolism. It increases nucleic acid and protein synthesis, decreases nitrogen excretion in the urine. It diminishes the amino acid content of the plasma by transferring it into the tissues and helps in the growth of tissue. In fat metabolism, it causes mobilisation of peripheral fat depot to the liver. In carbohydrate metabolism, its primary effect is to stimulate its storage. Administration of growth hormone produces hyperglycemia and glycosuria. In mineral metabolism, it increases intestinal absorption of calcium as well as its secretion.

The secretion of growth hormone by acidophil cells is ***regulated by*** the hypothalamic hormone, the growth hormone-releasing factor (GHRF). GHRF levels in the hypothalamus are reduced by corticosteroids and increased by thyroxine. Certain stimuli which can increase growth hormone secretion are insulin-induced hypoglycemia, fasting, physical exercise, amino acid administration. Stress and sleep also stimulate growth hormone release. Various hormones i.e., thyroxine and ACTH also stimulate growth.

Hyposecretion of pituitary **during childhood** leads to *'dwarfism'* which is of two type, Lorain type and Frohlich's type and is characterized by stunted growth of the skeleton with resultant 'dwarfism.'

Hyposecretion during adult life leads to ***'Simmond's disease'*** and is characterized by dry and wrinkled skin, grey hair and there is a atrophy of the sexual organs and cessation of menstrual cycle in the female.

Hypersecretion during childhood leads to ***'gigantism'*** and is characterized by excessive skeletal growth.

Hypersecretion during adult life leads to ***'acromegaly'*** and is characterized by excessive growth of facial bones, hands become large and spade like, thickening of facial and hand's skin etc.

Clinical Preparations

Human growth hormone is produced by recombinant DNA technique. The preparation available are:

Sometrem (PROTROPIN)	5 mg (13 IU) inj.
Somatropin (GENOTROPIN)	(12 & 16 IU per vial inj. and 1 mg contains 2.6 IU)

The main **use** of growth hormone is in the treatment of dwarfism.

Side effects include allergic reaction, pain at the site of injection, hypothyroidism and glucose intolerance. Water retention may also occur.

SOMATOSTATIN

It is a peptide containing 14 amino acids and inhibits the release of growth hormone, TSH and prolactin from the pituitary and insulin and glucagon in pancreas. It has a very short plasma half-life. Because of its shorter duration of action and lack of specificity in inhibiting only GH secretion, its use in the treatment of acromegaly is limited.

Another newer synthetic compound, ***octerotride*** is a longer acting analogue of somatostatin and is used in acromegaly.

THYROID STIMULATING HORMONE

This hormone controls the growth and activity of the thyroid gland. It influences the uptake of iodine, synthesis of thyroxine (T_4) and triiodothyronine (T_3) by the thyroid gland and their release into the blood stream.

Details are discussed in chapter 'Thyroid & antithyroid agents'.

ADRENOCORTICOTROPHIC HORMONE (ACTH)

It is a polypeptide of 39 amino acid residues of molecular weight approximately 4,500. It is secreted by basophil cells under the control of CRF (corticotropin releasing factor) from the hypothalamus. ACTH controls the growth of adrenal cortex and the synthesis of corticosteroids and is essential to life. The action of ACTH on adrenal cortex is mediated through cyclic AMP.

This hormone stimulates the cortex of adrenal gland to produce its hormones. The amount of ACTH secreted depends upon the concentration in the blood of the hormones from the adrenal cortex and on stimulation by hypothalamus.

The cortex of adrenal gland produces three types of hormones – the glucocorticoids, mineralocorticoids and the sex hormones.

Glucocorticoids

The secretion is stimulated by ACTH from the anterior lobe of pituitary gland. Cortisone and hydrocortisone are the main glucocorticoids and their main function is to regulate carbohydrate metabolism.

Mineralocorticoids

It is associated with the maintenance of the electrolyte balance in the body. Aldosterone is the main mineralocorticoid which stimulates the reabsorption of sodium by the renal tubules and when the amount of sodium reabsorbed is increased the amount of potassium excreted is increased. Angiotensin (vasopressor agent) produced by the renin (from kidneys) stimulates the secretion of aldosterone.

Sex Hormones

The secretion of estrogens in females and androgens in males by the adrenal cortex is controlled by ACTH. They are responsible for the development and maintenance of secondary sexual characters in both males and females. They also increase the deposition of protein in muscles and reduce the excretion of nitrogen in males.

Hyposecretion of hormones from the adrenal cortex leads to development of '*Addison's disease*' which is characterized by loss of appetite, muscular weakness, loss of weight due to loss of water, hypoglycemia, subnormal body temperature, decreased basal metabolic rate, increased blood potassium, decreased blood sodium and inability to maintain the normal protein deposition in the muscles.

Hypersecretion from the adrenal cortex leads to condition known as '*Cushing's syndrome*' which leads to '*feminism*' in males, which is the tendency to develop female sex characters and in females '*virilism*' develops, which is the tendency to develop male sex characters such as excess growth of hair on chest and pubic region, increase and darkening of facial hair, atrophy of mammary glands (breasts) and cessation of menstrual cycle (amenorrhoea).

ACTH is available as lyophilized powder which on reconstitution gives 40 IU/ml solution and is used mainly for the diagnosis of pituitary adrenal axis disorders.

GONADOTROPHIC HORMONES (GTH) OR GONADOTROPHINS

The basophil cells secrete gonadotrophins which control the growth and activity of the gonads and indirectly other processes connected with it. There are two gonadotrophins:

- Follicle stimulating hormone (FSH),
- Luteinising hormone (LH) or interstitial cell stimulating hormone (ICSH).

Both of them are glycoprotein in nature.

FSH

In females, the target organs are the ovaries where it increases the number and size (maturation, development and ripening) of Graafian follicles and prepare them for ovulation. During its development, the ovarian follicles secrete its own hormone estrogen. In males, it stimulates spermatogenesis. Under the influence of this hormone, seminiferous tubules produce spermatozoa.

LH

In females, it is responsible for:

- Complete development of the ovarian follicles to secretory stage and secretion of estrogen.
- Promotes the final maturation of ovarian follicles and ovulation and the formation of corpus luteum which secretes progesterone.

In males, the same hormone under the name of ICSH stimulates the development and functional activity of interstitial cells and ultimately the production of testicular androgen, testosterone.

Gonadotrophin secretion is under the control of hypothalamus and sex hormones. The hypothalamic nuclei secrete a specific releasing factor for the release of both FSH & LH.

This single releasing factor is a decapeptide and is designated as GnRH or gonadorelin. Frequency and amplitude of GnRH release pulses determine whether LH or FSH or both will be secreted as well the amount of each. Gonadal hormones from ovary and testis regulate the FSH and LH secretion by direct action on pituitary as well as through hypothalamus.

Gonadotrophins are **used** in the treatment of amenorrhoea, infertility, cryptorchidism and hypogonadotrophic hypogonadism in males. It is also useful in *in vitro* fertilization.

There are two types of gonadotrophins available:

- Obtained from urine of pregnant women, **chorionic gonadotrophin** as 1,000-10,000 IU (powder form, can be used after reconstitution by parenteral route).
- Obtained from urine of menopausal women, **menotrophin** (combination of FSH 75 to 150 IU and LH 75 to 150 IU).

Preparations of gonadotrophins have been used to treat infertility for the last several years.

MENOTROPHIN

Purified extract of human post-menopausal urine containing follicle stimulating hormone (FSH) and luteinising hormone (LH) is known as human menopausal gonadotrophin. The relative *in vivo* activity is designated as a ratio, the 1:1 ratio is also known as menotrophin.

Adverse reactions include polycystic ovary, edema, pain in lower abdomen and allergic reactions.

It is **used** in amenorrhoea and infertility, hypogonadism in males and females, follicle stimulation in IVH and cryptorchidism.

NAFARELIN ACETATE

It is potent analogue (200 times more potent) of gonadotrophin releasing hormones (GnRH).

It is rapidly absorbed into the systemic circulation following intranasal delivery. It **stimulates the release of LH and FSH from the anterior pituitary** resulting in a temporary increase of ovarian steroidogenesis. After 2 to 3 days of daily administration, the pituitary becomes refractory to further stimulation. LH/FSH release is inhibited within 10 days and is followed by a decrease in secretion of gonadal steroids within 2 to 6 weeks.

After intranasal administration maximum serum concentration are achieved within 10 to 45 minutes. It is 80% bound to plasma proteins.

Adverse effects include hot flushes, change in libido, vaginal dryness, headache. Incidents of emotional lability and depression are higher in infertile patients. Nasal mucosal irritation, migraine may also occur. Naferelin therapy for six to nine months may lead to three to five percent bone loss.

It is **indicated** in endometriosis, precocious puberty.

In infertile women choosing *in vitro* fertilization, naferelin in combination with gonadotrophins can be used for stimulating ovulation. It is also useful in management of uterine leiomyoma, benign prostatic hypertrophy, hirsutism and polycystic ovarian syndrome.

PROLACTIN OR LACTOGENIC HORMONE

It is a single chain peptide hormone, isolated in pure form and contains tyrosine, tryptophan, cystine, arginine, methionine of approximately 25,000 molecular weight. It has a direct effect upon the breasts immediately after the delivery of baby and in conjunction with other hormones, it stimulates the breast to secrete milk.

It also stimulates the proliferation of the glandular elements of the mammary glands during pregnancy and helps in complete development of breasts.

Prolactin secretion is under the inhibitory control of hypothalamus through prolactin inhibiting hormone (PRIH) which is a dopamine and acts on pituitary lactotrope D_2 receptor.

BROMOCRIPTINE (Bromoergocriptine)

It is a semisynthetic ergot alkaloid and dopamine receptor agonist.

It acts on pituitary lactotrophic cells to

inhibit the synthesis and release of prolactin by agonist action on dopaminergic receptors.

Adverse effects are nausea, vomiting, postural hypotension, behavioral alterations, mental confusion, psychosis.

It is **used** in hyperprolactinemia and for suppression of lactation and breast engorgement. It is also useful in parkinsonism because it has levodopa like actions and in the treatment of acromegaly. **Dose:** PROCTINAL 1.25 mg BD.

POSTERIOR LOBE OF PITUITARY GLAND

The posterior lobe secretes two hormone namely oxytocin and antidiuretic hormone (ADH or vasopressin).

ADH OR VASOPRESSIN

Discussed in detail in chapter 'Diuretics and antidiuretics'.

UTERINE STIMULANTS (OXYTOCICS, ABORTIFACIENTS)

OXYTOCIN

Oxytocin is an octapeptide synthesized in hypothalamus and transported down the axons into the posterior lobe of pituitary.

It promotes contraction of the uterine muscle. It also causes contraction of the myoepithelial cells of the lactating breast and squeezing milk into the large ducts situated behind the nipple of the mammary gland.

Oxytocin takes part in the onset of parturition, expulsion of the foetus and placenta. It also facilitates the transport of sperm in the female genital tract.

Oxytocin is **used** in induction of labour, in postpartum haemorrhage, abortion and in breast engorgement. It is used by IM/IV route (PITOCIN, 2-5 IU/ml inj).

ERGOMETRINE

It increase force, frequency and duration of uterine contractions. It is used to control and prevent postpartum haemorrhage. It is also used to prevent uterine atony after cesarean or instrumental delivery.

PROSTAGLANDINS

PGE_2, $PGF_{2\alpha}$ and 15-methyl $PGF_{2\alpha}$ are potent uterine stimulant (Other details are given in chapter 5.3).

❑❑❑

CHAPTER 8.2 Antidiabetic Agents

Diabetes mellitus (DM) is a chronic disorder characterized by altered metabolism of carbohydrates, proteins and fats. Epidemiological survey conducted in several developing countries show that prevalence rates of diabetes mellitus vary from two to four percent in different population groups. Roughly two percent of the world population suffers from diabetes mellitus.

Types of Diabetes Mellitus

- Insulin dependent or type I diabetes (IDDM). Formerly called juvenile onset, or ketone prone diabetes. It is an autoimmune disease of pancreatic β-cells. Arises due to insulin insufficiency.
- Non-insulin dependent or type II diabetes (NIDDM). Formerly called non ketotic or maturity onset diabetes. It arises due to insulin resistance in peripheral tissues.

INSULIN

Insulin (MW 5,800) a polypeptide hormone secreted from β-cells of islets of Langerhans in pancreas was discovered by Banting and Best in 1921. It was purified and crystallized by Abel and it's amino acid sequence was established by Sanger in 1960. It's formed from proteolysis of proinsulin to give rise to two peptide chains (A with 21 amino acid residues and B with 30) which are interconnected by disulphide bond.

Mechanism of Insulin Action

Insulin acts by binding to insulin receptors on cell membrane. The insulin receptor complex is internalized. By phosphorylation and dephosphorylation reactions there is stimulation or inhibition of enzymes involved in metabolic actions of insulin. Second messengers like phosphatidyl inositol glycan and DAG also mediate the action of insulin on metabolic enzymes.

Normally, insulin stimulates storage of glucose in liver as glycogen and in adipose tissues as triglycerides and storage of amino acids in muscle as protein. It also promotes utilization of glucose in muscle for energy. Insulin inhibits the breakdown of triglycerides, glycogen, and protein and conversion of amino acids to glucose (gluconeogenesis). Conversion of amino acids to glucose and glucose to fatty acids occur mainly in liver.

Table 8.2.1: *Classification of insulin preparations.*

I.	**Conventional preparations**	
	Regular (soluble) insulin (HUMINSULIN-R)	40, 80 IU/ml; SC/IV
	Insulin zinc suspension 'prompt' (Semilente)	40, 80 IU/ml; SC
	Insulin zinc suspension (Lente insulin; HUMINSULIN-L)	40-80 IU/ml; SC
	Isophane or Neutral Protamine Hagedorn (NPH) insulin (HUMINSULIN-N)	40 IU/ml; SC
	Globin zinc insulin	40 IU/ml; SC
	Insulin zinc suspension 'extended' (Ultralente; HUMINSULIN-U)	40 IU/ml; SC
	Protamine zinc insulin (PZI)	40 IU/ml; SC
II.	**Newer purified insulin preparations**	
i.	Regular-ILETIN (Purified by gel filtration)	
ii.	Regular-ILETIN-II (Purified by gel filtration and ion exchange chromatography)	
iii.	Single peak insulins (Purified by gel filtration and then recrystallization)	
	Pork regular insulin (ACTRAPID)	40 U/ml
	Pork lente insulin (LENTARD)	40 U/ml
	Pork regular and isophane insulin (in a ratio of 30:70; RAPIMIX)	40 U/ml
iv.	Monocomponent insulin (Purified by gel filtration and then by ion exchange chromatography; ACTRAPID MC and MONOTRAD MC)	40 U/ml
III.	**Biosynthetic human insulins (by recombinant DNA technique)**	
	Human soluble insulin (HUMAN ACTRAPHANE)	40 U/ml
	Human regular insulin (HUMAN ACTRAPID)	40 & 100 U/ml
	Human lente insulin (HUMAN MONOTRAD)	40 & 100 U/ml

In diabetes mellitus, there is either insulin deficiency or insulin resistance in peripheral tissues which lead to hyperglycemia and glycosuria. Insulin corrects the various abnormalities of carbohydrate metabolism by its action on various tissues.

Pharmacokinetics

Insulin is not given orally. After IV or SC injection, it circulates as free, monomer in blood and has a short plasma half life. Insulin is degraded mainly in liver, muscle and kidney.

Adverse Reactions

The most frequent and serious adverse reaction is hypoglycemia. It can occur in any diabetic patient due to heavy dose of insulin, failure to eat or missing a meal, performing extensive exercise or by consuming alcohol. The hypoglycemia caused by insulin is characterized by neuroglucopenic symptoms that include confusion, dizziness, behavioural changes, visual disturbances, fatigue, muscle incoordination and may be fall in blood pressure.

The other side effects include insulin allergy which consists of local itching, swelling, redness at the site of injection. Urticaria and anaphylactic reactions are rarely seen. Other rare side effects include insulin lipodystrophy (atrophy at the site of injection), insulin neuropathy and weight gain (obesity).

Therapeutic Uses

Insulin is used in:

- Insulin dependent diabetes mellitus (IDDM).
- Diabetic ketoacidosis or diabetic coma.

HUMINSULIN

Huminsulin 30/70 [biphasic isophane insulin injection (30% soluble insulin and 70% isophane insulin)] is a mixture of soluble human insulin injection, a short acting blood glucose lowering agent and isophane insulin human suspension, an intermediate acting blood glucose lowering agent.

Adverse Effects

Local allergy: Patients occasionally experience redness, swelling, and itching at the site of injection of insulin.

Systemic allergy: Less common, but potentially more serious, is generalized allergy to insulin, which may cause rash over the whole body, shortness of breath, wheezing, reduction in blood pressure, fast pulse, or sweating. Severe cases may be life threatening.

ORAL ANTIDIABETIC AGENTS

These are the agents which are effective orally and lower the elevated blood glucose levels. They are classified as in table 8.2.2.

SULFONYLUREAS

These drugs **stimulate insulin secretion from pancreatic β-cells** (so called 'sulfonylurea receptors') which cause depolarisation by reducing conductance of

Table 8.2.2: *Classification of oral antidiabetic agents.*

I. **Sulfonylureas**	
i. ***First generation***	
Tolbutamide (RASTINON)	0.5-2 g/day
Chlorpropamide (COPAMIDE)	100-500 mg/day
Tolazamide	0.125-1.0 g/day
ii. ***Second generation***	
Glibenclamide (BETANASE)	5-20 mg/day
Glipizide (DIBIZIDE)	5-20 mg/day
Gliclazide (GLIZID)	160-320 mg BD
Glimepiride (GLIMER)	1-6 mg OD
II. **Biguanides**	
Metformin (GLYCOMET)	250 mg to 3.0 g/day
III. **Meglitinides**	
Repaglinide (RAPILIN)	0.25-4 mg/day
Nateglinide (GLINATE)	60 mg/day
IV. **Thiazolidinediones**	
Rosiglitazone (ENSELIN)	4-8 mg OD-BD
Pioglitazone (GLIZONE)	15-45 mg OD
V. **α-Glucosidase inhibitors**	
Acarbose (GLUBOSE)	50-200 mg TDS

ATP sensitive K^+ channels. They lower down the blood sugar level in type II diabetics and non-diabetic individuals. They also decrease the elevated plasma free fatty acid levels. They also sensitize the target tissues to action of insulin by increasing the number of insulin receptors.

Sulfonylureas inhibit neoglucogenesis and glycogenolysis. Sulfonylureas are rapidly absorbed from the gastrointestinal tract after oral administration and are more than 90 percent bound to plasma proteins and excreted unchanged in urine.

CHLORPROPAMIDE

After oral administration, it is rapidly absorbed and has long plasma half life and excreted by kidney slowly.

Adverse effects include nausea, vomiting, cholestatic jaundice, skin rash, anaemia, leucopenia, hypoglycemia and intolerance to alcohol (disulfiram like reaction).

It is **indicated** in the treatment of maturity onset non ketotic diabetes mellitus unresponsive to diet and neurogenic diabetes insipidus.

TOLBUTAMIDE

It is a short acting, less potent oral hypoglycemic agent and after administration it is readily metabolized in liver.

Adverse effects include, nausea, vomiting, skin rash and epigastric distress. It is mainly **used** in maturity onset diabetes mellitus.

GLIBENCLAMIDE

Glibenclamide is a second generation sulfonylurea. There are two mechanisms of action for the lowering of the blood glucose:

1. The **pancreatic effect**, in the case of failure of β-cell function together with an existing but inadequate insulin secretion, gives rise to an intensified insulin secretion as a result of a greater response of the β-cells to glucose.
2. The **extrapancreatic effect,** in the case of resistance to insulin due to a reduced sensitivity of the peripheral tissue to insulin, there is intensification of the insulin effect as a result of:

Adverse reactions include visual disturbances (transient, at the beginning of therapy), nausea and epigastric bloating (rare) and diarrhoea. Hypersensitivity including allergic skin reactions, thrombocytopenia, leucopenia, agranulocytosis, haemolytic anaemia, vasculitis, cholestatic jaundice and hepatitis.

It is **indicated** in non-insulin dependent diabetes mellitus (type II, maturityonset diabetes) whenever treatment by diet alone proves to be inadequate.

GLIPIZIDE

It is an oral blood glucose lowering drug of sulfonylurea class.

It is fast acting and post prandial insulinemic action persists even after prolonged use.

Glipizide is completely and rapidly absorbed ensuring prompt and constant activity.

It is **indicated** in management of type II diabetes where diet control alone is not effective in controlling the hyperglycemia.

Adverse effects include hypoglycemia, GIT disturbances, allergic reactions include urticaria and erythema.

GLICLAZIDE

Gliclazide **reduces blood glucose levels by correcting both defective insulin secretion and peripheral insulin resistance**. Gliclazide also has been reported to reduce plasma cholesterol and triglyceride levels after repeated administration.

Adverse effects include nausea, diarrhoea, gastric pain, vomiting, skin rash, pruritus, flushing, erythema, headache and dizziness with low incidence of hypoglycemia.

It is **indicated** in non-insulin dependent diabetes mellitus, diabetes with or without obesity in adults, diabetes in the elderly and diabetes with vascular complications.

GLIMEPIRIDE

It is a very potent sulfonylurea with long duration of action **indicated** in non-insulin dependent (type II) diabetes, whenever blood sugar levels can not be controlled adequately by diet, physical exercise or reduction in body weight.

Adverse effects include hypoglycemia, temporary visual impairment, gastrointestinal disturbances. Rarely leucopenia, haemolytic anaemia. Occasionally allergic or pseudoallergic reactions like itching, urticaria or rashes. In isolated cases allergic vasculitis, photosensitivity or a decrease in serum sodium may occur.

BIGUANIDES

They lower the blood sugar levels in all types of diabetes mellitus but like sulfonylureas they do not lower the blood sugar level in normal individuals. They **act by increasing peripheral anaerobic glycolysis** (stimulate peripheral utilization of glucose), **inhibit absorption of carbohydrates in gut and suppresses hepatic gluconeogenesis**.

Metformin improves glucose tolerance in NIDDM subjects by lowering both basal and postprandial plasma glucose. Metformin decreases hepatic glucose production, decreases intestinal absorption of glucose and improves insulin sensitivity (increases peripheral glucose uptake and utilization).

They are rapidly absorbed from gastrointestinal tract and show adequate plasma levels and excreted unchanged in urine.

Adverse effects include anorexia, nausea, bitter or metallic taste in mouth, abdominal discomfort, tolerance and lactic acidosis which is the most serious complication and more common with phenformin.

They are **indicated** in maturity onset non-insulin dependent diabetes mellitus and diabetes mellitus not responding adequately with dietary restrictions or with sulfonylureas.

Biguanides are **contraindicated** in hypotension, alcoholics (can precipitate lactic acidosis), respiratory, hepatic, cardiovascular and renal diseases.

MEGLITINIDES

REPAGLINIDE

Repaglinide is a novel insulin secretagogue. It **lowers postprandial blood glucose as well as fasting blood glucose** in patients with type II diabetes mellitus by acting on the beta cells of pancreas. It stimulates insulin release only during meal time. It is taken with or just before each meal, thus introducing the concept of 'one meal one dose, no meal no dose' and flexibility of meal times.

Adverse effects include mild or moderate hypoglycemia. Other adverse effects are nausea, vomiting, arthralgia, back pain, and headache.

It is **indicated** in the management of type II diabetes mellitus in patients who are not responding to diet and exercise.

NATEGLINIDE

Nateglinide is a novel drug designed for the management of postprandial hyperglycemia in type II diabetes. Nateglinide belongs to the meglitinide class of oral hypoglycemic agents. **It restores the first phase of insulin secretion in type II diabetes.** It is well tolerated and appears to have a significantly lower likelihood of inducing hypoglycemia than sulfonylureas.

Adverse reactions include dizziness, URTI, back pain, flu-like symptoms, bronchitis, cough and hypoglycemia.

It is mainly **indicated** in the management of postprandial hyperglycemia in type II diabetes mellitus.

THIAZOLIDINEDIONES

ROSIGLITAZONE

Rosiglitazone, a member of the thiazolidinedione class of antidiabetic agents, improves glycemic control by improving insulin sensitivity.

The oral bioavailability of rosiglitazone is 99%. Peak plasma concentrations are observed about one hour after dosing. Rosiglitazone plasma concentration increases in a dose-proportional manner over the therapeutic dose range.

Adverse reactions include weight gain, edema, increase of total cholesterol and reduction in haemoglobin content.

It is **indicated** in the management of type II diabetes mellitus as monotherapy or in combination.

PIOGLITAZONE

Pioglitazone hydrochloride, a thiazolidinedione, **acts primarily by decreasing insulin resistance**. It improves sensitivity to insulin in muscle and adipose tissue and inhibits hepatic gluconeogenesis. It also improves glycemic control while reducing circulating insulin levels.

α-GLUCOSIDASE INHIBITORS

ACARBOSE

It is a pseudo-tetrasaccharide derived from the fermentation process of the fungus *Actinoplanes utahensis*.

It acts by competitively inhibiting pancreatic alphaamylase and intestinal alpha glucosidase hydrolase enzymes. Thus, it delays carbohydrate digestion, prolongs digestion time and reduces the rate of glucose absorption thereby lowering postprandial hyperglycemia.

Given orally less than 2% is absorbed as the oral drug. It is metabolised in the GI tract primarily by intestinal bacteria and to a lesser degree by digestive enzymes.

Adverse effects include flatulence, soft stools, diarrhoea, abdominal distention and pain, rarely abnormal liver function tests and skin reactions.

It is **used** as first line therapy in NIDDM inadequately controlled by diet and as adjunct to existing conventional oral hypoglycemic agents where hypoglycemic control is inadequate.

❑❑❑

CHAPTER 8.3 Glucocorticoids & Sex Hormones

GLUCOCORTICOIDS

As discussed in previous chapters, secretion of adrenocortical steroids is controlled by the pituitary release of corticotrophin (ACTH). The adrenal gland has two main parts, **adrenal medulla**, which is responsible for the release of catecholamines and **adrenal cortex** which secretes glucocorticoids, mineralocorticoids and sex hormones. The glucocorticoids and mineralocorticoids are twenty one carbon compounds having a cyclopentanoperhydro-phenanthrene nucleus. Both these hormones are synthesised in the adrenal cortex from cholesterol (see Fig. 8.3.1).

The important glucocorticoid secreted in human being is hydrocortisone (10 mg/ day). They are listed in table 8.3.1.

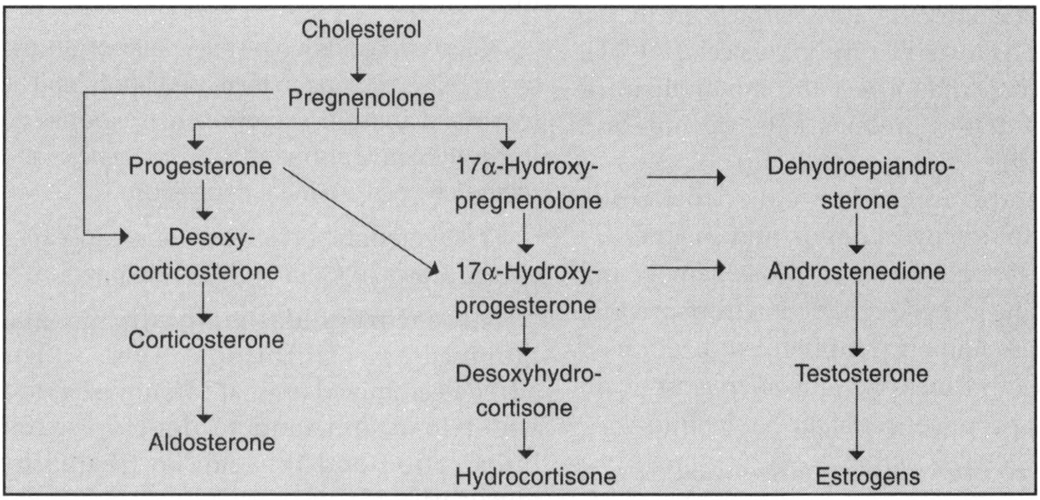

Fig. 8.3.1: Biosynthesis of various steroid hormones.

Table 8.3.1: *Classification of glucocorticoids and mineralocorticoids.*

Glucocorticoids	
Hydrocortisone (Cortisol; HYCOSON)	100 mg IM used as hydrocortisone sodium succinate injection. Also used as intraarticular inj. as hydrocortisone acetate & 1-2.5% topical (skin, ear & eye; WYCORT)
Prednisolone (EMSOLONE)	5-60 mg/day oral, 10-40 mg intramuscular/intra articular inj. and 0.25% topical (skin, eye)
Triamcinolone (TRICORT)	8-32 mg/day oral, intraarticular (2.5-15 mg), intradermal and deep intramuscular injection. 0.1% topical cream (as acetonide; LEDERCORT)
Dexamethasone (DEXONA)	0.5-5 mg/day oral, 4-20 mg/day IM/IV, 0.1% topical (skin cream) as dexamethasone sodium phosphate and trimethyl acetate
Betamethasone (BETNESOL)	0.5-5 mg/day oral, 4-20 mg/day IM/IV, 0.1 topical cream as betamethesone benzoate (TOPICASONE) and betamethasone valerate (BETNOVATE)
Beclomethasone (as dipropionate; BECLATE)	0.025% topical (cream)
Fluocinolone (as acetonide; FLUCORT)	0.025% topical (ointment)
Mineralocorticoids	
Desoxycorticosterone acetate (DOCA)	10-20 mg IM (once or twice in a week), 0.25 mg SL.
Flurdocortisone (FLORICORT)	0.2-2 mg/day
Aldosterone: It is a mineralocorticoid. Its actions are retention of sodium and reduction of serum potassium. It acts on distal tubules of kidney to increase sodium reabsorption (details are discussed in chapter 'Diuretics and antidiuretics').	

Pharmacological Actions

Corticosteroids are synthesized in the adrenal cortex under the influence of ACTH. Glucocorticoids affect the metabolism of carbohydrates, proteins, fats, calcium and electrolytes.

Metabolic effects: Glucocorticoids promote glycogen deposition in liver by stimulating glycogen synthetase activity and increasing glucose production from protein. They also inhibit peripheral utilization of glucose and increase glucose release from liver. It produces resistance to insulin.

Glucocorticoids also cause breakdown of protein and amino acid mobilization from peripheral tissues. They stimulate the conversion into glucose (neoglucogenesis) in the liver.

Glucocorticoids inhibit the uptake of glucose by fat cells, resulting in increased lipolysis. The increased insulin secretion in response to hyperglycaemia also stimulates lipogenesis and ultimately increase in fat deposition.

The catabolic effect on bone can cause osteoporosis in Cushing's syndrome.

Glucocorticoids maintain normal glomerular filtration rate. The adrenalectomized animal can not excrete a water load and tend to develop water intoxication and this can be treated by glucocorticoids.

Glucocorticoids also inhibit calcium

absorption from intestine and enhance renal excretion of Ca^{2+}.

Antiinflammatory and immunosuppressive effects: Glucocorticoids suppress all types of inflammation, hypersensitization and allergic reactions. They suppress the edema, capillary dilatation, migration of leukocytes, capillary permeability in the inflamed area.

Glucocorticoids inhibit the functions of leukocytes and tissues macrophages. They also stabilize lysosomal membranes, thereby reducing the concentration of proteolytic enzymes at the site of inflammation.

Glucocorticoids also inhibit the production of plasminogen activator by neutrophils.

They also influence the inflammatory response by reducing the prostaglandin and leukotriene synthesis that results from activation of enzyme phospholipase A_2.

Effect on CNS: Large doses of glucocorticoids cause euphoria, mood elevation, nervousness, restlessness, which are reversible type of actions. They often produce behavioural disturbances in human being and also increase intracranial pressure.

Effect on CVS and blood: Glucocorticoids inhibit capillary permeability and maintain myocardial contractility and also the tone of arterioles.

Glucocorticoids cause decrease in number of circulating lymphocytes, basophils and eosinophils in blood. They increase the number of neutrophils, platelets and erythrocytes.

Effect on GIT: Glucocorticoids stimulate production of acid and pepsin in the stomach and facilitate the development of peptic ulcer.

Effect on kidney: In deficiency of glucocorticoids, the glomerular filtration rate is impaired.

Effect on endocrine system: Glucocorticoids suppress the pituitary release of ACTH and betalipotropin and reduce secretion of FSH and TSH.

Mechanism of Action

Most of the established pharmacological effects of glucocorticoids are mediated by cytoplasmic glucocorticoid receptors. After binding to the receptor, the steroid-receptor complex binds to chromatin and stimulate the formation of mRNA. The mRNA stimulates the synthesis of enzymes which produce various pharmacological actions.

Pharmacokinetics

They are given by oral, parenteral and topical route. Oral bioavailability of synthetic cortico-steroids is high. Hydrocortisone after oral administration undergoes extensive first pass metabolism in liver.

They are metabolised in liver and after conjugation are excreted in urine. The synthetic derivatives are metabolised slowly and have longer duration of action.

Adverse Reactions

GIT: Acute erosive gastritis and haemorrhage. Peptic ulcer risk is increased.

Endocrine system: Cushing's habitus, hirsutism, retardation of growth, suppression of hypothalamopituitary-adrenal axis.

Metabolic disorders: Hyperglycemia, glycosuria and diabetes mellitus may be precipitated, osteoporosis,

Eye: Glaucoma, cataract may develop.

CNS: Psychiatric disturbances, euphoria.

Other side effects include muscular weakness, delayed healing of wounds, alopecia, hyperglycemia, susceptibility to infections etc.

Therapeutic Uses of Glucocorticoids

Glucocorticoids are used in the following physiological and clinical conditions:

1. Adrenocortical insufficiency:
   - **Acute:** Hydrocortisone/dexamethasone IV inj.
   - **Chronic:** Addison's disease; congenital adrenal hyperplasia (genetic disorder due to deficiency of steroidogenic enzymes).
2. Rheumatology:
   a. **Intraarticular injection:** Rheumatoid arthritis, osteoarthritis, gouty arthritis, joint sequelae of fractures and dislocations.

   b. **Periarticular/soft tissue injection:** Scapulohumeral periarthritis, periarthritis of hip, bursitis, tendinitis, synovitis, tenosynovitis, tarsalgia, metatarsalgia, epicondylitis, Dupuytren's contracture, Peyronie's disease, cystic tumors of aponeurosis or tendon (ganglia).
3. Severe allergic reactions such as urticaria, serum sickness, anaphylaxis.
4. Bronchial asthma, in acute and severe chronic asthma, aspiration pneumonia and pulmonary edema.
5. Autoimmune haemolytic anaemia, thrombocytopenia etc.
6. Ear disorders:
   a. Allergic rhinitis, nasal polyposis.

   b. Allergic sinusitis.

   c. Cicatrizing lesions of the middle ear.
7. Dermatology: Topical steroids are useful in keloids, hypertrophic scars, other localised hypertrophic, infiltrated, inflammatory lesions of lichen planus, psoriatic plaques, granuloma annulare and lichen simplex chronicus; discoid lupus erythematosus, necrobiosis lipoidica diabeticorum and alopecia areata.
8. Neurology: Lumbago, sciatica, cervicobrachial neuralgia and other painful radiculopathies; selected cases of inflammatory disorders such as tuberculous meningitis and multiple sclerosis.
9. **GIT:** Ulcerative colitis, Crohn's disease etc.
10. **Malignant diseases:** Corticoids are used in combination with other therapy in the treatment of Hodgkin's disease, acute lymphatic leukemia and other lymphomas.
11. **Miscellaneous uses:** Corticoids in higher dose can be given along with other immunosuppressants in certain organ transplantation cases to prevent rejection reaction.

PREDNISOLONE

It is more potent (4 times) than hydrocortisone. It has intermediate duration of action.

Adverse effects include peptic ulceration, myopathy, steroid psychosis. On prolonged use posterior subcapsular cataract, glaucoma, osteoporosis, hyperglycemia, increased susceptibility to infection, delayed wound healing and Cushing habitus.

It is **indicated** in suppression of inflammatory and allergic disorders, inflammatory bowel disease, asthma, immunosuppression and rheumatic disease.

TRIAMCINOLONE

It is a highly, selective glucocorticoid **used** in asthma, allergic disorders, rheumatoid arthritis and dermatoses.

DEXAMETHASONE

It is a selective and very potent long acting glucocorticoid. It causes suppression of pituitary adrenal axis. Used in shock due to trauma, allergic emergencies, rheumatoid arthritis, asthma, nephrotic syndrome and suppression of inflammation in eye and skin disorders.

BETAMETHASONE

It is a glucocorticoid similar to dexamethasone. Used in status asthmaticus, acute allergic reactions, anaphylactic allergic reactions, anaphylactic reaction to drugs, severe shock arising from surgical or accidental trauma or overwhelming infection; Addison's disease, Simmond's disease, hypopituitarism following adrenalectomy, tennis elbow, tenosynovitis and bursitis; rheumatological disease, ulcerative colitis, regional enteritis, TB meningitis and subarachnoid bleed.

SEX HORMONES

ESTROGENS

Estrogens are produced mainly by the ovary and the placenta and the synthesis of estrogens takes place from cholesterol (as discussed in section on 'glucocorticoids'). Estrogens are classified into two main groups (see table 8.3.2).

Estradiol is the major secretory product of ovary. Estrogens are required for normal maturation of the female. They stimulate the development of secondary sexual characters e.g. stimulate stromal development, ductal growth in the breast, growth of axillary and pubic hair and alter the distribution of body fat to produce typical female body contours.

Table 8.3.2: *Classification of estrogens and antiestrogens.*

I. **Natural**	
Estradiol (as benzoate/cypionate/ enanthate/valerate; ESTRADERM)	2.5-10 mg IM
II. **Synthetic**	
Ethinyl estradiol (EVALON)	0.1-1 mg/day
Mestranol	0.1-0.2 mg/day
Diethylstilbestrol	0.5-5 mg/day, oral/IM
Tibolone (LIVIAL)	2.5 mg/day
III. **Antiestrogens**	
Clomiphene citrate (CLOMID)	50 mg/day × 5 days
Tamoxifen citrate (TAMODEX)	20-40 mg/day

It also stimulates the development of skin pigmentation particularly in the region of the nipples and areolae and in the genital regions.

Estrogens also play a role in stimulation of the proliferative or preovulatory phase of endometrium and vasodilatation of endometrial capillaries.

Estrogens are anabolic but weaker than testosterone. Estrogens also cause retention of nitrogen, sodium and fluid in tissues. Estrogens also protect from osteoporosis in postmenopausal women, which occur as a result of estrogen deficiency.

Pharmacological Actions

Estrogens act by interacting with the specific estradiol receptors in the cytoplasm of the target cells and mediate the transcription of the relevant mRNA by attaching itself to the appropriate gene.

Estrogens produce proliferative changes in the endometrium. On chronic administration, estrogen suppresses the secretion of FSH and somewhat LH resulting in inhibition of ovulation. In testes it may reduce the secretion of androgens and inhibit spermatogenesis.

Estrogens suppress lactation without affecting the prolactin level in plasma.

On chronic administration it may inhibit the growth of epiphyseal cartilage.

Pharmacokinetics

Natural estrogens are inactive orally due to rapid metabolism in liver. Synthetic estrogens are well absorbed after oral administration as well as by transdermal application. Estradiol is metabolized to estrone and estriol. All these are conjugated and excreted in urine and bile. Synthetic estrogen are metabolized very slowly and are more potent.

Adverse effects include breast discomfort, pruritus, exanthema, thrombophlebitis and local skin irritation, increased risk of gall stones.

Therapeutic Uses

The most common use of estrogen are as oral/parenteral contraceptive and for hormone replacement therapy.

- **Primary hypogonadism:** Estrogens have been used for replacement therapy in estrogen deficient patients (treatment of amenorrhoea).
- **In post menopausal hormonal therapy:**
  - Estrogen have been used in prevention and treatment of osteoporosis.
  - Improve the general physical, mental and also sexual activity.
  - Maintain calcium balance.
  - Decreases the risk of cardiovascular (coronary artery) disease.

Transdermal estradiol is equally effective:

- In atrophic vaginitis.
- In atrophic urethritis.
- For the treatment of vaginal complaints such as dyspareunia, dryness and itching.
- Pre and postoperative therapy in postmenopausal women undergoing vaginal surgery.
- Infertility due to cervical hostility.
- As a diagnostic aid in case of doubtful atrophic cervical smear.

TIBOLONE

It is a synthetic steroid which combines oestrogenic and progestogenic activity with weak androgenic activity. It needs to be given continuously without cyclical progestogen.

It restores plasma endorphin level in postmenopausal women and act centrally to affect the thermoregulatory system.

Adverse effects include weight changes, ankle edema, dizziness, headache, abdominal pain, GI disturbances, vaginal bleeding, arthralgia, myalgia, migraine, visual disturbances, liver function changes, increased facial hair, depression, skin rash and pruritus.

It is **indicated** in vasomotor symptoms in estrogen deficiency and osteoporosis prophylaxis.

ANTIESTROGENS

Also known as estrogen antagonists or ovulation inducing agents. They act by binding to estrogen receptors.

CLOMIPHENE CITRATE

It is a triphenyl ethylene compound and a competitive partial agonist inhibitor of endogenous estrogen. It can produce regression of estrogen induced proliferative endometrium. It can also prolong the luteal phase in normal menstruating women.

Due to its probable direct effect on ovaries, it may increase the gonadotrophin secretion. It also exerts a weak estrogenic action on endometrium.

It is well absorbed after oral administration, metabolized and excreted in bile and main **side effects** include hot flushes, ovarian enlargement and cyst formation which may be due to overstimulation and can also lead to rupture and bleeding.

Clomiphene is mainly **used** in the treatment of female infertility due to ovulatory failure and is also found useful to aid *in vitro* fertilization.

It is also used to promote spermatogenesis in male due to oligospermia and asthenospermia.

TAMOXIFEN

It is a competitive partial agonist inhibitor of estradiol at the estrogen receptor and is **used** mainly in the treatment of advanced breast cancer in postmenopausal women. It is also used in male infertility due to its weaker estrogen effect and lesser side effects.

It is effective on oral administration and is excreted in bile.

Adverse effects include hot flushes, vaginal bleeding, menstrual irregularities, anorexia, depression and dermatitis.

PROGESTINS

Progesterone is naturally secreted by the corpus luteum and placenta and functions to maintain pregnancy after conception. Their derivatives are of two types, which are classified as in table 8.3.3.

PROGESTERONE

The physiological functions of progesterone include:

- Induction of secretory phase of the menstrual cycle.
- Development of alveolar system of breasts.
- Preparation of endometrium for the implantation of fertilized ovum for further pregnancy.

Table 8.3.3: *Classification of progestins and antiprogestin.*

I.	**Progesterone derivatives**	
	Progesterone (MICROGEST)	10-50 mg OD/wk IM
	Medroxyprogesterone (PROVERA)	5-20 mg oral, 50-400 mg IM
II.	**19-Nortestosterone derivatives**	
	Norethisterone (NORGEST)	5-10 mg OD
	Lynoestrenol (Ethinylestrenol)	5-10 mg OD
	Allylestrenol (NIDAGEST)	10-40 mg/day
	Levonorgestrel (OVRAL-G)	0.5-1 mg OD
III.	**Antiprogestin**	
	Mifepristone	600 mg single dose

- Induction of certain changes in the vaginal epithelium and secretion.
- Increases the basal body temperature and inhibit uterine contractions by decreasing sensitivity of myometrium to oxytocin.

Pharmacological Actions

Progesterone prolongs the luteal phase and induce decidual changes in the endometrial stroma. It prevents the cornification of the vaginal epithelium and brings about increased glycogen deposition. It changes the watery cervical secretion to viscid, thick and scanty secretion for sperm penetration.

Progesterone causes proliferation of acini in the breasts and with the help of estrogen, prepare them for lactation.

It causes slight rise in body temperature and this is seen during the luteal phase.

Administration during follicular phase suppresses the preovulation LH and prevents ovulation.

After reaching cell nucleus it binds to progesterone receptors and influences the transcription of a limited set of genes.

After oral administration progesterone undergoes extensive first-pass metabolism in liver to pregnanediol, which is conjugated and excreted in urine. It has a short plasma half life.

Adverse effects include acne, urticaria, fluid retention, weight changes, GI disturbances, change in libido, breast discomfort, premenstrual symptoms, irregular menstrual cycles, chloasma, depression, pyrexia, insomnia, somnolence, alopecia, hirsutism and rarely jaundice. Injection may be painful.

It is **indicated** as contraceptive, in hormone replacement therapy, primary and secondary amenorrhoea, dysfunctional uterine bleeding, endometriosis, postponement of menstruation, premenstrual syndrome, uterine hypoplasia, threatened or habitual abortion and premenstrual tension. It is also useful in endometrial carcinoma.

MEDROXYPROGESTERONE

It is a synthetic progestogen structurally related to progesterone given orally or by IM injection.

Adverse effects include skin rash, urticaria, pruritus, depression, nausea, alopecia, acne, hirsutism, galactorrhoea, anaphylaxis, thromboembolic disorders, insomnia, fatigue, dizziness, headache, tenderness of breast and somnolence.

It is **used** in dysfunctional uterine bleeding, secondary amenorrhoea and endometriosis.

NORETHISTERONE

Norethisterone and its acetate and enanthate esters are synthetic progestogens given orally in the treatment of abnormal uterine bleeding and endometriosis.

Adverse effects include breakthrough bleeding, amenorrhoea, spotting, exacerbation of epilepsy and migraine.

It is **indicated** in primary and secondary amenorrhoea of long duration, metropathia haemorrhagica, menorrhagia, dysmenorrhoea, polymenorrhoea and premenstrual syndrome.

LYNOESTRENOL

It is an oral synthetic progestogen.

Adverse effects include nausea, vomiting and epigastric discomfort, breakthrough bleeding or spotting, headache, nervousness, migraine, dizziness, edema and breast pain.

It is **indicated** in dysfunctional uterine bleeding, amenorrhoea, dysmenorrhoea, hypo and hypermenorrhoea, delay of menstrual period, oligo and polymenorrhoea, benign breast disease, endometriosis, metrorrhagia and endometrial carcinoma.

ALLYLESTRENOL

It stimulates placental progesterone synthesis and increases the secretion of placental hormones.

Adverse effects include nausea, vomiting and epigastric discomfort.

It is **indicated** in habitual abortion, failure of nidation, threatened abortion, premenstrual tension, metrorrhagia and threatened premature labour.

ANTIPROGESTIN

MIFEPRISTONE

It is 19-norsteroid partial agonist that binds to the progesterone receptor and inhibits the activity of progesterone. If given during the follicular phase it slows down the follicular development and failure of ovulation. It also stimulates uterine contraction and induces menstruation. Oral bioavailability is 25%. It is metabolized in liver and excreted in bile. Its major **use** is to terminate pregnancy. It can be used alone or in combination with vaginal pessary of prostaglandin E_1 (1 mg) or oral misoprostol to terminate the pregnancy.

It is also used as contragestational agent and for induction of labour.

ANDROGENS AND ANABOLIC STEROIDS

Androgens are substances which cause development of secondary sex characters in males. The most important androgen secreted by testes is testosterone. Testosterone is synthesized from the cholesterol in testes mainly, under the influence of LH from pituitary. In peripheral tissues testosterone is partly converted into more active dihydrotestosterone.

Adrenal cortex also produces small quantities of weak androgens (androstenedione and dehydroepiandrosterone) which are partially converted to testosterone in peripheral tissues. In females, ovaries also secrete small quantities of testosterone.

Follicle stimulating hormone is responsible for the growth of testes. It promotes spermatogenesis. Along with LH, FSH plays an essential role in maintaining the normal testicular functions such as development of male sex organs e.g. penis, scrotum; development of secondary sexual characters e.g. growth of facial,

Table 8.3.4: *Classification of androgens, anabolic steroids and antiandrogens.*

I. **Natural**	
Testosterone (as propionate, cypionate undecanoate, enanthate; NUVIR)	Propionate 25-200 mg IM per day to bimonthly; undecanoate 40 mg OD-TDS
II. **Synthetic**	
Methyltestosterone	25 mg/day SL
III. ***Anabolic steroids***	
Nandrolone (as decanoate, phenyl propionate; DURABOLIN)	10-100 mg IM once a wk to every 3 wks
Stanozolol (NEURABOL)	2-6 mg/day
Mesterolone (PROVIRONUM)	25-50 mg/day
IV. ***Antiandrogens***	
Danazol (DANOGEN)	200-800 mg/day
Cyproterone acetate	
Flutamide (PROSTAMID)	250 mg TDS

axilla, chest and pubic hair and change in voice; development of accessory sexual organs e.g. seminal vesicles, prostate and epididymis and development of male skeletal musculature.

Androgens and anabolic steroids are classified as in table 8.3.4.

TESTOSTERONE

It is a natural androgen secreted by testis. The secretion is regulated by LH hormone secreted by pituitary gland.

It is responsible for development of sex organs and secondary sex characters in males at puberty. It leads to growth of genitals, growth of hair (pubic, axillary, beard, moustache, body hair), thickening of skin, larynx grows and voice deepens and also behavioural changes. It is also needed for normal spermatogenesis and maturation of spermatozoa. It is also responsible for pubertal spurt of growth in boys leading to increased bony and skeletal muscles growth.

Pharmacokinetics

Testosterone is not given orally as it is extensively metabolised in liver and the bioavailability is low. Testosterone is converted by 5a-reductase in target tissues to more potent dihydrotestosterone.

It is metabolized in liver to glucuronic acid and sulfate conjugates and excreted in urine.

Adverse effects include menstrual irregularities, deepening of voice in women, edema, cholestatic jaundice, virilization, priapism, increased libido, acne, precocious puberty, premature epiphyseal closure, gynaecomastia and hepatic carcinoma and reduction in spermatogenesis.

The capacity of androgens to enhance the epiphyseal closure in children may persist for as long as several months after discontinuation of the drug. In children androgens should be used with great caution.

It is **indicated** in replacement therapy to maintain sex characteristics in adults with testicular failure, accidental castration; in hereditary angioneurotic edema, infertility due to defective spermatogenesis, osteoporosis, refractory anaemia, breast carcinoma, menopausal syndrome, endometriosis; to improve nitrogen balance in catabolic states; certain types of infertility due to disorders of spermatogenesis.

NANDROLONE

It is closely related to androgen testosterone having both lower androgenic and higher anabolic properties.

Adverse effects include virilism, edema and hypercalcaemia.

It is **used** in debilitating illness, postmenopausal osteoporosis, burn or major illness, postmenopausal metastatic mammary carcinoma, haemolytic, hypoplastic or malignancy associated anaemias.

STANOZOLOL

It is a synthetic steroid with anabolic and androgenic properties. Used in prophylactic treatment of hereditary angioedema, vascular manifestations of Behcet's syndrome.

Adverse effects include liver damage, virilism, nausea, skin rash, headache and epigastric discomfort.

MESTEROLONE

It provides oral therapy and does not cause liver damage. It is **indicated** in hypogonadism and male infertility. **Adverse effects** include frequent erection of penis and priapism.

ANTIANDROGENS

DANAZOL

It is an isoxazole derivative of ethisterone (17α-ethinyl testosterone) with weak progestational and androgenic activities used to inhibit ovarian and testicular function.

It inhibits gonadotrophin secretion from pituitary in both men and women thus inhibiting both testicular/ovarian function.

It is **used** in menorrhagia, gynaecomastia, fibrocystic breast disease, treatment of visually proven endometriosis or symptomatic control when surgery is contraindicated. It is also used in infertility in women and precocious puberty in boys.

Adverse effects include skin rash, nausea, flushing, headache, weight gain, acne, hirsutism, loss of libido and amenorrhoea.

CYPROTERONE ACETATE

It has a potent antiandrogen and mild progestional activity. It can also inhibit gonadotropin secretion in larger dose and also suppresses spermatogenesis and Leydig cell function. It is **used** in precocious puberty in males, acne, carcinoma prostate and hirsutism and virilization in women.

FLUTAMIDE

Non-steroidal drug having specific antiandrogen activity. Active metabolite, 2-hydroxyflutamide competitively blocks androgen action on accessory sex organs and pituitary. It leads to increased LH secretion by blocking feedback inhibition. It is **used** in advanced carcinoma prostate, female hirsutism.

Bicalutamide is a congener of flutamide, causing less hepatotoxicity and can be given once daily.

❑❑❑

CHAPTER 8.4

Thyroid Hormone & Antithyroid Agents

Thyroid gland secretes two important hormones, ***thyroxine*** (T_4) and ***triiodothyronine*** (T_3). The third hormone, ***calcitonin*** secreted from interstitial cells is physiologically different and is responsible for the regulation of calcium metabolism.

Thyroid hormones exert their effect by binding to nuclear receptors in target organs. Both the thyroid hormones are well absorbed after oral administration. They are conjugated with sulfuric acid in liver and excreted in bile.

The various preparation used are:

Preparation	Dose
Thyroxine (l-thyroxine sodium) (ELTROXIN)	50-300 µg/day
Liothyronine sodium (TETROXIN)	20-60 µg/day
Thyroglobulin (PROLOID)	32.5-195 mg/day

Therapeutic Uses of Thyroid Hormones

- Infant hypothyroidism (cretinism).
- Adult hypothyroidism (myxoedema).
- Myxoedema coma: It is an emergency. Liothyronine 100 µg IV can be used and maintained by thyroxine 500 µg IV.
- In the treatment of non-toxic goitre.
- Papillary thyroid carcinoma: It is often responsive to TSH.

Adverse reactions include palpitation, angina, tremors, thyrotoxicosis, allergic reactions, headache, tachycardia, diarrhoea, sweating, restlessness, loss of weight and muscle weakness.

ANTITHYROID AGENTS

These are **used to inhibit the functional activity of hypersecretive thyroid gland**. The hypersecretion leads to the development of thyrotoxicosis. The antithyroid agents acts by interfering with the synthesis and release of thyroid hormones. They are classified as in table 8.4.1.

Drugs Inhibiting Hormone Synthesis

The thioamides which include propyl thiouracil and methimazole are the major drugs for the treatment of thyrotoxicosis. In India carbimazole is most commonly used drug. They bind to thyroid peroxidase and

Table 8.4.1: *Classification of antithyroid agents.*

I. **Agents which inhibit hormone synthesis**	
Propyl thiouracil	50-100 mg/day (initial) and maintained at 20-30 mg/day
Carbimazole (THYROZOLE)	5-15 mg/day (initial) and maintained at 2.5-20 mg/day
Methimazole	5-10 mg/day (initial) maintained at 2.5-15 mg/day
II. **Agents which inhibit iodide trapping**	
Thiocyanates, perchlorates and nitrates	
III. **Agents which inhibit hormone release**	
Iodine (Lugol's solution: 5% iodine in 10% KI; Colloid iodine: 10% solution)	
Sodium and potassium iodide	
Organic iodide	
IV. **Agents which destroy thyroid gland tissue**	
Radioactive iodine (^{131}I)	3-5 mcurie.

prevent the oxidation of iodide and iodotyrosyl residue which subsequently inhibits the formation of tyrosine residue in thyroglobulin and coupling of iodotyrosine residues to T_3 and T_4.

CARBIMAZOLE

It inhibits oxidation of iodide, inhibits iodination of tyrosine residue and inhibits the coupling of iodotyrosine residue. After oral administration, it is rapidly absorbed and metabolised to **methimazole** which is active form and crosses the placental barrier.

Adverse reactions include agranulocytosis, transient leucopenia, arthralgia, nausea, fever, loss of hair and hepatic damage.

It is **used** in hyperthyroidism due to Graves' disease, prior to surgical treatment of hyperthyroidism i.e., thyroidectomy. It is also used in the treatment of paroxysmal tachycardia and intractable congestive cardiac failure.

Agents Which Inhibit Iodide Trapping

Monovalent anions such as thiocyanates, perchlorates and pertechnetate can block the uptake of iodide by the gland through competitive inhibition of iodide transport mechanism. But it requires higher dose which can cause aplastic anaemia and due to this major drawback they are not used clinically.

Agents Which Inhibit Hormone Release

Iodine inhibits hormone release. They inhibit organification and hormone release and also decrease the size and vascularity of hyperplastic gland on regular administration. Peak antithyroid affect is seen in two weeks after which thyrotoxicosis may reoccur. It is well absorbed orally and crosses the placental barrier.

Adverse effects include angioedema, fever, thrombocytopenia, arthralgia, lymphadenopathy, salivation, sneezing and swelling of lips and eyelids.

Iodine is **used** in thyroid storm, hyperthyroidism, preoperatively before thyroidectomy and prophylaxis of endemic goitre. Iodine is also useful as antiseptic and in expectorants.

The iodinated contrast agents, ipodate and iopanic acid are used in the treatment of hyperthyroidism. These drugs rapidly inhibit the conversion of T_4 to T_3 in the liver, kidney, brain and pituitary gland.

Agents Which Destroy Thyroid Gland Tissue

^{131}I is the only radioisotope of iodine used in the treatment of thyrotoxicosis. The other isotopes ^{123}I and ^{125}I are used only in diagnosis. ^{131}I emits gamma and beta radiations. It is available as sodium solution. When taken orally, it is rapidly absorbed, concentrated by the thyroid and incorporated into the storage follicles. Beta radiation penetrates up to 3 to 5 mm into the soft tissue, they destroy some of the thyroid follicles and produce fibrosis.

Adverse reactions include hypothyroidism, thyroid carcinoma, damage to foetal thyroid and possibility of genetic damage, so contraindicated during pregnancy.

Radioactive iodine is **indicated** in hyperthyroidism due to Graves' disease or toxic nodular goitre and also used as palliative therapy after thyroidectomy for papillary carcinoma of thyroid.

❑❑❑

CHAPTER 8.5 Hormonal Contraceptives

Hormonal contraceptive are the most effective spacing methods of contraception. They are used for reversible suppression of fertility.

Oral Contraceptives

The oral hormonal contraceptive can be classified as in table 8.5.1.

COMBINED PILLS

It is a combination of estrogen and progestin given together for remarkable efficacy, safety and ease in administration. It has total 21 pills, each pill is given orally for 21 consecutive days beginning on the 5th day of menstrual cycle (when the bleeding occurs this is considered the first day of cycle). The pill is to be taken everyday at a fixed time, preferably before going to bed at night.

PHASED PILLS

This is a combined pill but biphasic or triphasic in nature e.g. the estrogen level is kept constant but the progestin amount is low in early phase and increasing in subsequent phases of menstrual cycle.

Fifth day to tenth day menstrual cycle (ethinyl estradiol 30 µg + levonorgestrel 50 µg), eleventh to fifteenth day (ethinyl estradiol 30 µg + levonorgestrel 75 µg), sixteenth to twenty fifth day (ethinyl estradiol 30 µg + levonorgestrel 125 µg). They are supplied in one pack of different

Table 8.5.1: *Classification of oral contraceptives.*

Estrogen		Progestins
Ethinyl estradiol (20, 50 µg)	+	Norethindrone (1, 3 and 4 mg) (ANOVLAR)
Ethinyl estradiol (50 µg)	+	Norgestrel (0.5 mg) (OVRAL-G)
Ethinyl estradiol (30 µg)	+	Norgestrel (0.5 mg) (PRIMOVLAR-30)
Ethinyl estradiol (30 µg)	+	L-Norgestrel (0.3 mg) (OVRAL-L)
Mestranol (100 µg)	+	Ethynodiol diacetate (1 mg) (OVULEN)
Mestranol (50 µg)	+	Ethynodiol diacetate (1 mg) (OVULEN-50)
Ethinyl estradiol (50 µg)	+	Lynestrenol (1 mg) (LYNDIOL)

coloured pills starting from fifth day of menstrual cycle to twenty-fifth day and next pack can be started after a gap of seven days as in case of combined pills.

MINIPILL

It is also known as progestin only pill (POP). It contains only progestins, which is given in small amount throughout the menstrual cycle (without interruption) but because of lower efficacy rate, it is not much popular.

Norgestrel (OVRETTE)	0.075 mg
Norethindrone (MICRONOR)	0.35 mg

POSTCOITAL CONTRACEPTION

The postcoital (morning after) contraception is recommended within 48 hours after an unprotected intercourse, rape or contraceptive failure.

Diethylstilbestrol 5 mg per day is given for five days.

Other regimens used are combination of ethinyl estradiol 0.1 mg + levonorgestrel 0.5 to 1 mg. Two tablets are taken 12 hours apart within three days of intercourse. Levonorgestrel 0.75 mg (1 tablet) is also used and is taken as early as possible (within 72 hrs) and second tablet after 12-24 hours of first tablet. Withdrawal bleeding occur within 3-7 days.

INJECTABLE FORMULATIONS

They are usually given by IM route. They lead to higher incidence of menstrual irregularities and amenorrhoea.

- Norethindrone enanthate (NORISTERAT) 200 mg given once in two months.
- Depot medroxyprogesterone acetate (DEPOT PROVERA) 150 mg given once in 3 month and 400 mg given once in 6 month.

Some subcutaneous and intrauterine implants of progesterone have also been used which are prepared in biodegradable polymeric matrices.

Mechanism of Action of Oral Contraceptives

The oral contraceptives act by the different mechanisms.

- **Inhibiting ovulation** by blocking the release of follicle stimulating hormone and luteinising hormone from the anterior lobe of pituitary gland.
- **Increasing the thickness of cervical mucus** due to progestins and producing an unfavourable environment for penetration of sperm and further conception.
- Inducing other changes in the uterine mucosa which may be unfavourable for the implantation of fertilized ovum. This action is important in minipills and postcoital pills.

Adverse Effects

The most common side effects are nausea, vomiting, headache, dizziness, fatigue, weight gain and breast fullness. The other side effects which appear after sometime of therapy are acne, increased body hair, pigmentation of cheeks, nose and forehead (chloasma).

The other serious side effects include high blood pressure, increased risk of myocardial infarction, thromboembolic diseases like thrombophlebitis, venous thrombosis, cerebral thrombosis.

They were suspected to lead to increased risk of cancer of breast and carcinoma of cervix and endometrium.

CENTCHROMAN

Its a nonsteroidal estrogen antagonist, which acts by preventing implantation due to embryouterine asynchrony, accelerated tubal transport and suppression of decidualization. It has no effect on pituitary or ovarian functions. It is taken 30 mg twice weekly for 12 weeks followed by once a week as long as fertility is to be suppressed.

MALE CONTRACEPTIVE

The main research focus is different approaches e.g. agent which prevent spermatogenesis, interfering with sperm storage and maturation and preventing sperm transport in vas deferens. But the hormones which suppress sperm production tend to lower testosterone and affect the potency and libido.

The one product obtained from cottonseed oil, **Gossypol** which is categorized as non-hormonal selective spermatogenesis suppressant, is effective in producing azoospermia or severe oligospermia but it is not widely used as male contraceptive. Mechanism of action is not known. Adverse effects are edema, diarrhoea, hypokalemia, neuritis.

❑❑❑

Section 9

Chemotherapy

CHAPTER 9.1

Sulfonamides, Nitrofurans and Quinolones

CHEMOTHERAPY

Chemotherapy is the use of chemical compounds for the treatment of infectious diseases by killing or inhibiting the growth of causative organisms without damaging the host tissues or cells.

Paul Ehrlich demonstrated the effective use of methylene blue in the treatment of malaria. He also synthesized arsenical compounds (neoarsphenamine) effective in the treatment of syphilis. The synthesis of newer and powerful antibacterial substances gave the recognition to **Paul Ehrlich** as '**the father of modern chemotherapy**' and awarded the Nobel prize of medicine in 1909.

In 1928, Sir Alexander Fleming found that a diffusible substance was elaborated by *Penicillium notatum* (a fungus) which prevented the growth of surrounding bacterial colonies in culture plate. He named this as 'penicillin' but this discovery remained a scientific curiosity for more than a decade. This work was followed up by Chain, Falk and Florey who established the efficacy of penicillin in 1941 and in 1945, Fleming, Chain and Florey were awarded the Nobel Prize.

The general mechanism of action of antimicrobial agents is listed in table 9.1.1.

Antimicrobials can be classified according to type of action into:

a. **Primarily bactericidal**: Penicillin, cephalosporins, aminoglycosides, vancomycin, polypeptides, INH, cotrimoxazole, rifampicin, fluoroquinolones, nalidixic acid.
b. **Primarily bacteriostatic**: Ethambutol, erythromycin, chloramphenicol, tetracyclines, sulfonamides.

Beta lactam antibiotics having a β-lactam ring, which includes penicillin, in which a thiazolidine ring is attached to a betalactam ring that carries a secondary amino group. Other similar compounds are cephalosporins, monobactams and carbapenems.

ANTIMICROBIALS USED IN DENTISTRY

Various antimicrobials agents is used in dentistry for prevention of local oral wound infection and prevention of distant infection i.e., bacterial endocarditis. Generally, prophylaxis by the use of antibiotics is not required for routine type of dental surgery

Table 9.1.1: *Mechanism of action of antimicrobial agents.*

1. **Inhibit cell wall synthesis**	Penicillins, cephalosporins, bacitracin, vancomycin and cycloserine.
2. **Damage to the cytoplasmic membrane**	
Polypeptides	Polymyxin, bacitracin, colistin.
Polycines	Nystatin, amphotericin B, hamycin.
3. **Inhibit protein synthesis & impairment of functions of ribosomes**	Tetracyclines, chloramphenicol, aminoglycosides, erythromycin, clindamycin and other macrolide antibiotics.
4. **Inhibit DNA gyrase**	Fluoroquinolones i.e. ciprofloxacin, ofloxacin.
5. **Interfere with DNA function**	Rifampicin, metronidazole.
6. **Interfere with DNA synthesis**	Acyclovir, idoxuridine, zidovudine.
7. **Antimetabolite action**	Sulfonamides, sulfones, INH, ethambutol, trimethoprim, PAS, pyrimethamine.

as simple extraction and other minor peridental procedures are associated with very low risk of any wound infection. Prophylaxis is recommended when the procedure in which a prosthesis is inserted into bone or soft tissue (e.g., dental implants), or in other extensive reconstructive surgery.

In dentistry, the antimicrobials agents which should be active against gram positive cocci and oral anaerobes and which yields peak blood levels higher than minimum inhibitry concentration for the common oral pathogens is recommended. Amoxycillin, safe & bactericidal in nature is generally the drug of choice. Antiseptic rinse (chlorhexidine 0.2%) is also used as an adjuvant to reduce the bacteraemia following dental extraction. The detail pharmacology of antimicrobial agents are given in individual chapters.

SULFONAMIDES

Chemically, all sulfonamides may be considered to be derivatives of sulfanilamide (p-aminobenzene sulfonamide). Sulfonamides were the first antimicrobial agents effective against pyogenic bacterial infections. The antimicrobial compounds containing a sulfonamido (SO_2 NH_2) group are called sulfonamides and a free amino group at the para position is required for its antibacterial activity. The same sulfonamido group is also present in other non-bacterial compounds such as tolbutamide (oral antidiabetic drug), chlorothiazide, furosemide and acetazolamide (diuretics) etc.

The sulfonamides can be classified according to their therapeutic utility and pharmacokinetic parameters (table 9.1.2). However, because of bacterial resistance and discovery of many safer and more effective antibiotics, the utility of sulfonamides is limited to few infections which are of clinical interest.

Pharmacological Actions

The most important pharmacological action of sulfonamides is its antibacterial activity against variety of gram positive and

Table 9.1.2: *Classification of sulfonamides.*

I. **Highly absorbed sulfonamides**	
a. ***Short acting***	
Sulfadiazine	2 g initially then 1 g 4-6 hourly
Sulfadimidine	2 g initially then 0.5 g 6-8 hourly
Sulfafurazole (GANTRISIN)	2 g initially then 1 g 4-6 hourly
Sulfamethizole (UROLUCOSIL)	1.0-2 g 4-6 hourly
b. ***Intermediate acting***	
Sulfamethoxazole (used in combination with trimethoprim; SEPTRAN: Sulfamethoxazole 400 mg + Trimethoprim 80 mg)	160 mg of trimethoprim & 800 mg of sulfamethoxazole every 12 hourly
c. ***Long acting***	
Sulfadimethoxine (MADRIBON)	1 g initially then 0.5 g OD
Sulfamethoxine (SULFADOXINE)	1 g initially then 0.5 g OD
Sulfamethoxypyridazine (LEDERKYN)	1 g initially then 0.5 g OD
Sulfamethopyrazine (used in malaria; METAKELFIN)	
II. **Poorly absorbed sulfonamides (for GIT local action)**	
Phthalyl sulfathiazole (THALAZOLE)	3-6 g/day
Succinyl sulfathiazole (SULFASUXIDINE)	3-6 g/day
Sulfaguanidine	3-6 g/day
III. **Special purpose sulfonamides**	
Sulfacetamide (ALBUCID)	10-30% eye drops
Sulfacetamide (NEBASULF)	6% powder used externally
Sulfasalazine (for autoimmune bowel disease; SALAZOPYRIN)	1-2 g QID initially then 0.5 g TDS-QID
Silver sulfadiazine (burn etc. local application; SILVIRIN)	1% local cream
Mafenide propionate (MARFANIL)	1% local cream

gram negative organisms (mainly bacteriostatic) and certain species of chlamydia infections such as:

- Streptococci, staphylococci, pneumococci, gonococci, meningococci, *Haemophilus influenzae, H. ducreyi, Calymmatobacterium granulomatis, Vibrio comma, Vibrio cholerae, E. coli, Pasteurella pestis, Shigella.*
- *Actinomyces, Nocardia* and *Toxoplasma.*
- *Chlamydia* causing lymphogranuloma venereum, psittacosis, trachoma and inclusion conjunctivitis.

Mechanism of Action

The compound sulfanilamide exhibits a structural similarity to para-amino benzoic acid (PABA). Woods and Fields proposed the theory that sulfonamides, being structurally similar to PABA, **inhibit bacterial folate synthetase so that folic acid is not formed** which is needed for a number of metabolic reactions. Folic acid derived from PABA is essential for bacterial metabolism. Sulfonamides inhibit the enzyme folic acid synthetase which is involved in the conversion of PABA to folic acid, which causes folic acid deficiency and ultimately cause injury to the bacterial cell.

Pharmacokinetics

After oral administration, sulfonamides are rapidly and completely absorbed from gastrointestinal tract and approximately 70 to 90 percent of oral dose reaches to the blood stream, but the binding with plasma proteins differ considerably among different groups. The highly plasma protein bound sulfonamides have longer action. The main site of absorption is small intestine.

Adverse Reactions

The common side effects are nausea and vomiting. The others are allergic symptoms including drug fever, skin rash, urticaria, eosinophilia, photosensitization reactions, serum sickness like syndrome. Stevens-Johnson syndrome and exfoliative dermatitis are also common with longer acting agents.

The uncommon allergic reactions include acute toxic hepatitis, toxic nephrosis and acute haemolytic anaemia.

Sulfonamides also cause renal irritation and may precipitate renal colic. Crystalluria, haematuria and albuminuria can also occur which may lead to the development of oliguria and anuria.

The hematopoietic toxicity includes agranulocytosis, thrombocytopenia and rarely aplastic anaemia and in patients with glucose-6-phosphate dehydrogenase (G-6-PD) deficiency, sulfonamides may cause intravascular haemolysis.

The other CNS effects include depression, confusion, tinnitus, fatigue etc.

Therapeutic Uses

Because of development of resistance and availability of more advanced antimicrobial agents, the use of sulfonamides is limited. However they are used in combination with trimethoprim. The important therapeutic uses are:

i. **Urinary tract infection:** Used in chronic suppressive therapy in various UTI conditions e.g. acute cystitis.
ii. **Acute bacillary dysentery**.
iii. **Ulcerative colitis,** mainly sulfasalazine (a chemical combination of sulfapyridine and 5-amino salicylic acid) is used in the treatment of ulcerative colitis.
iv. **Streptococcal pharyngitis,** prophylaxis of rheumatic fever and tonsillitis.
v. **Trachoma and inclusion conjunctivitis:** Sulphacetamide (10-30%) local eye drops are used.
vi. **Chancroid:** Sulfadimidine may be used.
vii. In the treatment of **meningococcal meningitis**.
viii. Sulfonamides in combination with pyrimethamine are used in the treatment of **chloroquine resistant malaria**.
ix. **Toxoplasmosis:** Sulfadiazine and pyrimethamine combination is used.
x. **Burns:** Topical silver sulfadiazine or mafenide is used.

TRIMETHOPRIM

Trimethoprim is a pyrimidine derivative (diaminopyrimidine) related to antimalarial drug pyrimethamine, which selectively **inhibits its bacterial dihydrofolate reductase, necessary for the conversion of dihydrofolate to tetrahydrofolic acid**. Sulfonamides act by inhibiting the incorporation of PABA into dihydrofolate by bacteria. A combination of trimethoprim and sulfamethoxazole (cotrimoxazole) act sequentially in the same metabolic pathway in the synthesis of nucleotides.

Adverse Effects

All those side effects seen with sulfonamides.

Therapeutic Uses

Used in all types of infection caused by *Salmonella typhi*, *Klebsiella*, *Enterobacter*, *Pneumocystis carinii* etc. and many other sulfonamide resistant stains of *S. aureus*, *Strep. pyogenes*, *Shigella*, *E. coli*, *H. influenzae*, meningococci and gonococci etc. It is particularly effective as a second line agent in penicillin allergic patients and also in patients where newer antibiotics are contraindicated or can't be used.

The common indications are:

i. **Urinary tract infection**: Acute cystitis.
ii. **Bacterial diarrhoea and dysentery**.
iii. **Respiratory tract infection** such as chronic bronchitis and otitis media etc.
iv. In the treatment of **typhoid**.
v. **Chancroid**.
vi. **Sexually transmitted diseases**.
vii. Prophylaxis and treatment of certain **HIV associated infections**.
viii. For the prophylaxis of **certain concurrent bacterial infections** e.g. organ transplantation patients receiving immunosuppressants.
ix. **Nosocomial infections**.

Despite development of resistance to this combination in certain microorganisms, it has been used widely for several clinical indications. The combination is cheaper than newer antibiotics.

NITROFURANS

It possesses antimicrobial action against gram positive and negative organisms including staphylococci, streptococci, *E. coli*, *Salmonella* and *Shigella* species.

NITROFURANTOIN

Bacteriostatic drug. It is effective against a variety of gram positive and negative organisms including *E. coli* and *Aerobacter*. It is most commonly used as urinary antiseptic for prophylaxis and treatment of urinary tract infections.

Adverse effects are nausea, diarrhoea, haemolytic anaemia in persons with G-6-PD deficiency and peripheral neuritis (on long-term use).

Dose: FURADANTIN; 50-100 mg TDS-QID.

NITROFURAZONE

Bactericidal drug for both gram positive and negative bacteria. Acts by inhibiting enzymes necessary for carbohydrate metabolism in bacteria. It is available as ointment. Used for the topical treatment of superficial wounds and skin infections. FURACIN; 0.2% ointment/cream.

FURAZOLIDONE

This is mainly employed for the treatment of gastrointestinal infections e.g. bacillary dysentery, giardiasis, bacterial enteritis etc.

Dose: FUROXONE; 100-200 mg TDS-QID.

QUINOLONES

Quinolones, are synthetic antimicrobial agents effective against gram negative bacteria. Although newer compounds (second generation quinolones – the fluoroquinolones) are also effective against gram positive bacteria.

The important quinolones are synthetic fluorinated analogs of nalidixic acid (which was introduced in mid 1960s and had limited use in UTI and GIT infections). They are active against a variety of gram positive and gram negative bacteria. Quinolones **block bacterial DNA synthesis by inhibiting bacterial topoisomerase II (DNA gyrase) and topoisomerase IV**. Inhibition of DNA gyrase prevents the relaxation of positively supercoiled DNA that is required for normal transcription and replication.

The important quinolones are listed in table 9.1.3.

NALIDIXIC ACID

It is 4-quinolone derivative effective against gram negative bacteria mainly *E. coli* and *Shigella*. It is less effective against *Klebsiella* and *Aerobacter* species and very rarely against *Pseudomonas*. Acts by inhibiting bacterial DNA gyrase.

It is mainly **used** as urinary antiseptic and in diarrhoea caused by *E. coli, Shigella, Salmonella*.

The main **side effects** are GIT upset, headache, drowsiness, vertigo, visual disturbances and on prolonged use can produce parkinsonism like symptoms. In individuals with G-6-PD deficiency can cause haemolysis.

FLUOROQUINOLONES

These are quinolone antimicrobial agents having one or more fluorine substitutions, relatively broad spectrum of action and effective against gram positive and gram negative organisms. They are highly effective against *E. coli, Klebsiella, Proteus mirabilis, Shigella, Salmonella* species, *H. ducreyi* etc. The **fluoroquinolones inhibit bacterial enzyme DNA gyrase**.

The presence of a 6-fluoro and 7-piperazine substitution greatly enhances their antimicrobial efficacy as compared to nalidixic acid. The fluorine atom is responsible for increased potency against gram negative organisms and broadens the spectrum of their activity including gram

Table 9.1.3: *Classification of quinolones.*

Nalidixic acid (GRAMONEG)	0.5-1.0 g QID
Ciprofloxacin (CIPLOX)	250-750 mg BD
Norfloxacin (NORFLOX)	400 mg BD
Pefloxacin (QUCIN)	400 mg BD
Sparfloxacin (SPARFLOX)	200-400 mg OD
Ofloxacin (OFLIN)	200-400 mg BD
Levofloxacin (LOXOF)	500 mg OD
Gatifloxacin (GATILOX)	400 mg OD, eye drop (0.3%)

positive organism. The piperazine moiety imparts antipseudomonal activity.

After oral administration, the fluoroquinolones are well absorbed with the bioavailability of 80 to 95 % and distributed widely in body fluids and tissues. Depending upon the newer compound, the different dose regimen have been adopted. The fluoroquinolones are excreted mainly by tubular secretion and by glomerular filtration.

Fluoroquinolones are well tolerated. The most common **adverse effects** are nausea, vomiting, diarrhoea, headache, insomnia, skin rash and occasionally abnormal liver function tests (with trovafloxacin). Phototoxicity has been particularly reported with pefloxacin, lomefloxacin, sparfloxacin and ofloxacin. Tendinitis is a serious side effect rarely reported in adults. Because of cartilage damage in children it must be used under close supervision.

Therapeutic Uses

The most common conditions in which fluoroquinolones may be useful is:

- Urinary tract infections.
- Bacterial gastroenteritis.
- Typhoid fever.
- In septicemia.
- In otitis media.
- Respiratory infections e.g. acute pneumonia etc.
- Ocular infections and
- Other infections caused by *E. coli*, *K. pneumoniae*, *Enterobacter*, *Salmonella typhi*, *N. gonorrhoeae*, *N. meningitidis*, *H. influenzae*, *H. ducreyi*, *Shilgella*, *Vibrio cholerae*, *Pseudomonas aeruginosa*, *Staph. aureus* etc.

CIPROFLOXACIN

It is the most potent first generation fluoroquinolone, effective against a broad range of microorganisms. The most susceptible one are the aerobic gram negative bacilli.

It attains several times higher concentration in the urine than plasma. Ciprofloxacin produces rapid and complete clinical relief in nosocomial bronchopneumonia patients. It has been successfully used prior to cardiac surgery and has attained levels higher than MICs for the commonly susceptible pathogens for at least 8 hours. The bone, soft tissue and skin infections, bacterial gastroenteritis, severe/ complicated UTI will respond to ciprofloxacin. It has been used widely as a drug of first choice for typhoid fever, however, resistance has also been reported. It is also **useful** in respiratory infections due to *Mycoplasma*, *Legionella*, multidrug resistant tuberculosis and as topical agent in conjunctivitis.

The drug has been used alone as well as in combination.

NORFLOXACIN

It is less potent than ciprofloxacin and is primarily **used** in genitourinary tract infections. It is relatively more potent than ciprofloxacin in above condition. It is not useful in respiratory and systemic infections due to gram positive cocci.

PEFLOXACIN

It is a methyl derivative of norfloxacin which penetrates tissues better and attains higher plasma concentration. Concentration in CSF is higher than other fluoroquinolones, therefore is preferred drug for meningeal infections. It is **used** in the treatment of gonorrhoea and typhoid. Genotoxicity has been reported at higher concentration of pefloxacin.

SPARFLOXACIN

It is difluorinated quinolone effective against gram positive bacteria, anaerobes and mycobacteria. It is **used** in the treatment of pneumonia, chronic bronchitis, sinusitis etc.

OFLOXACIN

It is more potent than ciprofloxacin for gram positive organisms. It also inhibits *Mycobacterium tuberculosis* and *Mycobacterium leprae* and used as alternative in multidrug resistant therapeutic regimens. It is also used in the treatment of chronic bronchitis and other ENT infections. Also used in gonorrhoea, gonococcal urethritis and urinary tract infections due to *E. coli, K. pneumoniae, P. mirabilis, Citrobacter diversus* or *paeruginosa. Mycoplasma pneumoniae, U. urealyticum* are also susceptible. The anaerobes like *Bacteroides fragilis, Clostridium perfringens, B. intermedium, C. welchii, Peptococcus niger, Peptostreptococcus* sp. respond well to ofloxacin *in vitro*. It does not inhibit the cytochrome P450.

LEVOFLOXACIN

It is the levoisomer of ofloxacin and having better activity than ciprofloxacin and ofloxacin against *S. pneumoniae*. It is also **used** in chronic bronchitis, sinusitis, pyelonephritis, and other related infections of soft tissues. Due to high oral bioavailability, patient can be shifted from IV to oral therapy. It can be administered just once a day regimen as an alternate to other fluoroquinolones in the treatment of respiratory infections.

GATIFLOXACIN

The antibacterial action of gatifloxacin result from **inhibition of DNA gyrase and topoisomerase IV**. DNA gyrase is an essential enzyme that is involved in the replication, transcription and repair of bacterial DNA. Topoisomerase IV is an enzyme known to play a key role in the partitioning of the chromosomal DNA during bacterial cell division.

Gatifloxacin ophthalmic solution is the first FDA approved fourth generation fluoroquinolone and is available in Indian market.

❑❑❑

CHAPTER 9.2 Tetracyclines, Chloramphenicol and Chemotherapy of UTI

TETRACYCLINES

The tetracyclines are a group of drugs with a common basic chemical structure and pharmacological activity. The first tetracycline, chlortetracycline was isolated from *Streptomyces aureofaciens,* then oxytetracycline was derived from *Streptomyces rimosus* and then tetracycline was obtained by catalytic dehalogenation of chlortetracycline. They are classified as in table 9.2.1.

Mechanism of Action

The tetracyclines are primarily **bacteriostatic** and are thought to exert their antimicrobial **effect by the inhibition of protein synthesis**. The tetracyclines, including doxycycline, have a similar antimicrobial spectrum of activity against a wide range of gram positive and negative organisms. Cross-resistance of these organisms to tetracyclines is common.

Antimicrobial Spectrum of Activity

Tetracyclines has one of the widest spectrum amongst antimicrobials. The microbes that are sensitive to tetracycline include *Staph. aureus, Staph. epidermidis, Strep. pyogenes, Strep. viridans, Strep. pneumoniae, Strep. faecalis (UTI), Listeria monocytogenes, Bacillus anthracis, Clostridium* sp., *Actinomyces* sp., *T. pallidum, T. pertenue, Borrelia recurrentis, Fusobacterium fusiforme, Brucella* sp. and bacteroides sp. Commonly occurring gram negative organisms e.g. *H. influenzae, H. ducreyi, Neisseria gonorrhoeae,*

Table 9.2.1: *Classification of tetracyclines.*

• Tetracycline (SUBAMYCIN)	250-500 mg/day, 1-3% topical (eye/ear drop, skin oint)
Oxytetracycline (TERRAMYCIN)	250-500 mg/day, 1-3% topical (skin, eye ointment)
Chlortetracycline (AUREOMYCIN)	250-500 mg/day, 1-3% topical (skin, eye ointment)
Demeclocycline (LEDERMYCIN)	300 mg BD, 0.5% skin oint.
Doxycycline (BIODOXI)	200 mg OD
Minocycline (CANOMYCIN)	100 mg BD

V. cholerae, E. coli, Enterobacter aerogenes, Shigella sp. are also highly *sensitive.* Atypical bacteria e.g. *Chlamydia* sp., *Mycoplasma* sp., *Ureaplasma urealyticum* as well as *Rickettsia* are extremely sensitive to tetracycline. Besides being highly effective against a wide range of gram positive and negative organisms, tetracycline is effective against all bacteria responsible for sexually transmitted diseases viz. syphilis, gonorrhoea, chancroid and nongonococcal urethritis. It is effective/synergistic with specific drugs against even protozoa and fungi. Though effective against a number of anaerobes it can not be relied upon as sole therapy of anaerobic infections. Tetracycline is not effective against viruses, *Pseudomonas, Proteus* and *Klebsiella.*

Pharmacokinetics

The absorption of tetracycline administered orally is variable and depend upon the type of tetracycline used. The tetracycline form insoluble complexes i.e. chelation with calcium, magnesium, milk and antacids reduce their absorption. Administration of iron also interferes with the absorption of tetracycline. Doxycycline is rapidly and virtually completely absorbed after oral administration and its absorption is not affected by presence of food or milk.

The tetracyclines are widely distributed in the body and diffuse into various body fluids.

Adverse Effects

Because of virtually complete absorption of doxycycline and minocycline side effects pertaining to the lower bowel, particularly diarrhoea have been infrequent. The following side effects have been observed with the use of tetracycline including doxycycline.

Anorexia, nausea, vomiting, diarrhoea, glossitis, dysphagia, maculopapular and erythematous rashes and photosensitivity; **hypersensitivity reactions** including urticaria, angioneurotic edema, anaphylaxis, anaphylactoid reactions. They also cause discoloration of deciduous teeth.

Therapeutic Use

1. **Orodental infection** caused by mixed aerobic, anaerobic bacteria including Vincent's infection caused by *Fusobacterium.* Tetracycline also prove to be beneficial in peridontal inflammation by scavenging free radicals. Its use in pregnancy, lactation and in children is contraindicated. Its use in dentistry is very much restricted due to its chelating effect on teeth and bones.
1. **Respiratory tract infection**: Bronchitis, pneumonia and other lower respiratory tract infections due to susceptible strains of *Strep. pneumoniae, H. influenzae, K. pneumoniae* and other organisms including *Mycoplasma pneumoniae.* Upper respiratory tract infections including sinusitis, otitis, mastoiditis.
2. **Urinary tract infection**: Caused by susceptible strains of *Klebsiella* sp., *Enterobacter* sp., *Strep. faecalis* and other organisms.
3. **Sexually transmitted diseases**: Uncomplicated urethral, endocervical and rectal infections. Non gonococcal urethritis (NGU) caused by *Ureaplasma urealyticum*, chancroid caused by *H.*

ducreyi, granuloma inguinale caused by *Calymmatobacterium granulomatis*.

As an alternative drug in the treatment of gonorrhoea and syphilis in patients allergic to penicillin.

4. **Dermatological infections**: Acne vulgaris, when antibiotic therapy is considered necessary.
5. **Ophthalmic infections**: Due to susceptible strains of *N. gonorrhoeae*, staphylococci, *H. influenzae* and in the treatment of trachoma.
6. Prophylaxis and treatment of Traveller's diarrhoea.
7. **Miscellaneous infections** caused by susceptible strains of bacteria causing psittacosis, cholera, melioidosis, leptospirosis, brucellosis, bartonellosis, plague, tularemia, *Campylobacter fetus* infection, rickettsial infections including typhus and Q fever, relapsing fever due to *Borrelia recurrentis* and actinomycosis in penicillin allergic patients.
9. As an adjunct in acute intestinal amoebiasis.
10. Prophylaxis of malaria due to *P. falciparum*.

CHLORAMPHENICOL

It is a broad spectrum antibiotic originally derived from *Streptomyces venezuelae* and later on became the first completely synthetic antibiotic. It is used as palmitate and sodium succinate salt in given dosage.

Dose: 250-500 mg QID oral, 1-2 g IM injection, 0.5-1.0% topical (eye ointment/drops/applicap and ear drops).

Chloramphenicol is a **potent inhibitor of microbial protein synthesis. It acts by binding reversibly to the 50S submit of the bacterial ribosome. It inhibits the peptidyl transferase step of protein synthesis**. It is bacteriostatic broad-spectrum antibiotic active against gram positive and negative organisms, *Rickettsia*, the *Chlamydia* of the psittacosis, lymphogranuloma group and *Mycoplasma pneumoniae*. The other organisms sensitive to chloramphenicol are *E. coli*, *K. pneumoniae*, *Shigella*, and certain strains of *Brucella*, *Pasteurella*, *Proteus* and *Vibrio comma*. It exerts bactericidal against *H. influenzae*, *Strep. pneumoniae* and *N. meningitidis*.

Pharmacokinetics

Chloramphenicol is completely absorbed after oral administration, bound to plasma protein (approximately 60%) and widely distributed in body. It crosses the blood-brain and placental barrier and shows its presence in CSF, bile and milk. It is conjugated with glucuronic acid in liver and excreted in urine. Small amount is excreted in urine in unchanged form.

Adverse Effects

Allergic reaction includes skin rashes, drug fever, dermatitis, angioneurotic edema.

Bone marrow depression includes aplastic anaemia, leukopenia, agranulocytosis, thrombocytopenia.

Gray baby syndrome: Premature babies develop vomiting, hypothermia, abdominal distension, shallow irregular respiration and further leading to gray cyanosis, vascular collapse, shock and death.

CNS toxicity includes headache, mental confusion, internal ophthalmoplegia, peripheral neuritis, depression, optical neuritis.

Other adverse effects include superinfection, hepatotoxicity and typhoid shock.

Therapeutic Uses

Because of bone marrow toxicity of chloramphenicol, its use is restricted to the treatment of infection caused by *S. typhi* and *paratyphi* (treatment of typhoid fever).

Other indications in which chloramphenicol can be used are *H. influenzae* meningitis, urinary tract infections, anaerobic infections caused by *Bacteroides fragilis* and locally in eye and external ear infections.

CHEMOTHERAPY OF URINARY TRACT INFECTIONS

URINARY ANTISEPTICS

Urinary antiseptics are orally administered agents that exert antibacterial activity in the urine but have no systemic antibacterial activity. Urinary antiseptics are listed as in table 9.2.2.

NITROFURANTOIN

It is bacteriostatic and but bactericidal against many gram positive and negative organisms in higher concentration and acidic urine. *Pseudomonas aeruginosa* and various strains of *Proteus* are resistant. It antagonizes the action of nalidixic acid and its activity is enhanced by lower pH. After oral administration it is rapidly and completely absorbed from GIT, metabolized in liver and less than half is excreted unchanged in urine.

It is used exclusively for urinary tract infections. The **side effects** include nausea, vomiting, diarrhoea, anorexia, leukopenia, haemolytic anaemia, jaundice, dizziness and headache. On chronic use can lead to peripheral neuritis and interstitial pulmonary fibrosis.

METHENAMINE

Methenamine mandelate is a salt of mandelic acid and methenamine and both of these possess property of urinary antiseptic. It is rapidly absorbed in gastrointestinal tract and excreted unchanged in urine, where it broken down in acidic pH (< 5) of urine and formaldehyde is released, which inhibits most of the bacteria. It is administered with sodium biphosphate, mandelic acid or ascorbic acid to keep the urinary pH below 6. Its **use** is restricted to chronic, resistant type of UTI.

Adverse effects are gastritis, hematuria, chemical cystitis and skin rash. It is contraindicated in renal failure and hepatic insufficiency.

Table 9.2.2: *Classification of urinary antiseptics.*

Nitrofurantoin (FURADANTIN)	50-100 mg QID
Methenamine (as mendelate & hippurate)	1 g TDS-QID
Phenazopyridine (PYRIDIUM)	200-400 mg TDS
Other antimicrobial agents used in urinary tract infection e.g. sulfonamides, quinolones, penicillins, cephalosporins etc. (details are discussed in respective sections).	

PHENAZOPYRIDINE

It is used for symptomatic relief of urinary burning sensation and urgency due to cystitis. It is a orange dye and excreted in urine. It has no antibacterial property.

URINARY ALKALINIZERS AND ACIDIFIERS

Certain antimicrobial agents used to treat urinary tract infections act better in acidic pH i.e. nitrofurantoin, tetracycline, methenamine, cloxacillin. Certain other antimicrobial agents such as gentamicin, cephalosporins, fluoroquinolones, cotrimoxazole act better in alkaline medium. In specific cases, where urine of desired reaction (acidic or alkaline), some acidifying or alkalinizing agents is sometimes used to get a desired clinical result. Urinary pH can be increased by carbonic anhydrase inhibitors (e.g. acetazolamide) and prolonged therapy requires bicarbonate administration. In treatment of drug poisoning, the excretion of some drugs can be hastened by acidification and alkalinization of the urine. Ammonium chloride is used to acidify urine and potassium acetate/citrate is used to alkalinize urine.

❑❑❑

CHAPTER 9.3 Beta Lactam Antibiotics

PENICILLINS

Penicillin was originally extracted from the mould *Penicillium notatum* but now it is extracted from its related mould *Penicillium chrysogenum* due to its high yield. Penicillin consists of thiazolidine ring fused with a beta lactam ring which is essential for its antibacterial activity. These two rings forms a nucleus named as 6-aminopenicillanic acid.

Mechanism of Action

The bacterial cell wall is a rigid outer layer that completely surrounds the cytoplasmic membrane. Penicillin and other betalactam antibiotics **inhibit bacterial growth by interfering with a specific step in bacterial cell wall synthesis**. Penicillins are classified as in table 9.3.1.

BENZYL PENICILLIN

It is the most potent β-lactam antibiotic and inhibits the growth of susceptible microorganism *in vitro* in lowest concentration and is available in water soluble sodium and potassium salts.

Penicillin is effective against gram positive and negative cocci and some gram positive bacilli. Among the cocci, streptococci are highly sensitive. Gonococci, pneumococci and meningococci are sensitive to penicillin.

Among the bacilli, gram positive *Bacillus anthracis, Corynebacterium diphtheriae, Clostridium* species are highly sensitive. Among the spirochetes, *Treponema pallidum* is highly sensitive to penicillin.

Gram negative bacilli, fungi, protozoa, rickettsiae, chlamydiae, viruses and *Mycobacterium tuberculosis* are totally insensitive to penicillin.

Pharmacokinetics

After oral administration, benzyl penicillin is destroyed by gastric acid. It is mainly absorbed from the duodenum. It is absorbed in aqueous solution rapidly after intramuscular or subcutaneous administration. Penicillin is widely distributed in the body after absorption and approximately 60% of plasma penicillin is bound to albumin. The major

Table 9.3.1: *Classification of penicillins.*

I. **Penicillinase sensitive penicillins**	
Benzyl penicillin (Penicillin G; sodium and potassium salt)	0.5-5 MU* IM/IV
Procaine penicillin G	0.5-1 MU IM
Benzathine penicillin G (PENIDURE)	0.6-2.4 MU IM
Phenoxymethyl penicillin (Penicillin V; KAYPEN)	250-500 mg/day
II. **Penicillinase resistant penicillin**	
Cloxacillin (BIOCLOX)	250-500 mg 6 hourly oral/IM/slow IV
III. **Broad spectrum penicillins**	
Ampicillin (BIOCILIN)	0.25-2 g 6 hourly, oral/IM/slow IV
Amoxycillin (NOVAMOX)	0.25-1 g/day
IV. **β-Lactamase Inhibitors**	
Clavulanic acid	125-250 mg/day oral, IV
Sulbactam	0.25-1 g/day IM/IV
V. **Antipseudomonal penicillins**	
Carbenicillin (BIOPENCE)	1-2 g/day IM, 1-5 g IV 4-6 hourly
Piperacillin (PIPRACIL)	25-50 mg/kg IM/IV 6 hourly
Ticarcillin	200-300 mg/kg/day IV 4-6 hourly

* IU of crystalline sod. benzyl penicillin = 0.6 mg of standard preparation (1 MU = 0.6 g or 1 g = 1.6 million units).

portion is rapidly excreted by the kidney mainly by tubular secretion and small amounts appear in bile, saliva, and milk.

Adverse Effects

The penicillins are nontoxic and remarkably safe drug. The hypersensitivity reaction leading to anaphylaxis is only major problem which is seen in approximately 5 to 10% of the patients taking penicillin.

The minor **adverse effects** include nausea, vomiting, pain and inflammation at the site of injection after intramuscular administration has been reported. After intrathecal administration (which is a contraindication) it may lead to convulsions, arachnoiditis and encephalopathy.

The *major side effect is allergic reactions and anaphylaxis* which is characterized by skin rash, pruritus, serum sickness like syndrome, eosinophilia, angioneurotic edema, asthma, haematuria, albuminuria, haemolytic anemia, granulocytopenia and anaphylaxis.

To avoid that, a ***skin test*** using a 10,000 U of benzyl penicillin per ml is to be done and if any local edema or wheal occurs within 15 minutes, it is considered to be as a positive test and in that person penicillin should not be used.

Therapeutic Uses

Penicillin G is the drug of choice for the following categories of infection:

- **Dental infections:** Penicillin G is effective in majority of infections caused by both aerobic and anaerobic bacteria in dentistry. It is used in acute suppurative pulpits, pericoronitis, oral cellulitis, necrorotizing ulcerative gingivitis etc. But due to penicillin resistance, its use in dentistry is restricted.

- **Streptococcal infections:** Pharyngitis, rheumatic fever, otitis media and even for subacute bacterial endocarditis.
- **Staphylococcal infections:** Penicillinase resistant penicillin can be used.
- **Meningococcal infections:** Meningitis & other infections caused by meningococci.
- **Pneumococcal infections:** Pneumonia and meningitis.
- **Gonococcal infection:** Procaine penicillin along with probenecid can be used.
- **Sexually transmitted diseases:** Penicillin is a drug of choice in the treatment of syphilis.
- In the treatment of **actinomycosis** and **anthrax**.
- In the treatment of **diphtheria**, **tetanus** and **gas gangrene**.
- Penicillins are also used in the **prophylaxis of rheumatic fever, sexually transmitted diseases** e.g. gonorrhoea and syphilis and **bacterial endocarditis**.

SEMISYNTHETIC PENICILLINS

Semisynthetic penicillins are produced by combining the specific side chains in place of benzyl side chain. They have been produced to overcome the shortcomings of benzyl penicillin like poor bioavailability, susceptibility to penicillinase and narrow spectrum of activity.

PHENOXYMETHYL PENICILLIN

It has an antibacterial spectrum similar to benzyl penicillin but is less active. It is gastric acid stable and effective on oral administration.

Adverse effects include urticaria, fever, rashes, angioedema, anaphylaxis, haemolytic anemia, neutropenia, thrombocytopenia, coagulation disorders, diarrhoea etc.

It is **used** in tonsillitis, otitis media, erysipelas, prophylaxis of rheumatic fever and pneumococcal infections.

PENICILLINASE RESISTANT PENICILLIN

It is resistant to degradation by penicillinase. Mainly it exhibits activity against gram positive microorganisms and is useful against penicillinase producing *Staph. aureus*.

CLOXACILLIN

It has an isoxzalyl side chain and has weaker antibacterial activity than benzyl penicillin. It is absorbed after oral administration partially and elimination occurs mainly by kidney and partly by liver. It is devoid of any serious side effect but can cause hypersensitivity reaction in some patients.

Other analogs of cloxacillin are dicloxacillin and flucloxacillin. They are relatively less protein bound, however, dicloxacillin gives approximately double the blood level than cloxacillin.

BROAD SPECTRUM PENICILLINS

They have broad antibacterial spectrum and are effective against both gram positive and gram negative organisms. They are hydrolysed by penicillinase.

AMPICILLIN

It is a broad spectrum penicillin which is not destroyed by gastric acid but is penicillinase susceptible. It is more effective than benzyl penicillin against a variety of gram negative microorganisms.

After oral administration it is readily but incompletely absorbed and food interferes with its absorption. Peak plasma level are reached within two hours after oral administration and one hour after IM administration. It is excreted in urine in unchanged form and high amount is also present in the bile.

Adverse effects include skin rash, nausea, epigastric distress, diarrhoea, drug fever, urticaria etc.

It is **used** in infection caused by susceptible gram positive and gram negative organisms (respiratory tract, soft tissue, gonococcal, GI and genitourinary infections), septicaemia, meningitis, chronic bronchitis, otitis media, sinusitis, invasive salmonellosis and cholecystitis.

AMOXYCILLIN

Amoxycillin is a semisynthetic penicillin, a close congener of ampicillin and active against gram positive and negative organisms. Its absorption is more complete than ampicillin. Food does not interfere with its absorption. Its absorption after oral administration is complete hence less incidence of diarrhoea. It is eliminated in urine in unchanged form.

Adverse effects include nausea, epigastric distress, diarrhoea, skin rash, urticaria, serum sickness, thrombocytopenia, leucopenia, eosinophilia etc.

It is **used** in respiratory, genitourinary, skin and soft tissue, ENT infections caused by pneumococci, streptococci, staphylococci, *H. influenzae, E. coli* and other susceptible organisms. Also useful in *Chlamydia trachomatis* in pregnancy, meningitis due to susceptible strains of gram negative microorganisms, enteric fever, gonococcal urethritis, bacteriaemia and septicaemia. Amoxycillin is also used in chemoprophylaxis during dental procedures.

Amoxycillin is also used in combination with clavulanate potassium. The formulation of amoxycillin with clavulanic acid protects amoxycillin from degradation by beta lactamase enzymes and effectively extends the antibiotic spectrum of amoxycillin to include β lactamase producing bacteria normally resistant to amoxycillin and other betalactam antibiotics.

Amoxycillin along with bromhexine and carbocisteine is used in bronchitis, bronchopneumonia, bronchiectasis, sinusitis and otitis media.

Amoxycillin along with cloxacillin is used in lower respiratory tract, skin and soft tissue, urinary tract and postoperative infections, osteomyelitis, gynaecological infections, septicaemia, bacterial endocarditis and bacterial meningitis.

Amoxycillin along with probenecid is used in bacterial septicaemia, skin and soft tissue infection, acute and chronic respiratory tract infections.

β-Lactamase Inhibitors

CLAVULANIC ACID

It 'progressively' inhibits a wide variety of β-lactamases produced by gram positive and negative organisms and is obtained from *Streptomyces clavuligerus*. It has no antibacterial activity of its own.

It is used along with amoxycillin in various infections as discussed above.

SULBACTAM

It is another semisynthetic β-lactamase inhibitor used along with ampicillin. It is related to clavulanic acid both chemically and in activity.

Adverse effects include diarrhoea, rash, pain at site of injection and thrombophlebitis of injected vein.

It is **indicated** in gynaecological, intra-abdominal, skin and soft tissue infections.

Antipseudomonal Penicillins

These are indicated mainly to treat gram negative bacilli infection by pseudomonas, proteus and enterobacter.

CARBENICILLIN

It is a penicillinase susceptible and is principally indicated for serious infection caused by *Pseudomonas aeruginosa*. It is effective against certain other gram negative bacilli including *Proteus* species and *Bacteroides fragilis*.

Adverse effects include platelet dysfunction, hypokalemia and hypersensitivity reaction.

It is **indicated** in bacteriaemia, septicaemia, genitourinary and respiratory tract infections, endocarditis and postoperative infections caused by pseudomonas or proteus.

PIPERACILLIN

The unique advantages of piperacillin are broad spectrum of antibacterial activity and excellent antipseudomonal activity.

They have a synergistic effect with aminoglycosides (e.g. gentamicin or netilmicin) and hence should be given concomitantly in pseudomonas septicaemia. They should however, not be mixed in the same syringe. Owing to the sodium content, high doses may lead to hypernatremia.

Adverse effects include platelet dysfunction leading to bleeding, superinfection, local pain and thrombophlebitis.

It is **indicated** in systemic and local infections, gynaecological infections, UTI, RTI, neonatal and lifethreatening paediatric infections, burns and septicaemia caused by susceptible organisms.

TICARCILLIN

It is derived from penicillin nucleus 6-aminopenicillanic acid. It has broad spectrum of activity against both gram positive and negative organisms. It is more potent than carbenicillin against *Pseudomonas.*

Adverse effects include hypersensitivity, thrombocytopenia, neutropenia, leucopenia, pain at the site of injection and GI disturbances.

It is **indicated** in bacterial septicaemia, skin and soft tissue infections, acute and chronic respiratory tract infections.

CEPHALOSPORINS

Cephalosporins are important bactericidal broad spectrum β-lactam antibiotics used for the treatment of septicaemia, pneumonia, meningitis, urinary tract infections, peritonitis and biliary tract infections. They are obtained from fungus *Cephalosporium acremonium* and are chemically related to penicillin. It consists of beta lactam ring fused to a dihydrothiazine ring.

All cephalosporins **act by inhibiting bacterial cell wall synthesis and are bactericidal**. Also the autolytic enzymes in cell wall may be activated leading to bacterial death.

They are widely distributed after administration throughout body fluids. Cephalosporins are mainly excreted by the kidneys and dose should be altered in patients with renal disease.

Cephalosporins are classified as in table 9.3.2.

Antibacterial activity: Cephalosporins are active against a wide range of gram positive and negative bacteria which includes pneumococci, *C. diphtheriae, E. coli, N. gonorrhoeae, Proteus mirabilis, S. typhi* and *paratyphi*. The newer cephalosporins are effective against *Pseudomonas aeruginosa*. In dentistry, cephalosporins is used only as alternative to penicillin or amoxycillin in patients who are allergic to penicillins. The second generation cephalosporins are having good activity against oral anaerobes and are generally preferred in dentistry.

Pharmacokinetics

Cephalosporins are distributed in the body after oral or parenteral administration in same manner as penicillin is distributed. The majority are not metabolized and are eliminated by kidney.

Table 9.3.2: *Classification of cephalosporins.*

I. **First generation cephalosporins**	
Cephalexin (SPORIDEX)	1-4 g QID
Cefazolin (AZOLIN)	1-4 g/d IM/IV
Cefadroxil (ODOXIL)	0.5-1 g BD
II. **Second generation cephalosporins**	
Cefuroxime (CEFTUM)	250-500 mg BD
Cefaclor (KEFLOR)	250-500 mg TDS
Cefoxitin	1-2 g/day IM/IV
III. **Third generation cephalosporins**	
Cefotaxime (OMNATAX)	1-2 g TDS, IM/IV
Ceftriaxone (CEFAXONE)	0.5-2 g OD IM/IV
Ceftizoxime (CEFIZOX)	1-3 g BD-TDS
Cefixime (BIOTAX-O)	200-400 mg OD-BD
Cefoperazone (CEFOMYCIN)	1-2 g TDS IM/IV
IV. **Fourth generation (Newer) cephalosporins**	
Cefpirome (FORGEN)	1-2 g BD
Cefepime (KEFAGE)	1-2 g BD-TDS IV

Adverse Reactions

Cephalosporins are generally well tolerated and various side effects include pain at the site of injection and can also cause thrombophlebitis. Allergic reactions include skin rash, fever, serum sickness, eosinophilia, neutropenia and rarely anaphylactic reaction.

CNS side effects include nystagmus and hallucinations and some of the newer compounds can cause disulfiram like reaction.

Larger doses can cause nephrotoxicity.

First Generation Cephalosporins

Highly active against gram positive but weaker against gram negative bacteria.

CEPHALEXIN

It is orally active first generation cephalosporin and less active against penicillinase producing staphylococci.

Adverse effects include skin rash, urticaria, nausea, vomiting, diarrhoea and neutropenia.

It is excreted unchanged in urine. It is **indicated** in respiratory, genitourinary, skin and soft tissue infections, bone and joint infections, dental and ENT infections.

CEFAZOLIN

It is a semisynthetic potent cephalosporin for parenteral administration. It can be administered less frequently because of its long half life. It is **used** in infections of genitourinary tract, bone, joint and soft tissue infections, septicaemia, endocarditis, gonorrhoea, postoperative chest infections, biliary tract infection and surgical prophylaxis.

CEFADROXIL

It has good tissue penetration. Excreted unchanged in urine. **Used** in soft tissue and skin infection caused by staphylococci or streptococci, pharyngitis, tonsillitis, ENT infections and urinary tract infections.

Second Generation Cephalosporins

CEFUROXIME

It is effective against a wide range of gram positive and negative organisms. It is **indicated** in:

- Lower respiratory tract infections e.g., pneumonia, acute bronchitis and acute exacerbations of chronic bronchitis.
- ENT infections, such as otitis media, sinusitis, tonsillitis and pharyngitis.
- Genitourinary tract infections e.g., pyelonephritis, cystitis and urethritis.
- Skin and soft tissue infections e.g., furunculosis, pyoderma and impetigo.
- Enteric fever.
- Gonorrhoea, acute uncomplicated gonococcal urethritis, and cervicitis.

Adverse reactions to cefuroxime have been generally mild and transient in nature. As with other cephalosporins there have been rare reports of erythema multiforme, Steven-Johnson syndrome, toxic epidermal necrolysis (exanthematic necrolysis) and hypersensitivity reactions including skin rashes, urticaria, pruritus, drug fever, serum sickness and very rarely anaphylaxis.

CEFACLOR

The antibacterial spectrum of cefaclor includes the following organisms: Staphylococci (coagulase-positive, coagulase-negative and penicillinase producing strains), *Streptococcus pyogenes, Streptococcus pneumoniae, Moraxella catarrhalis, H. influenzae* including beta-lactamase producing strains, *E. coli, P. mirabilis, Klebsiella* sp., *N. gonorrhoeae.*

Cefaclor is well absorbed after oral administration. The presence of food may delay the absorption of cefaclor but the total amount absorbed remains unchanged. About 25 percent of the drug is protein bound. Cefaclor is widely distributed in the body. It is rapidly excreted by the kidneys, up to 85% appears unchanged in the urine within two hours.

It is **indicated** in:

- Pneumonia, acute bronchitis and acute exacerbation of chronic bronchitis.
- Otitis media, pharyngitis, tonsillitis and sinusitis.
- Urinary tract infections.
- Skin and soft tissue infections.

Cefaclor is generally well tolerated. However the reported **adverse effects** include mild gastrointestinal reactions (nausea, vomiting, abdominal cramps and diarrhoea). Symptoms of pseudomembranous colitis may appear either during or after antibiotic treatment. The other side effects are allergic in nature viz. skin rash, itching, bronchospasm, hypotension, erythema multiforme, Steven-Johnson syndrome. Other side effects viz. haemolytic anaemia, hypoprothrombinemia, seizures and thrombophlebitis have been rarely reported.

CEFTAZIDIME

It is a broad spectrum cephalosporin having anti-pseudomonal activity. **Used** in serious infections of respiratory tract, ENT and soft tissue infection, septicaemia, meningitis, GI and biliary tract infections.

CEFOXITIN

It is produced by an *Actinomyces.* **Used** in the treatment of anaerobic and mixed surgical infections and lung abscess.

Third Generation Cephalosporins

CEFOTAXIME

A broad spectrum cephalosporin, effective against staphylococci, *Haemophilus influenzae, Salmonella, Shigella, Serratia, Citrobacter, Neisseria and Proteus.*

The drug is given by parenteral route and is deacetylated in body to active metabolite which acts synergistically with parent drug.

Adverse effects include skin rash, drug fever, anaphylaxis, nausea, vomiting, diarrhoea, thrombocytopenia and leucopenia. Local reaction and pain at injection site, pseudomembranous colitis and headache.

It is **used** in respiratory, genitourinary infections including gonorrhoea, septicemia, meningitis, endocarditis; surgical, abdominal, bone and joint infections; preoperative prophylaxis in those at increased risk of infection and CNS infections.

CEFTRIAXONE

It is a broad spectrum cephalosporin having a long half life and administered once daily and **indicated** in meningitis, septicaemia, typhoid, urinary tract infections, prophylaxis in surgical infections, pneumonia, STD, bacteremia and pelvic inflammatory disease.

Adverse effects include diarrhoea, nausea, vomiting, skin rash, urticaria, drug fever, pruritus, dizziness, hypersensitivity reactions, hematological disorders.

It is **indicated** in respiratory tract infections, gonorrhoea, otitis media, urinary tract infection and typhoid fever.

CEFTIZOXIME

It is a parenteral, semisynthetic third generation cephalosporin. It is not metabolised and approximately 90 percent of drug is excreted by the kidney in unchanged form. It is **indicated** in lower respiratory tract, skin and soft tissue infection, septicaemia, urinary tract infection and gonorrhoea.

CEFIXIME

Cefixime is an orally active third-generation cephalosporin antibiotic which has marked *in-vitro* bactericidal activity against a wide variety of gram positive and negative organisms. It is indicated for the treatment of urinary tract, infection, respiratory tract infection and biliary tract infection etc.

Cefixime given orally is about 40 to 50 percent absorbed whether administered with or without food. However, time to maximum absorption is increased approximately 0.8 hours when administered with food. It is excreted unchanged in the urine in 24 hours.

CEFOPERAZONE

It is broad spectrum cephalosporin with anti-pseudomonal activity. It is more susceptible to β-lactamases and is primarily excreted in bile. **Used** in severe susceptible infections of respiratory, urinary, GIT, skin and soft tissues, meningitis, septicaemia, gonorrhoea, bacteremia and peritonitis.

Cefoperazone is also used in combination with sulbactam.

FOURTH GENERATION CEPHALOSPORINS

CEFPIROME

It is fourth generation cephalosporin **used** mainly in serious infections including septicaemia and respiratory tract infections and infections acquired from hospitals. It is resistant to many β-lactamases.

CEFEPIME

Its antibacterial spectrum is similar to that of third generation cephalosporins. It is highly resistant to β-lactamases.

It is **indicated** in bacteremia, septicaemia, febrile neutropenia and hospital acquired infections.

❑❑❑

CHAPTER 9.4

Aminoglycosides Antibiotics

Aminoglycosides are group of **bactericidal antibiotics** originally obtained from various *Streptomyces* species.

All aminoglycosides **act by inhibiting protein synthesis of bacteria by directly combining with ribosomes**. They penetrate the outer cytoplasmic membrane and inhibit protein synthesis. Streptomycin combines with the bacterial 30S ribosomes and inteferes with the mRNA-ribosome combination. Other aminoglycosides bind to additional sites on 50S subunit as well as to 30S-50S interface.

All aminoglycosides are poorly absorbed after oral administration, are more active in alkaline pH and are excreted unchanged by glomerular filtration. Since excretion is principally via the kidney, accumulation occurs in renal impairment.

All the aminoglycosides produce cochlear and vestibular damage (ototoxicity) which is a dose and duration of treatment related side effect. Another serious side effect is nephrotoxicity. Aminoglycosides also reduce the acetylcholine release from the motor nerve endings and cause neuromuscular blockade.

Aminoglycoside antibiotics are classified as in table 9.4.1.

STREPTOMYCIN

The aminoglycoside antibiotic, obtained from *Streptomyces griseus* is the first antitubercular drug.

Table 9.4.1: *Classification of aminoglycoside antibiotics.*

Streptomycin (AMBISTRYN-S)	0.75-1 g/day IM
Gentamicin (TAMIACIN)	3-5 mg/kg/day IM; 0.1-0.3% topical (eye drop, skin ointment/cream)
Tobramycin (TOBACIN)	3-5 mg/kg/day IM/IV
Amikacin (NOVACIN)	15 mg/kg/day IM
Kanamycin (KANSIN)	0.5-1 g/day IM
Neomycin (as sulphate)	0.3-0.5% topical (eye/ear drop, ointment/powder)
Framycetin (SOFRAMYCIN)	0.5-1.0% topical (eye drop/ointment, skin cream)

It is bactericidal drug and **exerts its action by combining with bacterial ribosome and induces misreading of mRNA codons**. Also in sensitive bacteria, disruption of cytoplasmic membrane occurs resulting in leakage of amino acids, ions, leading to bacterial death.

After oral administration it is not absorbed. After IM injection the absorption is rapid. It is excreted unchanged in urine. Half life is prolonged in patients of renal failure.

Adverse effects include pain at injection site, ototoxicity, nephrotoxicity, skin rash, fever, exfoliative dermatitis and eosinophilia. Anaphylaxis is rarely seen. Optic nerve dysfunction.

It is **used** in all forms of tuberculosis along with other antitubercular drugs. Other **indications** are tularemia, plague, brucellosis, bacterial endocarditis, enterococcal endocarditis. Used concomitantly with penicillin G for synergistic effect in the treatment of enterococcal endocarditis when other antibiotics are ineffective or contraindicated.

GENTAMICIN

It is obtained from *Micromonospora pupurea.* It has broader spectrum of action and is effective against *Pseudomonas aeruginosa, E. coli, Klebsiella, Enterobacter* and *Proteus.* Streptococci and enterococci are relatively resistant to it owing to failure of the drug to penetrate into the cell. Following parenteral administration, it defuses mainly into extracellular fluids.

It is **valuable** in critically ill patients with impaired host defence; *Pseudomonas* or *Proteus* infections in burns, urinary tract infections, lung abscesses, osteomyelitis, middle ear infection, septicaemia; meningitis caused by gram negative bacilli, peritonitis, in skin and soft tissue infections and postoperative infection.

Topical administration in the form of drop and ointment have been **used** for the treatment of infected burns, wounds and the prevention of intravenous catheter infections and in the treatment of ocular infections.

Adverse effects include ototoxicity (incidence is related to dose and duration of therapy), nephrotoxicity, hypersensitivity reactions, skin itching, headache, neuromuscular junction blockade, anorexia, nausea, vomiting, superinfection, photosensitivity, drowsiness, weakness, thrombocytopenia, agranulocytosis.

TOBRAMYCIN

It belongs to family nebramycins, is isolated from *Streptomyces tenebrarius*. Its antibacterial activity is similar to gentamicin and slightly more active than gentamicin against *Pseudomonas aeruginosa* and *Proteus*.

It is **used** in the treatment of infection of gastrointestinal and respiratory tract, skin and soft tissue infections, septicaemia and urinary tract infection.

Adverse effects include skin rash, ototoxicity, nephrotoxicity, phlebitis, nausea, vomiting, urticaria and headache. Ototoxicity and nephrotoxicity is lower than gentamicin.

AMIKACIN

It is semisynthetic derivative of kanamycin. It is active against gentamicin resistant organisms e.g. *Pseudomonas aeruginosa, Klebsiella, E. coli* and *Proteus.* It is resistant to bacterial aminoglycoside inactivating enzymes.

It is **indicated** in bacteriaemia, septicaemia; respiratory tract, bones and joints, CNS (including meningitis), skin, soft tissue, intraabdominal infections (including peritonitis); burns and postoperative infections.

Adverse effects include hypersensitivity reactions, nausea, vomiting, nephrotoxicity, ototoxicity, headache and neuromuscular blockade.

KANAMYCIN

It is derived from *Streptomyces kanamyceticus.* It is active against *Pseudomonas,* but due to severe ototoxicity and nephrotoxicity, it is replaced by other aminoglycosides and occasionally used in multidrug resistant cases of tuberculosis.

NEOMYCIN

It is isolated from *Streptomyces fradiae* and is effective against most gram negative bacilli and some gram positive cocci. Because of its high ototoxicity and nephrotoxicity, it is not used systemically and **used** locally in various skin and eye infections.

FRAMYCETIN

It is derived from *Streptomyces lavendule.* It is similar to neomycin and **used** locally in various skin infections and eye/ear infections.

❑❑❑

CHAPTER 9.5 Macrolide and Polypeptide Antibiotics

MACROLIDE ANTIBIOTICS

Macrolides, as their name indicates are characterized by a large or macrocyclic lactone ring with attached sugar residue(s). They are classified as in table 9.5.1

ERYTHROMYCIN

Erythromycin was the first macrocyclic antibiotic which was isolated from *Streptomyces erythreus*. Erythromycin is widely used antibiotic both in children as well as in adults.

It acts by binding with 50S ribosomal subunit of bacteria and inhibit protein synthesis.

It is a **narrow spectrum antibiotic**, low concentration are **bacteriostatic**, however high concentrations are **bactericidal**. The spectrum of activity also depends on the concentration of drug at the desired site and sensitivity of the target microorganisms. It is more active in alkaline medium.

Erythromycin is effective against gram positive and few gram negative organisms which mainly includes pneumococci, streptococci, staphylococci, *Neisseria* and some strains of *C. diphtheriae, H. influenzae, Rickettsiae* and *Treponema.* It is also effective against penicillin resistant staphylococci,

Table 9.5.1: *Classification of macrolide antibiotics.*

Erythromycin	250-500 mg QID
as stearate (RESTOMYCIN)	
as estolate (ALTHROCIN)	
also as ethyl succinate,	0.4-0.6 g every 6 hourly (drop & syrup)
and gluceptate	0.5-1.0 g IV 6 hourly
Roxithromycin (ROXID)	150 mg BD
Azithromycin (ZATHRIN)	500 mg OD
Clarithromycin (CLAMYCIN)	250-500 mg BD
Clindamycin (DALACIN-C)	150-300 mg QID oral, 200-600 mg TDS IV
Lincomycin (LYNX)	500 mg TDS-QID oral, 600 mg IV 6-12 hourly
Vancomycin (FORSTAF)	250-500 mg 6 hourly

Mycoplasma, Campylobacter, Legionella, Gardnerella vaginalis are also highly sensitive.

Adverse effects include gastrointestinal side effects like nausea, epigastric pain are common. Diarrhoea occurs occasionally. Skin rashes, hypersensitivity reaction, hepatotoxicity (hepatitis alongwith cholestatic jaundice, especially with estolate ester), oral candidiasis, thrombophlebitis and fever have been reported.

Erythromycin is **used** as a substitute to penicillin in allergic patients for upper respiratory tract infections, e.g. tonsillitis, pharyngitis and mastoiditis, pneumococcal infection and prophylaxis of rheumatic fever. It is drug of choice in treatment of atypical pneumonia due to *Mycoplasma pneumoniae,* Legionnaire's pneumonia and whooping cough. It is also useful in wound and burn infections and severe impetigo not responding to topical antibiotics.

ROXITHROMYCIN

Roxithromycin is a semisynthetic macrolide antibiotic.

It is effective against *Streptococcus pyogenes, Streptococcus viridans, Streptococcus pneumoniae, Staphylococcus mitis, S. aureus* and coagulase negative staphylococci, *Neisseria meningitidis, Bordetella pertussis, Moraxella catarrhalis, Corynebacterium diphtheriae, Listeria monocytogenes, Clostridium, Mycoplasma pneumoniae, Pasteurella multocida, Chlamydia trachomatis/psittaci/pneumoniae, Ureaplasma urealyticum, Legionella pneumophila, Helicobacter pylori, Gardnerella vaginalis.*

It is more stable in acid media than other macrolides. Roxithromycin is found in the serum after 15 minutes of administration. It is more than 90% plasma protein bound and more than half the dose is excreted unchanged in urine and faeces.

Adverse effects include gastrointestinal symptoms like nausea, vomiting, epigastric pain, diarrhoea, hypersensitivity reactions like rash, urticaria, angioedema, exceptionally bronchospasm, anaphylactic shock; dizzy sensations (caution in driving or use of machinery); moderate increase in ASAT, ALAT and/or alkaline phosphatases; cholestatic or more rarely acute liver injury.

AZITHROMYCIN

Azithromycin is an azalide antibiotic, a sub-class of the macrolides. Azithromycin differs chemically from erythromycin in that a methyl substituted nitrogen atom is incorporated into the lactone ring.

Following oral administration, azithromycin is rapidly absorbed and widely distributed throughout the body. Rapid distribution into tissues and high concentration within cells result in significantly higher azithromycin concentration is tissues than in plasma or serum.

Azithromycin is **indicated** for the treatment of following infections caused by sensitive organisms:

1. **Lower respiratory tract infections:** Community-acquired pneumonia, acute bacterial exacerbations of chronic obstructive pulmonary disease, acute bronchitis due to *Haemophilus influenzae, Moraxella catarrhalis* or *Streptococcus pneumoniae.*
2. Ear, nose and throat infections like tonsillitis, sinusitis, otitis media and pharyngitis.

3. **Skin/skin structure infections:** Furunculosis, pyoderma and impetigo due to *Staphylococcus aureus, S. pyogenes* or *S. agalactiae.*

Adverse reactions include vomiting, dyspepsia, flatulence, jaundice, palpitations, chest pain. Allergic reactions include rash, photosensitivity and angioedema. CNS side effects are headache, dizziness, vertigo and fatigue.

CLARITHROMYCIN

It is a macrolide antibiotic obtained by substitution of hydroxyl group by a CH_3O group in the erythromycin lactone ring. It is found to be 2 to 10 times more active than erythromycin.

Clarithromycin is readily and rapidly absorbed after oral administration and is metabolized significantly in liver. Active metabolite is excreted by kidney and other routes.

It is **indicated** in the treatment of lower respiratory tract infection e.g. bronchitis and pneumonia, upper respiratory tract infections e.g. pharyngitis and sinusitis, infections due to chlamydia, legionella and mycoplasma, skin and soft tissue infections and eradication of *H. pylori* with acid suppressants.

The most frequently reported **side effects** are GI-related complaints i.e. nausea, dyspepsia, abdominal pain and diarrhoea. Other side effects include headache, skin rash and transient elevation of liver enzymes, hepatic dysfunction with or without jaundice and psychosis.

CLINDAMYCIN

It is a lincosamide and **act by binding exclusively to 50S submit of the bacterial ribosomes and hence suppresses protein synthesis**. It is 7-chloro-7-deoxylincomycin, a semisynthetic derivative of lincomycin.

It inhibits most of the gram positive cocci e.g. streptococci, staphylococci and pneumococci, *C. diphtheriae, Actinomyces, Nocardia* and *Toxoplasma.*

It is **used** in the treatment of severe anaerobic infections caused by bacteroides and other anaerobes. It is also used in combination with aminoglycoside in the treatment of abdomen and GIT wounds, infections of female genital tract, pelvic abscesses, aspiration pneumonia and septic abortion. It is also used for prophylaxis of endocarditis. It is also used along with primaquine in *Pneumocystis carinii* pneumonia in AIDS patients and with pyrimethamine for toxoplasmosis.

Oral absorption is good. It is largely metabolized and metabolites are excreted in urine and bile.

Adverse effects include pain at injection site, stomatitis, glossitis, angioneurotic edema, serum sickness, vertigo, tinnitus, aplastic anaemia. Hypotension and cardiac arrest after rapid IV use. Anorexia, metallic taste, oesophagitis, abdominal pain.

LINCOMYCIN

It is mainly **bacteriostatic** and inhibits the growth of gram positive organisms which includes staphylococci, streptococci, pneumococci, *C. diphtheriae* and *B. anthracis.* Like erythromycin it **act by interfering with protein synthesis**.

Adverse effects include nausea, vomiting, diarrhoea, abdominal pain, pseudomembranous colitis, dizziness, rash, headache, pruritus, jaundice, leucopenia etc.

It is **indicated** in upper and lower respiratory tract infections, skin infections, septicaemia, bone and joint infection including acute haematogenous osteomyelitis.

VANCOMYCIN

It is a glycopeptide antibiotic and primarily active against gram positive bacteria, strains of *Staph. aureus* which are resistant to methicillin are inhibited by vancomycin. It is also effective against *Strep. viridans*, enterococcus, *Clostridium difficile* and diphtheroids.

It is **bactericidal** drug and it exerts it **action by inhibiting the synthesis of the cell wall in sensitive bacteria**.

After oral administration it is poorly absorbed. It is given by parenteral route and high concentration of drug may accumulate when renal function is impaired.

It is **indicated** in serious life threatening staphylococcal infections resistant to other antibiotics, in severe staphylococcal infections in patients who are allergic to penicillin and cephalosporin.

Adverse effects include skin rash, anaphylaxis, nephrotoxicity, ototoxicity like other aminoglycosides. Other side effects are local pain and phlebitis at the site of injection, fever, eosinophilia and hypotension.

POLYPEPTIDE ANTIBIOTICS

They have bactericidal activity against gram negative bacteria only and are low molecular cationic polypeptide antibiotics.

They are listed in table 9.5.2.

POLYMYXIN B

Has **detergent like action on cell membrane** and **have high affinity for phospholipids. They penetrate into and disrupt the structure of cell membranes**, as a result of which amino acids and ions leak out.

After oral administration negligible or no absorption occurs.

It is **used** systemically in enteric infections caused by gram negative organisms and topically for pseudomonal infections of conjunctiva and cornea, burns and skin.

Adverse effects include nausea, vomiting, diarrhoea after oral administration. Parenteral administration (IM) cause pain, flushing, ototoxicity, nephrotoxicity and neurotoxicity.

COLISTIN

Also known as polymyxin E, is also a cationic detergent used only orally. Side effects and uses are similar to polymyxin B.

Table 9.5.2: *Classification of polypeptide antibiotics.*

Polymyxin B (AEROSPORIN)	15,000-25,000 U/kg daily for 7-10 days
Colistin (as sulphate) (WALAMYCIN)	25-100 mg TDS
Bacitracin	250 μ/g powder, skin/eye ointment
Tyrothricin	(0.5 mg/kg skin cream, 0.2 mg/ml solution (topical), 0.05% as otic solution with benzocaine

BACITRACIN

This antibiotic is obtained from *Bacillus subtilis*. It is effective against gram positive (cocci and bacilli), *Neisseria* and *H. influenzae*. It is used only topically as antibacterial powder, skin and eye ointment and **acts by inhibiting the cell wall synthesis**. It is bactericidal.

TYROTHRICIN

It is obtained from *Bacillus bravis* and effective against gram positive and some gram negative organisms. It **acts on bacterial cell membrane causing leakage and uncoupling of oxidative phosphorylation.** Used topically as skin cream and solution.

❑❑❑

CHAPTER 9.6 Antiviral Agents

Viruses have no cell wall and made up of nucleic acid core enclosed in a protein coat which consists of identical subunits. Viruses are of two types, **DNA (deoxyribonucleic acid)** viruses and **RNA (ribonucleic acid)** viruses. DNA viruses are herpes simplex, small pox, hepatitis B, varicellazoster etc. and RNA viruses are rabies, measles, dengue, rubella, yellow fever, poliomyelitis and HIV etc.

In viral infections, replication of viruses are at peak, at or before the manifestation of clinical symptoms. So, the treatment generally depends either on early initiation of therapy or prevention of infection i.e. chemoprophylaxis.

The various antiviral agents are classified as under (the doses for specific infections is given in text) in table 9.6.1.

ANTI-HERPES AGENTS

IDOXURIDINE

It is chemically related to thymidine and acts by **competing with it in the synthesis of DNA** and **ultimately preventing the utilization of thymidine**. It **prevents the replication of DNA viruses** and its clinical use is limited to **herpes simplex keratitis.**

Toxicity includes alopecia, leucopenia, thrombocytopenia and liver damage.

It is **used** in herpes simplex keratoconjunctivitis in 0.1 to 0.5% solution/eye ointment applied one to two hourly.

ACYCLOVIR

Acyclovir is a synthetic purine nucleoside analogue with *in vitro* and *in vivo* inhibitory activity against human herpes viruses.

Acyclovir triphosphate **interferes with the viral DNA polymerase and inhibits viral DNA replication** with resultant chain termination following its incorporation into the viral DNA.

Acyclovir is only partially (20%) absorbed from the gut.

Most of the drug is excreted unchanged by the kidney by tubular secretion and glomerular filtration.9-Carboxymethoxymethylguanine is the only significant metabolite of acyclovir recovered from the urine.

Adverse reactions include nausea, vomiting, fatigue, diarrhoea and abdominal pain, rashes including photosensitivity, urticaria, pruritus, increase in blood urea and creatinine, reversible rise in bilirubin and liverrelated enzymes. **Neurological adverse effects** are headache, dizziness, confusional state, hallucinations, somnolence and convulsions.

Indications

- Treatment of herpes simplex virus infection of the skin and mucous membrane, including initial and recurrent genital herpes.
- For the prevention of recurrences of herpes simplex infection in immunocompetent patients.
- Prophylaxis of herpes simplex infection in immunocompromised patients.
- Treatment of varicella (chickenpox) and herpes zoster (shingles) infections. Early treatment of shingles with acyclovir can reduce the incidence of post-herpetic neuralgia (zosterassociated pain).

Dosage

For treatment of herpes simplex in adults: 200 mg five times daily for five days.

Table 9.6.1: *Classification of antiviral agents.*

I.	**Antiherpes agents**
	Idoxuridine (RIDINOX)
	Acyclovir (ZOVIRAX)
	Famciclovir (FAMTRAX)
	Valacyclovir
	Ganciclovir
II.	**Antiretroviral agents**
a.	***Nucleoside reverse transcriptase inhibitors***
	Zidovudine (RETROVIR)
	Lamivudine (HEPITEC)
	Stavudine (STAVIR)
	Didanosine (DINEX)
b.	***Nonnucleoside reverse transcriptase inhibitors***
	Nevirapine (NEVIMUNE)
	Efavirenz (EFAVIR)
c.	***Retroviral protease inhibitors***
	Indinavir (INDIVIR)
	Ritonavir
	Saquinanir
	Nelfinavir
III.	**Antiinfluenza virus agents**
	Amantadine
	Rimantadine
	Zanamavir
	Ribavarin (RIBAVIN)
	Interferons

In severely immunocompromised patients or in patients with impaired absorption from the gut the dose can be doubled to 400 mg or IV dose can be given.

Dosage for suppression of herpes simplex in adults: In immunocompetent patients, 200 mg four times daily six hourly.

Dosage for prophylaxis of herpes simplex in adults: 200 mg four times daily at six hourly intervals.

In severely immunocompromised patients or in patients with impaired absorption from the gut the dose can be doubled to 400 mg or IV dosing can be given.

Dosage for treatment of varicella and herpes zoster in adults: 800 mg five times daily four hourly intervals for seven days.

IV dose can be given in severely immunocompromised patients or in patients with impaired absorption from the gut.

Dosage for management of severely immunocompromised patients: 800 mg four times daily at six hourly intervals.

FAMCICLOVIR

Famciclovir is an orally administered prodrug of the antiviral agent penciclovir. Famciclovir is indicated for the treatment of acute herpes zoster (shingles), treatment or suppression of recurrent genital herpes in immunocompetent patients, treatment of recurrent mucocutaneous herpes simplex infections in HIV-infected patients.

Adverse reactions are headache, paresthesia, migraine, nausea, diarrhoea, vomiting, flatulence, abdominal pain, fatigue, pruritus, rash and dysmenorrhoea.

DOSAGE AND ADMINISTRATION

Herpes Zoster

- *Immunocompetent patients*: 750 mg once daily for 7 days or 250 mg every 8 hours for 7 days.
- *Immunocompromised patients*: 500 mg three times daily for 10 days. Famciclovir should be initiated immediately upon diagnosis of herpes zoster, preferably within 48 hours of the onset of the rash.

Genital Herpes

First episode of genital herpes:

- *Immunocompetent patients*: 250 mg famciclovir three times daily for 5 days, initiated as soon as possible after lesion onset.
- *Immunocompromised patients*: 500 mg twice daily for 7 days.

Episodic treatment of recurrent genital herpes:

- *Immunocompromised patients*: 125 mg twice a day for 5 days.

Acute recurrent genital herpes infection:

- *Immunocompromised patients*: 500 mg twice daily for 7 days.

Suppressive treatment of recurrent genital herpes:

- *Immunocompetent patients*: 250 mg BD for up to one year.
- *In HIV-infected patients*: Famciclovir is to be given 500 mg BD orally.

VALACYCLOVIR

It is the L-valyl ester of acyclovir and rapidly converted into acyclovir after oral admnistration. Its mechanism of action and pharmacokinetics are similar to acyclovir.

In genital herpes dose required is 1 g BD for 10 days and on recurrence 500 mg BD for 5 days. For herpes zoster infection 1 g TDS for 7 days is required. Dose of 2 g QID has also been used in preventing cytomegalovirus (CMV) disease after organ transplantation.

GANCICLOVIR

It is an acyclic guanosine analog which require triphosphorylation for activation prior to inhibition of viral DNA polymerase. It is active against cytomegalovirus (CMV), varicellazoster virus, Epstein-Barr virus and human herpes virus-8. It is almost 100 times more potent than acyclovir against CMV.

Its use is restricted in severe CMV infections in immunocompromised especially CMV retinitis, CMV pneumonia or colitis.

ANTI-RETROVIRAL AGENTS

ZIDOVUDINE

It is a thymidine analogue. After phosphorylation in body zidovudine triphosphate selectively **inhibits viral reverse transcriptase i.e. RNA dependent DNA polymerase**. It is effective against retrovirus only.

It has rapid oral absorption and 65% bioavailability. It can cross the placenta. It is eliminated primarily by renal excretion following glucuronidation in the liver.

Adverse effects include anorexia, nausea, headache, abdominal pain, myalgia, anaemia insomnia, neutropenia, convulsions and encephalopathy.

It is **used** in asymptomatic and symptomatic HIV disease in a dose range of 200 mg six times a day on initial basis and thereafter upto 500 to 1500 mg daily in four to five divided doses.

It decreases the rate of clinical progression and prolongs the survival in HIV infected patients. However, it does not protect individuals from contracting HIV infection even if started soon after inoculation. Thus, it can not be used as a prophylactic in health care workers who are accidently exposed to HIV infection.

LAMIVUDINE

It is synthetic nucleoside analogue active against HIV. It is phosphorylated to its active 5′-triphosphate metabolite (L-TP). Lamivudine triphosphate **inhibit HIV reverse transcription via viral DNA chain termination**.

It is rapidly absorbed after oral administration. The major part of the dose is excreted in unchanged form in urine.

Adverse effects include pancreatitis with symptoms of nausea, vomiting, severe abdominal or stomach pain and is more frequent in children. Paresthesia and peripheral neuropathy with tingling, burning, numbness or pain in the hands and feet are also more frequent in children.

Lamivudine may be **used** prophylactically in health care workers at risk of acquiring HIV infection after occupational exposure to the virus and in combination with zidovudine for treatment of HIV infection.

It is to be given in a dose of 150 mg BD in combination with zidovudine (in children 4 mg/kg BD, max 150 mg BD).

STAVUDINE

It is synthetic thymidine nucleoside analogue, active against HIV.

Stavudine rapidly enters cells by diffusion. Stavudine triphosphate acts as a **competitive inhibitor of reverse transcriptase with respect to deoxythmidine triphosphate and incorporation causes termina-**

tion of DNA chain elongation. It **inhibits replication of HIV** in human cells.

It is rapidly absorbed after oral administration. Approximately 40 percent of stavudine appears unchanged in the urine through tubular secretion and glomerular filtration. Nonrenal clearance mechanisms account for about 50 percent of elimination of a dose.

Adverse effects include peripheral neuropathy which is a major clinical toxicity. Other **side effects** include pancreatitis, anaemia, arthralgia, headache, fever, rash, nausea, vomiting, diarrhoea, elevated transaminase values.

It is **indicated** in the treatment of advanced HIV infection in a dose range 30 to 40 mg BD.

NEVIRAPINE

It is **non-nucleotide reverse transcriptase inhibitor** extensively metabolized by the CYP3A P450 isoform to hydroxylated metabolites and excreted in urine. It is **indicated** in combination with other anti-retroviral agents in a dose of 200 mg OD-BD for first 14 days. It is also been shown to be effective in the prevention of transmission of HIV from mother to new born.

The serious **side effect** is life threatening rash including Stevens Johnson syndrome and rarely toxic epidermal necrolysis. Other side effects are hepatitis, nausea, vomiting, fatigue, fever, headache, hypersensitivity reactions, urticaria, angioedema and anaphylactic shock.

EFAVIRENZ

It is also an **non-nucleotide reverse transcriptase inhibitor** having long half-life (40-55 hrs) and administered once daily. It is metabolised by CYP3A4 and CYP2B6 to inactive hydroxylated metabolites and eliminated in feces. It is **used** in combination with other retroviral drugs for the treatment of HIV infection in a dose of 600 mg once daily.

Adverse effects include drowsiness, insomnia, dizziness, agitation, confusion, depression, delusions, vomiting, diarrhoea, crystalluria, elevation in liver enzyme and total serum cholesterol. Serious side effect is skin rash including Stevens Johnson syndrome as in case of nevirapine.

INDINAVIR

It is an inhibitor of the enzyme HIV protease which is required for the proteolytic cleavage of the viral polyprotein precursors into the individual functional proteins found in infectious HIV.

Indinavir **binds to the protease active site** and **inhibits the activity of the enzyme HIV protease preventing cleavage of the viral polyproteins** resulting in the formation of immature noninfectious viral particles.

Adverse effects include nausea, vomiting, diarrhoea, abdominal discomfort, dry mouth, taste disturbances; headache, dizziness, insomnia; myalgia, rash, pruritus, dry skin, hyperpigmentation, nephrolithiasis, dysuria, haematuria, crystalluria, proteinuria; elevated liver enzymes and bilirubin, hepatitis; neutropenia, haemolytic anaemia and hyperglycaemia etc.

It is **indicated** in treatment of HIV infection and is used in combination with other anti-retroviral agents in a dose 800 mg every eight hourly.

RITONAVIR

It is inhibitor of HIV-1 and 2 proteases. The common **adverse effects** include GIT disturbances, hypertriglyceridemia and elevation of serum aminotransferase.

ANTI-INFLEUNZA VIRUS AGENTS

AMANTADINE AND ITS DERIVATIVES

It exerts its action by **inhibiting the replication of influenza virus**, by **inhibiting uncoating of viral RNA of influenza A** within infected host cells. It is used in a dose of 200 mg/day in prevention of influenza A virus infection.

After oral administration, it is excreted unchanged in urine.

Adverse effects include confusion, insomnia, anxiety, hallucinations, skin rash and retention of urine.

It is **used** in prophylaxis of influenza A virus, idiopathic parkinsonism and drug-induced extrapyramidal reactions.

Rimanditine is a more potent and longer acting congener of amantadine.

RIBAVIRIN

It is a guanosine analog which probably **interferes with the synthesis of guanosine triphosphate, inhibiting capping of viral mRNA** and to **inhibit the viral RNA-dependent RNA polymerase**.

Orally absorbed and bioavailability is about 50%. It is partly metabolized and eliminated in a multiexponential manner.

Adverse reactions include anaemia, gastrointestinal disturbances, headache and haemolysis.

It is **active against** influenza A and B, measles, paramyxoviruses, respiratory syncytial virus, HCV and HIV-1 in a dose of 200 mg four times per day.

INTERFERONS

Interferons are cellular glycoproteins produced by the host cells which exert complex antiviral, immunoregulatory and antiproliferative activities. After binding to interferon receptors it **acts through cellular metabolic processes which involves synthesis of viral RNA and proteins**. Interferon receptors are tyrosine protein kinase receptors which on activation phosphorylate cellular proteins. These then induce transcription of 'interferon induced proteins' which exert antiviral effects. There are three type of interferons – alpha, beta and gamma.

Interferons are **indicated** in chronic hepatitis B and C in a dose of 10 MU injection three times a week for six months.

Alpha interferon is also **effective** in the treatment of hairy cell leukaemia, condyloma acuminata (caused by papilloma virus), chronic myelogenous leukaemia and AIDS related Kaposi's sarcoma.

Interferons are not effective orally and is used only by IM or SC injection.

Adverse effects include fever, leucopenia, thrombocytopenia, alopecia, neurotoxicity and elevated aminotransferase levels. Other less common side effects include hypotension, cardiomyopathy and hyperglycaemia.

❑❑❑

CHAPTER 9.7 Antifungal Agents

Antifungal agents are used in the treatment of topical and systemic fungal infection. They can be classified as systemic or topical antifungal agents and some are used both systemically as well as topically in the form of powder, ointment and vaginal tablets etc. They are classified as in table 9.7.1.

ANTIFUNGAL ANTIBIOTICS

AMPHOTERICIN B

It is an antifungal antibiotic obtained from *Streptomyces nodosus* and chemically it is an amphoteric polyene macrolide. It has a highly double bonded structure. The cell membrane sterol 'ergosterol' is found in the cell membrane of fungi and the predominant sterol of bacteria and human cell is cholesterol. This antifungal antibiotic **binds to ergosterol** which alters the permeability of the cells by forming amphotericin-B associated pores in cell membrane, which **allows the leakage of intracellular ions and macromolecules which can lead to cell death**.

Amphotericin B has a wide spectrum of antifungal activity. It is active against *Histoplasma capsulatum, Cryptococcus neoformans, Candida albicans, Sporotrichum schenkii, Blastomyces brasiliensis, Coccidioides immitis, Rhodotorula, Aspergillus* etc. It is fungicidal at high and fungistatic at low concentration.

It is poorly absorbed from GIT and topically. After IV administration it is widely distributed in tissues. About 60% drug is metabolized in liver and excretion occurs slowly both in urine and bile.

Adverse effects include nausea, vomiting, headache, fever, breathlessness, anaemia, thrombophlebitis on IV administration. On long term use, dose related nephrotoxicity and anaemia occurs.

It is **used** orally for intestinal candidiasis, topically for oral, vaginal and cutaneous candidiasis and hospital treatment of progressive and potentially fatal systemic fungal infections. It is the gold standard of antifungal therapy. Flucytosine has supraadditive action with amphotericin B if the fungi is sensitive to both. It is also potentiated by rifampicin and minocycline.

Table 9.7.1: *Classification of antifungal agents.*

I. Antifungal antibiotics	
Amphotericin-B (FUNGIZONE)	50-100 mg QID, 200 µg to 1.5 mg/kg daily or on alternate days IV infusion, 3% topical (ear drops)
Nystatin (MYCOSTATIN)	5 lac U orally TDS, 1 lac U topical (ointment vaginal tablet)
Griseofulvin (DERMONORM)	0.5-1.0 g/day
Pimaricin	Topical (2% cream, 25 mg vaginal tablet, 5% ophthalmic ointment)
Hamycin	2-5 lac U (suspension & topically as vaginal tablet and ointment)
II. Antimetabolite	
Flucytosine (ALCOBON)	100-150 mg/kg/day
III. Imidazoles & triazoles	
Clotrimazole (CLOTRIN)	100 mg vaginal tablet, 1% topical (lotion, cream and powder)
Ketoconazole (NIZRAL)	200 mg OD-BD orally, topical 2% ointment and shampoo
Miconazole (DAKTARIN)	3-15 mg/kg with glucose & saline IV infusion, 1-2% topical (powder, lotion, vaginal gel, ointment & vaginal ovules)
Econazole	150 mg vaginal tablet, 1% topical (cream & ointment)
Itraconazole (CANDITRAL)	100-200 mg/day (the number of days depend upon the type of infection)
Fluconazole (FLUZON) Also used with tinidazole (AZOSTAT)	400 mg on 1st day, then 200-400 mg OD, for 28 days,
Terbinafine (LAMISIL)	250 mg OD for 6-12 wks.
IV. Miscellaneous agents (used topically)	
Tolnaftate (TINADERM)	1% solution cream
Selenium sulfide (SELSUN)	Shampoo
Cyclopirox olamine	1% solution, skin cream & vaginal cream
Benzoic acid	3-5% skin ointment
Sodium thiosulfate	20% solution
Quiniodochlor	3-8% skin cream

NYSTATIN

It is obtained from *Streptomyces noursei*. It has similar antifungal action as amphotericin but is highly toxic and used topically only. It is effective against *Candida, Histoplasma, Trichophyton, Blastomyces, Microsporum audouini* etc. It is **indicated** in *Candida albicans* especially oral moniliasis, monilial vaginitis, conjunctival, cutaneous and corneal candidiasis.

GRISEOFULVIN

It is isolated from *Penicillium griseofulvium*. It is active against *Epidermophyton, Trichophyton* and *Microsporum* causing superficial infection or dermatophytosis.

It is not effective against fungi causing deep/systemic infection.

It **interferes with mitosis** and also **causes abnormal metaphase configurations**. Griseofulvin gets deposited in keratin and persists for weeks. As it is fungistatic the newly formed keratin is not invaded by the fungus but fungus persists in already infected keratin, till it is shed off.

Oral absorption is irregular. It is largely metabolised by methylation and excreted in urine. It is ineffective topically.

Adverse effects include nausea, epigastric distress, vomiting, headache, peripheral neuritis, skin rash, photosensitivity, drowsiness and transient leucopenia. It can cause disulfiram like reaction.

It is **indicated** in fungal infections of skin, scalp and nails, tinea of hand and beard and athlete's foot.

PIMARICIN

It is obtained from *Streptomyces notalensis* and it is found effective against *Trichophyton violaceum, Trichomonas vaginalis* and *Aspergillus fumigatus.* It is **used** as eye ointment in keratitis due to *Fusarium* and *Cephalosporium* and as an inhalation in bronchopulmonary aspergillosis and candidiasis.

HAMYCIN

It is obtained from *Streptomyces pimprina* and effective against blastomycosis, cryptococcosis, vaginal and cutaneous candidiasis, *Trichomonas* vaginitis and *Aspergillus* otomycosis.

Adverse effects include diarrhoea, eosinophilia, nephrotoxicity and rise in SGOT levels after oral administration in the treatment of blastomycosis in man.

ANTIMETABOLITES

FLUCYTOSINE

It is a synthetic fluorinated pyrimidine anti-metabolite which acts by its conversion to anti-metabolite 5-fluorouracil which **inhibit DNA synthesis**.

It is effective against *Cryptococcus neoformans* and some *Candida* strains and dermatiaceous moulds which cause chromoblastomycosis.

Adverse effects include anaemia, leukopenia, thrombocytopenia, diarrhoea, GIT disturbances and liver dysfunction.

It is mainly **used** as an adjuvant drug to amphotericin.

IMIDAZOLES & TRIAZOLES

CLOTRIMAZOLE

Clotrimazole, is an imidazole derivative and has a broad antimycotic spectrum of action *in vivo*, which includes dermatophytes, yeasts, moulds etc.

Clotrimazole acts against fungi by **inhibiting ergosterol synthesis**. Inhibition of ergosterol synthesis leads to structural and functional impairment of the cytoplasmic membrane.

In addition, it also acts on *Trichomonas vaginalis*, gram positive microorganisms (streptococci/staphylococci) and gram negative microorganisms (*Bacteroides/ Gardnerella vaginalis*).

It is useful as topical application. It is **indicated** in infections of the genital region (vaginitis) caused by fungi (mostly *Candida*) and superinfections caused by clotrimazole sensitive bacteria; infectious leucorrhoea caused by yeast fungi.

It is well tolerated but some patients reported skin reactions including burning, stinging or redness.

KETOCONAZOLE

It is orally effective broad spectrum imidazole antifungal drug. It is **useful** in both dermatophytosis and deep mycosis. Oral absorption is facilitated by gastric acidity. It is highly protein bound, metabolised in liver and metabolites are excreted in urine and faeces. Its spectrum is similar to that of miconazole and is more active against *Coccidioides*.

Adverse effects include gastric irritation, nausea, vomiting, headache, paresthesia, rash, hair loss, allergic reaction and gynecomastia.

MICONAZOLE

It has broad spectrum antifungal and antibacterial activity and is effective against *Cryptococcus*, *Blastomyces*, dermatophytes, *Microsporum*, *Coccidioides* and *Candida*. Used topically as ointment, lotion, gel, ear drop and vaginal gel. **Adverse effects** include fever, chills, allergic reaction and even anaphylaxis.

It is **indicated** in vulvovaginal candidiasis, *Trichomonas* vaginitis, otomycosis, tinea and *Pityriasis versicolor*.

ECONAZOLE

It is similar to clotrimazole and is **effective** in dermatophytosis, otomycosis and oral thrush. It causes local irritation.

ITRACONAZOLE

It is a triazole antifungal drug closely related to ketoconazole and is meant for oral use. It is very effective in a wide range of superficial and deep seated fungal infections.

It **impairs the synthesis of ergosterol** in fungi.

After oral administration, it is widely distributed in the body. CSF and saliva contain negligible amounts of the drug. It is extensively metabolised in liver and the metabolites are excreted in urine.

It is **indicated** in dermatophytoses, tinea versicolor, onychomycoses, oropharyngeal candidiasis, cutaneous candidiasis, chronic mucocutaneous candidiasis, oculomycoses; *systemic mycoses* like cryptococcosis, candidiasis and aspergillosis; subcutaneous mycoses like sporotrichosis and chromomycosis.

Adverse effects include nausea, vomiting, skin rash, depression, dizziness, vertigo and loss of libido, hypokalemia and hypertriglyceridemia.

FLUCONAZOLE

It has broad range of antifungal activity. It is well absorbed orally (94%). It is primarily excreted unchanged in urine. Fungicidal concentration is achieved in nail, saliva and vagina and also penetrates brain. **Adverse effects** include nausea, vomiting, headache, abdominal pain, diarrhea and skin rash.

It is **indicated** in mucosal candidiasis, systemic candidiasis, crypttococcosis, prophylaxis of fungal infections following cytotoxic chemotherapy or radiotherapy; maintenance to prevent relapse of cryptococcal meningitis in patients with AIDS; sporotrichosis, histoplasmosis and vaginal candidiasis.

TERBINAFINE

It is a synthetic allylamine derivative, which exerts its antifungal effect by **inhibiting squalene epoxidase leading to deficiency of ergosterol** and corresponding accumulation of squalene which causes fungal cell death.

It is well absorbed from the GI tract, widely distributed in body. It is strongly plasma protein bound. It is metabolised in the liver to inactive metabolites which are excreted in the urine.

Adverse effects are irritation, burning, itching and dryness on topical application. Oral intake causes gastric upset, rash, taste disturbance and hepatic dysfunction.

Terbinafine is **used** in the treatment of dermatophytoses especially onchomycosis by oral therapy. Also useful in tinea and pityriasis versicolor.

MISCELLANEOUS AGENTS

Tolnaftate is effective in tinea cruris and tinea corporis. Used in the form of solution and cream used topically. Not useful in candidiasis and other types of superficial mycoses. **Adverse reaction** includes local irritation.

Selenium sulfide is used as shampoo and used in the treatment of scalp fungal infection.

Cyclopirox olamine is used in the treatment of tinea infections, dermal and vaginal candidiasis.

Benzoic acid has got antifungal and anti-bacterial activity and used in combination with salicylic acid (Whitfield's ointment). Salicylic acid by its keratolytic action helps to remove the infected tissue and promotes the penetration of benzoic acid into the lesion.

Sodium thiosulfate is effective against *Malassezia furfur*.

Quiniodochlor is found effective against dermatophytosis, infected eczema and seborrhoeic dermatitis. Orally it is used as luminal amoebicide.

❑❑❑

CHAPTER 9.8

Antimalarial Agents

Human malaria is caused by four species of *Plasmodium* namely *Plasmodium falciparum, P. vivax, P. malariae* and *P. ovale. P. vivax* is mainly responsible for most of the infections (70%) which results in **benign tertian malaria**. In *P. falciparum* and *P. vivax* infections, the patient has fever with rigors every third day and termed as **tertian**. The other two, *P. ovale* and *P. malariae* are mild in nature in which fever develops every fourth day and termed as **benign quartan**. Symptoms and complications in *P. falciparum* malaria are more severe than *P. vivax* malaria.

The antimalarial drugs can be classified as in table 9.8.1.

4-Aminoquinoline Derivatives

CHLOROQUINE

Chloroquine is a 4-aminoquinoline antimalarial agent used for the suppression and clinical cure of malaria. It is an excellent **erythrocytic schizontocide**. It does not prevent relapse in *P. vivax* and *P. ovale* malaria. It has no effect on pre and exoerythrocytic phase of the parasite. It also has antiinflammatory and local irritant properties.

It probably **influences haemoglobin degradation by parasitic lysosomes by raising intravesicular pH in malarial parasite cells**. It also **interferes with synthesis of nucleoproteins by the parasite**.

It is well absorbed (about 90%) from gastrointestinal tract. After IM injection absorption is rapid. Elimination is very slow and it may persist in tissue for months or years after discontinuation of therapy

Adverse reactions include nausea, vomiting, epigastric distress, headache, anorexia, difficulty in accommodation and chronic therapy may cause loss of vision due to retinal damage. On prolonged use it may also cause skin rash, photoallergy, myopathy, loss of hearing, greying of hair and mental disturbances.

Parenteral administration may cause hypotension, arrhythmia and CNS toxicity.

Therapeutic Uses

It is a drug of choice for clinical cure and suppressive prophylaxis of acute malaria but not for the resistant cases of *P. falciparum*. It can be safely used in preg-

Table 9.8.1: *Classification of antimalarial drugs.*

	Drug	Dose
I.	**4-aminoquinoline derivative**	
	Chloroquine (LARIAGO)	Initially 600 mg, after 6 hr 300 mg followed by 300 mg daily for 3 days, 200-400 mg IM 6 hourly
	Amodiaquine (CAMOQUIN)	25-35 mg/kg for 3 days
II.	**8-aminoquinolines**	
	Primaquine (MALIRID)	15 mg daily for 14 days
III.	**Quinoline-methanol derivatives**	
	Mefloquine (MEFLOC)	15 mg/kg single dose (for treatment, maximum 1 g); 5 mg/kg, up to 250 mg per wk (for prophylaxis in areas with multidrug resistance)
	Bulaquine (AABLAQUIN)	125 mg (used with chloroquine 500 mg)
IV.	**Acridine derivative**	
	Mepacrine (MALADIN)	900 mg 1st day, 600 mg on 2nd & 3rd day, 300 mg on 4th, 5th and 6th day in divided doses; 600 mg/wk for prophylaxis
V.	**Cinchona alkaloids**	
	Quinine (as sulphate)	600 mg/day, oral TDS or 10 mg/kg with 5% glucose IV infusion TDS (for cerebral malaria) for 7 days
VI.	**Biguanides**	
	Proguanil (Chloroguanide; LAVERAN)	100 mg daily during exposure and continued for 6 weeks after exposure
VII.	**Diaminopyrimidine & Sulfonamides**	
	Pyrimethamine (DARAPRIM)	25 mg (for prophylaxis)
	Pyrimethamine 25 mg + sulfadoxine 500 mg (MALARPRIM)	Once a week 3 tablets single dose
	Pyrimethamine 25 mg + sulfamethopyrazine 500 mg (METAKELFIN)	3 tablets single dose
VIII.	**Artemisinin derivatives**	
	Artesunate (FALCIGO)	100 mg BD on 1st day, followed by 50 mg BD for next four days (for cerebral malaria, chloroquine-resistant malaria & *P. falciparum* malaria).
	Artether (EMAL)	150 mg daily for 3 days IM
	Artemether (LARITHER)	160 mg BD on first day and 80 mg OD for next four days orally; 80 mg BD IM on first day and 80 mg OD IM for next four days IM

nancy. Apart from malaria, chloroquine in also used in:

- Rheumatoid arthritis.
- Giardiasis.
- Discoid lupus erythematosus.
- Infectious mononucleosis.
- Taeniasis.
- Lepra reactions.
- Hepatic amoebic abscess (used along with metronidazole).

AMODIAQUINE

Another 4-aminoquinoline and possesses antimalarial activity similar to that of chloroquine. It is useful in uncomplicated falciparum malaria but is not recommended for prophylaxis.

8-Aminoquinolines

PRIMAQUINE

Primaquine, a 8-aminoquinoline, is a poor **erythrocytic schizontocide**. It is highly effective against gametocytes and exoerythrocytic stages.

It disrupts the parasites mitochondria and binds to native DNA, resulting in inhibition of gametocytes and exoerythrocytic forms.

Adverse effects include nausea, vomiting, weakness, abdominal pain and methaemoglobinaemia. Haemolytic anaemia in patients with G-6-PD deficiency. Passage of dark urine is indication of haemolysis. In larger dose it can cause leucopenia.

It is effective in radical cure of *P. vivax* and *P. ovale* malaria.

Quinoline-Methanol Derivatives

MEFLOQUINE

It is a highly effective **erythrocytic schizonticide** especially against mature trophozoite and schizont forms of malarial parasite.

It behaves like quinine in many ways but does not inhibit haem polymerase. It probably **acts by forming toxic complexes with free haem that damages membranes and interacts with other plasmodial components**.

It is absorbed after oral administration and presence of food may enhance the absorption. It is extensively metabolised in liver and primarily secreted in bile.

Adverse reactions include nausea, vomiting, dizziness, diarrhoea, abdominal pain, anxiety disorder, sinus bradycardia, ataxia. It is reported that mefloquine is teratogenic in nature so should not be given in first trimester of pregnancy.

It is **used** in multiresistant *P. falciparum* malaria. It is not useful in complicated/ cerebral malaria.

BULAQUINE

Bulaquine is a mixture of 3{-1-4-6(-methoxy-8-quinolinyl) aminopentyl} ethylidenedihydro-2-(3H) furanone and it's tautomers.

The exact action is not fully elucidated. However, bulaquine **inhibits protein synthesis in protozoa and indirectly inhibits polymerisation of amino acids by the plasmodia**. Treatment prevents emergence of either primary or secondary liver stage parasitaemia and the disease.

Since bulaquine is a **tissue schizontocide** it is effective against the dormant hepatic stages of *P. vivax* only. It has to be combined with chloroquine which acts on the erythrocytic stage of the plasmodium. For convenience bulaquine is available along with chloroquine as an **anti-relapse treatment pack**.

It is an erythrocytic schizontocide used in the treatment and prevention of *P. vivax* malaria relapse.

Acridine Derivative

MEPACRINE

It is an erythrocytic schizontocide related to its ready intercalation into DNA.

Readily absorbed from the GI tract even in the presence of severe diarrhoea. It is widely distributed in the tissues and is eliminated very slowly.

Adverse effects include urticaria, exfoliative dermatitis, GI disturbances, dizziness and yellow discoloration of the skin on prolonged use.

It is **indicated** in drug resistant *P. falciparum* malaria and in the treatment of giardiasis.

Cinchona Alkaloids

QUININE

Quinine is a natural alkaloid obtained from cinchona bark.

It is **erythrocytic schizontocide** and is effective against all species of plasmodia. It has no effect on preerythrocytic stage and on hypnozoites of relapsing malaria. It kills the gametes of *P. vivax*.

It also has anaesthetic, local irritant action. Quinine causes hypotension, cardiac depression (IV injection), stimulates myometrium and rapid IV injection causes hypoglycaemia.

It is highly concentrated in the acidic food vacuoles of the parasite where it inhibits haem polymerase leading to the accumulation of haem which is cytotoxic.

Adverse effects include nausea, vomiting, epigastric discomfort, skin rash, itching, hypotension, haemolysis, blurred vision, vertigo, tinnitus and cinchonism.

It is **used** in the treatment of cerebral falciparum malaria and multidrug resistant strains of cerebral malaria. It is also used along with clindamycin in the treatment of babesiosis. It is also effective in myotonia congenita and nocturnal muscle cramps.

Biguanides

PROGUANIL

It is an effective **erythrocytic schizontocide** against *P. falciparum* and *P. vivax* but slower acting than chloroquine.

The active triazine metabolite, **inhibits plasmodial dihydrofolate reductase** and thus **disrupts the synthesis of nucleic acids in the parasite**.

It is slowly but adequately absorbed from the GI tract. It is metabolised in the liver to the active metabolite **cycloguanil**.

Adverse effects include gastrointestinal disturbances, nausea, vomiting, diarrhoea, abdominal pain and haematuria.

It is mainly **used** in prophylaxis of malaria in combination with chloroquine in areas with low chloroquine resistance among *P. falciparum*. It can be safely used in pregnancy.

Diaminopyrimidine & Sulfonamides

PYRIMETHAMINE

It is an **inhibitor of plasmodial**

dihydrofolate reductase. It is slow acting erythrocytic schizontocide. It can eliminate preerythrocytic phase of *P. falciparum* and the secondary tissue phase of *P. vivax*. Absorption of pyrimethamine from GIT is slow but good. It is concentrated in liver, spleen, kidney and lungs. It is metabolised and excreted in urine. If it is employed alone development of resistance occurs fast. Pyrimethamine alone is used for prophylaxis occasionally.

PYRIMETHAMINE-SULFONAMIDE COMBINATION

Ultra long acting sulfonamides in combination with pyrimethamine are used. The effect is supraadditive due to sequential block. It may be employed as a clinical curative. Another advantage of the drug combination is that the development of resistance is retarded.

Its action is based on differential requirement between host and parasite for nucleic acid precursors involved in growth as it **selectively inhibits plasmodial dihydrofolate reductase**.

It is very well absorbed after oral use and is metabolised in the liver.

Pyrimethamine is a safe drug and cause only nausea, vomiting, skin reaction e.g. skin rash, pruritus and higher dose can cause megaloblastic anaemia and granulocytopenia.

The combination is indicated in chloroquine resistant malaria and prophylaxis. Pyrimethamine-sulfadiazine combination is used for treatment of toxoplasmosis.

ARTEMISININ DERIVATIVES

Artemisinin is the active plant principle isolated from plant *Artemisia annua*, active against *P. falciparum* resistant strains.

ARTESUNATE

It is a new, potent antimalarial drug and is a water soluble synthetic analogue of artemisinin.

It is concentrated in parasitized erythrocytes, where it is activated by parasite haem, generating free radicals. Hence it **causes increase in oxidant stress on the infected red cells promoting cytotoxicity and death of parasites**. It rapidly clears parasitaemia, faster than any other antimalarial drug.

After administration it is rapidly absorbed and distributed in tissue e.g. liver, intestine and kidneys. It is metabolised in liver and converted to active metabolite dihydroartemisinin.

Adverse effects include nausea, vomiting, dizziness, anorexia, gastrointestinal disturbances and convulsions.

It is **indicated** in acute attack of multidrug resistant *P. falciparum* malaria where quinine is not effective.

ARTETHER

It is an ethyl ether derivative of dihydroartemisinin in sterile arachis oil. A racemic mixture of a, β-artether (30:70 ratio) has greater solubility and stability than artemisinin and is more cost-effective.

It shows rapid schizonticidal action and brings about quick clinical improvement in falciparum malaria with low recrudescence rate. It has some gametocidal action too.

It is **used** in the treatment of chloroquine resistant malaria and cerebral malaria.

ARTEMETHER

It is derivative of artemisinin. These agents produce a more rapid clearance of parasites than quinine, chloroquine and mefloquine in treatment of severe cerebral and falciparum malaria. It is a effective drug against all strains resistant to other antimalarial agents.

It is a schizonticidal drug and leads to **destruction of asexual erythrocytic forms** of *P. falciparum* and *P. vivax*. There is inhibition of protein synthesis during growth of trophozoites.

❑❑❑

CHAPTER 9.9 Antiamoebic and other Antiprotozoal Drugs

AMOEBIASIS

Amoebiasis is an infectious disease caused by *Entamoeba histolytica*. It can cause asymptomatic intestinal infection, colitis (mild to moderate), dysentery (severe intestinal infection), ameboma, liver abscess etc. The drugs used in chemotherapy of amoebiasis are classified as in table 9.9.1.

METRONIDAZOLE

It is a nitroimidazole. It has a broad spectrum of protozoal and antimicrobial activity. It shows antibacterial action against all anaerobic cocci, anaerobic gram negative bacilli including bacteroides species and anaerobic spore forming gram positive bacilli. It is very effective in infections due to *Entamoeba histolytica*, *Giardia lamblia* and *Trichomoniasis*. It also causes radio-sensitization.

In shows selective toxicity to anaerobic microorganisms, where it is converted to active form by reduction of its nitro group and this gets **bound to DNA and prevent nucleic acid formation**.

After oral administration it is rapidly and completely absorbed. It penetrates well into body tissues and fluids. It is metabolised in liver by oxidation and glucuronide conjugation and is excreted in urine.

Adverse effects include nausea, metallic taste, headache, dry mouth, abdominal distress, vomiting, diarrhoea, glossitis, stomatitis, vertigo, dizziness, ataxia, thrombophlebitis and very rarely convulsions. It shows disulfiram like effect.

It is drug of choice for all forms of amoebic infections **used** in trichomonas vaginitis, anaerobic postoperative infections, giardiasis, acute ulcerative gingivitis, *H. pylori* infection, pseudomembranous enterocolitis and anaerobic vaginosis.

TINIDAZOLE

It is similar to metronidazole and has long plasma half life and given once daily.

It is well absorbed after oral administration and penetrates well into the body tissues and fluids. Incidence of side effects in lower.

Table 9.9.1: *Classification of drugs used in amoebiasis.*

Drug	Dose
I. **Imidazole derivatives**	
Metronidazole (FLAGYL)	
Amoebiasis	400-800 mg TDS for 5-10 days; 7.5-15 mg/kg IV infusion BD-QID
Trichomonas vaginitis	400 mg TDS × 7 days
Giardiasis	200 mg TDS × 3 days
Tinidazole (TINIBA)	
Amoebiasis	2 g OD × 3 days
Trichomoniasis and giardiasis	2 g OD
Secnidazole (SECNIL)	2 g single dose
Ornidazole (DAZOLIC)	500 mg BD × 5-7 days
II. **Quinoline derivative**	
Iodochlorohydroxyquin (ENTEROQUINOL)	250-500 mg TDS
Diiodohydroxyquin (DIODOQUIN)	650 mg TDS
Chloroquine	600 mg × 2 days then 300 mg OD × 2-3 wks
III. **Emetine derivatives**	
Dehydroemetine (TILEMETIN)	10-20 mg TDS × 6-10 days
Emetine, emetine bismuth iodide	
IV. **Miscellaneous**	
Diloxanide furoate (FURAMIDE)	500 mg TDS × 5-10 days
Furazolidone (FUROXONE)	100 mg TDS-QID × 5-7 days
Paromomycin	500 mg TDS × 5 days
Tetracycline	250 mg QID

Side effects include nausea, epigastric discomfort, metallic taste, furred tongue, skin rash, urticaria and leucopenia.

It is **indicated** in giardiasis, amoebic liver abscess, intestinal amoebiasis, trichomoniasis, ulcerative gingivitis, treatment and prophylaxis of anaerobic infections.

It is also **used** in combination with diloxanide furoate and dicyclomine to eradicate intestinal and extraintestinal amoebiasis and also asymptomatic cyst passers.

SECNIDAZOLE

It is 5-nitroimidazole derivative with properties similar to metronidazole and having longer plasma half life and administered orally as single dose. It is **used** in intestinal amoebiasis, hepatic amoebiasis, giardiasis and trichomonal vaginitis.

Side effects include nausea, anorexia, epigastric pain, diarrhoea, skin rash, urticaria, headache and leucopenia.

ORNIDAZOLE

It is a 5-nitroimidazole derivative with the same antimicrobial profile as that of metronidazole, except that it has a much longer half-life.

Readily absorbed from the GI tract, widely distributed in body tissues and fluids including the CSF and metabolised in the liver. It is excreted mainly in the urine as conjugates and to a lesser extent in faeces.

Adverse effects include nausea, skin rash, abdominal pain and headache.

It is **indicated** in giardiasis, severe hepatic and intestinal amoebiasis, trichomoniasis of urogenital tract and bacterial vaginosis.

8-HYDROXYQUINOLINES

Diiodohydroxyquinoline, iodochlorohydroxyquin are effective against *E. histolytica, Trichomonas* and *Giardia.*

Diiodohydroxyquinoline is directly amoebicidal. It has activity against motile and cystic forms. It kills cyst forming trophozoites in intestine but has no tissue amoebicidal action. It is ineffective in extraintestinal amoebiasis. It is also effective in cyst passing patients.

Diiodohydroxyquinoline is partly and irregularly absorbed from the GI tract. Metabolised in liver and excreted in urine as glucuronide and sulfate conjugates.

Adverse effects include nausea, diarrhoea, abdominal discomfort, headache and goitre (so contraindicated in patients with intolerance to iodine). Prolonged use of iodochlorohydroxyquin causes subacute myelooptic neuropathy (SMON). They are **indicated** in giardiasis, trichomonas vaginitis, intestinal amoebiasis and amoebic colitis.

CHLOROQUINE

It kills trophozoites of *E. histolytica* and because of its selective concentration in liver, it is **used** in the treatment of hepatic amoebiasis concurrently or immediately after metronidazole for complete cure. It is not effective in amoebic dysentery and in cyst passers.

EMETINE DERIVATIVES

Emetine and dehydroemetine are natural alkaloid obtained from *Cephaelis ipecacuanha* and synthetic analog respectively. They are effective against tissue trophozoites of *E. histolytica*. It has no effect on cysts but effective in amoebic liver abscess also. **It acts by inhibiting protein synthesis by arresting intraribosome translocation of tRNA-amino acid complex**. Dehydroemetine is less toxic than emetine and very effective drug for tissue amoebiasis. It is more rapidly eliminated from the body than emetine.

Adverse effects include nausea, vomiting, diarrhoea, myalgias and because of its serious side effects including cardiac arrhythmia, CHF and hypotension, they have been almost completely replaced by metronidazole.

DILOXANIDE FUROATE

It is a dichloroacetamide derivative, very effective luminal amoebicide. Used alone for cyst passers or usually with metronidazole for other forms of amoebic infections.

It **directly kills trophozoites**. It has no antibacterial activity.

After oral administration it is rapidly absorbed and excreted rapidly in urine as glucuronide conjugate.

Adverse effects include flatulence, nausea, vomiting, anorexia and pruritus.

It is mainly indicated in mild intestinal amoebiasis and asymptomatic cyst passers.

It is also **used** in combination with tinidazole (TINIBA DF) and metronidazole (ENTAMIZOLE) in the treatment of intestinal amoebiasis, hepatic amoebiasis and other systemic diseases due to *E. histolytica*.

FURAZOLIDONE

It is effective against gram negative bacilli e.g. *Shigella, Salmonella* and also effective against *Trichomonas* and *Giardia*.

It is **indicated** in bacterial enteritis, diarrhoea, giardiasis and bacillary dysentery.

Adverse effects include nausea, vomiting, headache and dizziness.

PAROMOMYCIN

It is an aminoglycoside antibiotic used only as **luminal amoebicide** and has no effect against extra intestinal amoebic infections. It is less toxic than other agents, but it should be used cautiously in patients with significant renal disease and with gastrointestinal ulcer.

LEISHMANIASIS

Visceral leishmaniasis (kalaazar) is caused by *Leishmania donovani* and transmitted by *Phlebotomus* sandfly. In human being, it is found intracellularly within macrophages in the nonflagellate form. The important drugs used in leishmaniasis are pentamidine, sodium stibogluconate, antifungal antibiotics (amphotericin B and ketoconazole) and antigout agent (allopurinol).

PENTAMIDINE

Pentamidine is an aromatic diamidine formulated as an isoethionate salt used parenterally (4 mg/kg IM or slow IV injection). It has activity against trypanosomatid protozoans and against *Pneumocystis carinii*. It **probably interacts with kinetoplast DNA and inhibits topoisomerase II.**

It is **used** in the treatment of pneumocystosis (pulmonary and extrapulmonary disease caused by *P. carinii*), African trypanosomiasis (disease caused by *Trypanosoma brucei*) and leishmaniasis. Systemic pentamidine is highly toxic and can lead to severe hypotension, tachycardia, dyspnea, dizziness, hypoglycemia. Other **adverse effects** are skin rash, metallic taste, gastrointestinal symptoms, thrombocytopenia and cardiac arrhythmias.

SODIUM STIBOGLUCONATE

It is pentavalent antimonial. It **inhibits –SH dependent enzymes and block glycolytic & fatty acid oxidation pathways.** It is rapidly absorbed after IM injection and excreted unchanged in urine. **Used** in cutaneous and visceral leishmaniasis. It is given parenterally (20 mg/kg/day IM/IV) for three weeks in cutaneous leishmaniasis and for four weeks in visceral and mucocutaneous disease.

Adverse effects include metallic taste headache, fever, rash, myalgia and ECG changes.

TRYPANOSOMIASIS

It is caused by genus *Trypanosoma* which is characterized by skin eruptions, sustained fever, lethargy and lymphadenitis, progressive brain dysfunction.

Apart from imidazole derivative e.g. metronidazole, tinidazole, nimorazole etc. and other agents such as hydroxyquinolines, iodine preparation (povidoneiodine) and antifungal antibiotics e.g. clotrimazole (used mainly as vaginal pessaries), there are some other compounds which are mainly used in the treatment of trypanosomiasis. They are:

Suramin	1 g each wk for 5 wks IV or 1 g on day 1, 3, 7, 14, 21
Melarsoprol	3.6 mg/kg/day IV for 3-4 days
Eflornithine	100 mg/kg IV every 6 hrs for 14 days
Nifurtimox	8-10 mg/kg orally 3-4 months.

SURAMIN

It is a sulfated napthylamine and used as first line therapy for early hemolymphatic African trypanosomiasis (caused by *T. brucei gambiense*). It has very tight protein binding and having short initial half life but terminal half life is about 50 days and is excreted by kidney. It is also **used** for chemoprophylaxis against African trypanosomiasis.

Adverse effects include nausea, vomiting, fatigue, dermatitis, fever, photophobia, haemolytic anaemia, albuminuria and hematuria.

MELARSOPROL

Chemically it is trivalent arsenical used for advanced CNS African trypanosomiasis. It is administered IV in propylene glycol and after administration it is rapidly excreted. It is highly toxic and used only in advanced trypanosomiasis when no alternative is there.

Adverse effects include vomiting, fever, abdominal pain, renal and cardiac disease and encephalopathy characterized by cerebral edema, seizures, coma (even death).

EFLORNITHINE

It is an inhibitor of ornithine decarboxylase and is used as second line therapy for advanced CNS African trypanosomiasis. After oral or IV administration, peak plasma level is reached rapidly and elimination half life is approximately three hours.

It is **effective against** advanced *T. brucei gambiense* infection.

Adverse effects include vomiting, diarrhoea, leukopenia, thrombocytopenia, anaemia and seizures.

NIFURTIMOX

Chemically it is nitrofuran, **used** for American trypanosomiasis which is commonly known as 'Chagas disease.' After oral administration, it is well absorbed and plasma half life is about three hours.

Adverse effects include nausea, vomiting, fever, rash, abdominal pain, neuropathies and seizures.

TRICHOMONIASIS

It is caused by *Trichomonas vaginalis* and is mainly associated with vulvovaginitis which is characterized by greenish yellow and cheesy vaginal discharge.

The various agents used in trichomoniasis are metronidazole, tinidazole and secnidazole which are already described earlier. They produce 100% cure.

Other protozoal infection is **giardiasis** which is caused by *Giardia lamblia* and the drug of choice in its treatment are imidazole derivatives.

❑❑❑

CHAPTER 9.10 Anthelmintic Agents

Anthelmintic agents are used to eradicate (either kill or expel) the infesting helminths.

The important anthelmintic agents along with their specific uses and dosage are listed in table 9.10.1.

MEBENDAZOLE

It is a synthetic benzimidazole having a wide spectrum of anthelmintic activity. After administration it is poorly absorbed and approximately 90 percent of the drug is passed in faeces. Complete clearance of the parasites from the GIT may take up to three days.

Mebendazole binds to **microtubular protein 'β tubulin' of parasite and inhibits its polymerization**, thus irreversibly impairing glucose uptake.

Adverse effects include nausea, diarrhoea, abdominal pain. Alopecia and granulocytopenia may occur at high doses.

ALBENDAZOLE

Congener of mebendazole. It is given only as single dose.

Poorly absorbed from the GI tract, oral bioavailability being enhanced when given with a fatty meal (up to 5 fold). Its active sulphoxide metabolite is widely distributed throughout the body and is excreted in urine.

Adverse effects include nausea, vomiting, epigastric distress, abnormal LFTs, reversible alopecia.

THIABENDAZOLE

Apart from anthelmintic property, thiabendazole also possesses antiinflammatory, analgesic and antipyretic actions. It also **inhibits development of eggs of worms and kills the larvae**.

It is rapidly absorbed, metabolised by hydroxylation and conjugation to inactive metabolites and excreted through kidney.

Adverse effects include nausea, vomiting, skin rash, anorexia, giddiness, abdominal pain, diarrhoea, fever and headache.

LEVAMISOLE

It is a synthetic imidazothiazole derivative and is highly effective in

Table 9.10.1: *Classification of anthelmintic agents.*

Drug(s)	Uses and Dose
1. Mebendazole (MEBEX)	Ascariasis, ankylostomiasis: 100 mg BD × 3 days; Trichuriasis: 400 mg single dose; Pinworm: 100 mg OD & repeat after 2 & 4 weeks; Intestinal capillariasis: 400 mg/d × 21 days; Taeniasis: 300 mg BD × 3 days.
2. Albendazole (ZENTEL)	Ascariasis, ankylostomiasis and trichuriasis: 400 mg single dose; Taeniasis & strongyloidosis: 400 mg × 3 days; Neurocysticercosis: 15 mg/kg/daily × 1 month; Hydatid disease: 400 mg BD × 1 month (if required repeat after 2 wks).
3. Thiabendazole (MINTEZOL)	Trichinosis and strongyloidosis: 25 mg/kg/day in two divided doses × 2 days after meal (if required repeat after 2 days)
4. Levamisole (DECARIS)	Ascariasis and hook worm infestation: 50-150 mg single dose.
5. Niclosamide (NICLOSAN)	Taeniasis: 0.5-2 g (After breakfast 1 g to be chewed and swallowed with water followed by 1 g after 1 hr); For *H. nana* infestation: 2 g dose is repeated daily for 5 days.
6. Piperazine (as citrate)	Ascariasis: 4.5 g OD × 2 days; in children 0.75 g/year of age (max 4.5 g); Enterobiasis: 4.5 g OD, repeat after 3 weeks.
7. Pyrantel pamoate	For Ascaris, enterobius & ancylostoma: 10-15 mg/kg (max 1 g) single dose; Necator and strongyloides: 3 day course.
8. Diethyl carbamazine (HETRAZAN)	Tropical eosinophilia: 4-6 mg/kg BD-TDS × 7-10 days; Filariasis: 6-12 mg/kg OD-BD × 21 days; Also used in prophylaxis of filaria.
9. Ivermectin (IVERMECTOL)	Onchocerciasis: 150 μg/kg single dose. Also used in intestinal nematode infection and enterobiasis. For scabies and strongyloidiasis: 200 μg/kg single dose.
10. Praziquantel (CYSTICIDE)	Taeniasis: 10 mg/kg single dose; H. nana: 15-25 mg/kg single dose; Neurocysticercosis: 50 mg/kg in 3 divided doses × 15 days; Schistosome and other flukes except *Fasciola hepatica*: 75 mg/kg/day, can be repeated if needed.

eradicating ascariasis and ancylostomiasis. It **acts by stimulating ganglia of the worm which results in tonic paralysis**, which are subsequently eliminated from the intestines.

Adverse effects include nausea, epigastric discomfort, insomnia, dizziness, weakness and drowsiness.

If taken along with alcohol, it may produce disulfiram like reaction.

NICLOSAMIDE

It is salicylamide derivative, **act by inhibiting anaerobic phosphorylation of ADP by the mitochondria of the parasite**. It is devoid of any major toxicity except minor gastrointestinal disturbances.

PIPERAZINE CITRATE

It is an alternative drug for treatment of ascariasis and pinworms.

It possibly exerts its action by **antagonizing the action of acetylcholine** thus blocking neuromuscular transmission. Hence, **flaccid paralysis** occurs. It is considerably absorbed, partly metabolized in liver and excreted in urine. It can be safely used in pregnancy.

Adverse effects include nausea, vomiting, epigastric distress, skin rash, urticaria, headache and seizures.

PYRANTEL PAMOATE

It is a broad spectrum anthelmintic effective in pinworm, ascariasis and hook worm infestation. It exerts its action by **producing persistent nicotinic receptor activation which results in spastic paralysis of worms**.

It is poorly absorbed from GIT and is active against luminal organisms. It is excreted in urine as metabolites and in unchanged form. **Adverse reactions** include rash, nausea, vomiting, headache, dizziness, anorexia and elevation of SGOT levels.

DIETHYLCARBAMAZINE

It is the drug of choice for filariasis. It is effective against *W. malayi, W. bancrofti, Loa loa* and *Onchocerca volvulus*.

It has a dual action. Hyperpolarization effect of piperazine moiety **causes paralysis of the worms** and **alteration in microfilarial surface membrane** makes them susceptible to destruction by host defence mechanism.

It is absorbed after oral administration, distributed all over body, metabolized in liver and excreted in urine.

Adverse effects include anorexia, nausea, vomiting, skin rash, urticaria, fatigue, dizziness and headache.

It is **indicated** in filariasis and tropical eosinophilia.

IVERMECTIN

Semisynthetic derivative of drug obtained from *Streptomyces avermitilis*.

Ivermectin binds selectively and with high affinity to glutamate gated chloride ion channels in invertebrate nerve and muscle cells. This leads to an increase in the permeability of cell membrane to chloride ions with hyperpolarization of nerve of muscle cell, resulting in paralysis and death of the parasite.

Following the oral administration of ivermectin, peak plasma concentration is achieved in four hours. Ivermectin is absorbed well on an empty stomach. The bioavailability is 50 to 60%. It is mainly metabolized in the liver and the tissue concentration is maximum in liver and fat. Ivermectin and its metabolites are excreted mainly in faeces.

Adverse effects include nausea, vomiting, abdominal pain, constipation and fatigue.

It is mainly **indicated** in scabies, ascariasis trichuriasis, strongyloidiasis, enterobiasis, filariasis, onchocerciasis (River blindness) and elephantiasis. It is drug of choice for onchocerciasis producing long lasting reduction in microfilaria without affecting adult worm.

PRAZIQUANTEL

Effective against schistosomes, other trematodes, cestodes and their larval forms but not against nematodes.

It **causes spastic paralysis of worms due to leakage of intracellular calcium from membranes**. At high concentration it causes vacuolization of tegument and release of contents of worms and their destruction by host defence mechanism.

It is rapidly absorbed from intestine, undergoes high hepatic first pass metabolism. It readily crosses the blood brain barrier.

Adverse effects are nausea, abdominal pain, headache, dizziness.

Suramin	(1 gm. each wk for 5 wk. IV or 1 gm. on day 1, 3, 7, 14, 21)
Melarsoprol	3.6 mg/kg/day IV for 3-4 days
Eflornithine	100 mg/kg IV every 6 hrs. for 14 days
Nifurtimox	8-10 mg/kg orally 3-4 months.

SURAMIN

It is a sulfated napthylamine and used in first line therapy for early hemolymphatic African trypanosomiasis. (caused by *T. brucei gambiense*). It is very tight protein binding and having short initial half life but terminal half life is about 50 days and is excreted by kidney. It is also used for chemoprophylaxis against African trypanosomiasis. Adverse effects include nausea, vomiting, fatigue, dermatitis, fever, photophobia, haemolytic anaemia, albuminuria and hematuria.

MELARSOPROL

Chemically it is trivalent arsenical used for advanced CNS African trypanosomiasis. It is administered intravenously in propylene glycol and after administration it rapidly excreted. It is highly toxic and used only in advanced trypanosomiasis when no alternative is there, these effects include vomiting, fever, abdominal pain, renal and cardiac disease and encephalopathy characterized by cerebral edema, seizures, coma (even death).

EFLORNITHINE

It is an inhibitor of ornithine decarboxylase and is used as second therapy for advanced CNS African trypanosomiasis. After oral or intravenous administration, peak plasma level reached rapidly and elimination half life is approximately 3 hours.

It is effective against advanced *T. brucei gambiense* infection. Adverse effect includes vomiting, diarrhoea, leukopenia, thrombocytopenia, anemia and seizures.

❑❑❑

CHAPTER 9.11 Chemotherapy of Tuberculosis

Tuberculosis is a chronic infectious disease caused by various species of mycobacteria. The important human mycobacterium pathogens are *Mycobacterium tuberculosis* and *Mycobacterium bovis*. According to WHO, about one third of the world's population is infected with tuberculosis. Due to spread of HIV virus, there is increased prevalence of tuberculosis, infection with *Mycobacterium avium* complex and multidrug resistant tuberculosis. The chemotherapeutic agents used in the treatment

Table 9.11.1: *Classification of antitubercular drugs.*

I.	**First line or standard drugs**	
	Isoniazid (Isonicotinic acid hydrazide – INH; ISONEX)	300-450 mg/day
	Rifampicin (R-CIN)	450-600 mg/day
	Streptomycin (AMBISTRYN-S)	0.75-1 g IM
	Pyrazinamide (PZA-CIBA)	1.5-2 g/day
	Ethambutol (MYCOBUTOL)	15-25 mg/kg/day
	Combination of rifampicin & isoniazid (R-CINEX), combination of rifampicin, INH & pyrazinamide (MYCOCOX-Z)	
II.	**Second line or reserved drugs**	
	Ethionamide (MYCOTUF)	0.5-1.0 g/day
	Para-amino salicylic acid (PAS; INAPAS)	10-12 g/day
	Cycloserine (CYCLORINE)	0.5-1.0 g/day
	Thiacetazone	150 mg/day
	Kanamycin (KANSIN)	0.75-1 g/day IM
	Capreomycin (KAPOCIN)	0.75-1 g/day IM
	Amikacin (AMICIN)	0.75-1 g/day IM
	Fluoroquinolones like ciprofloxacin, ofloxacin; Macrolide antibiotics like clarithromycin, azithromycin.	
	Newer drugs	
	Rifabutin (Ansamycin)	450 mg/day
	Rifapentine	600 mg once or twice in a wk

of tuberculosis are classified as in table 9.11.1.

First Line or Standard Drugs

ISONIAZID

It is the most active drug used in the treatment of tuberculosis. It is a hydrazide of isonicotinic acid. It is a **bactericidal drug**, effective against *Mycobacterium tuberculosis* and ineffective against atypical mycobacteria.

Isoniazid possibly exerts its action **by inhibiting the synthesis of mycolic acid which is an essential component of mycobacterial cell wall.** It is also postulated that the ability of isoniazid to suppress the formation of DNA and RNA and also inhibition of various oxidative mechanisms may be responsible for its action.

Isoniazid is completely absorbed on oral administration and penetrates all tissues of the body. Peak plasma levels are reached within one hour and persists for 24 hours. It penetrates intracellularly and diffuses into macrophages and the necrotic centres. It is metabolized in liver by acetylation and isoniazid metabolites and a small amount of unchanged drug is excreted mainly by kidney.

Adverse effects include skin rash, fever, peripheral neuritis, nausea, vomiting, weakness, dizziness, lethargy, slurred speech, blurred vision, agranulocytosis, hepatitis (which is dose related, common in old people but rare in children), optic neuritis, optic atrophy and convulsions.

RIFAMPICIN

It is a semisynthetic derivative of rifamycin isolated from *Streptomyces mediterranei*. It is bactericidal against *Mycobacterium tuberculosis* and also against many gram positive and negative organisms such as *Staph. aureus*, pneumococci, *Bacillus anthracis*, *N. gonorrhoeae*, *C. diphtheriae*, meningococci, *H. influenzae* and *Streptococcus faecalis*.

It **acts by inhibiting DNA-dependent RNA polymerase and stopping the expression of bacterial genes**.

After oral administration, it is absorbed well and distributed to different body tissues and penetrates meninges, caseous masses and placental barrier. It is metabolized in liver to active deacylated metabolite and induces the microsomal enzymes in liver. It is excreted mainly in bile and urine.

Adverse effects include skin rash, drug fever, nausea, vomiting, peripheral neuropathy, fatigue, hepatitis and jaundice, haemolytic anaemia, diarrhoea, drowsiness, ataxia, headache, flu like syndrome and stomatitis.

Apart from its main use in tuberculosis, it is also **used** in leprosy and prophylaxis of meningitis due to *H. influenzae* and meningococci. It is also used with doxycycline in treatment of brucellosis.

STREPTOMYCIN

Detailed pharmacology is discussed in chapter 'Aminoglycoside antibiotics'.

PYRAZINAMIDE

It is chemically related to nicotinamide and thiosemicarbazone. It is bactericidal. It is effective against *Mycobacterium tuberculosis* resistant to INH and streptomycin. **It is converted to pyrazinoic acid (active**

form) by mycobacterial pyrazinamidase. Pyrazinamide is a first line drug. Resistance develops fast, if given alone, hence it is used in conjunction with isoniazid and rifampicin for shortcourse therapy.

It is absorbed after oral administration and has good penetration in CSF and is metabolised in liver and excreted in urine.

Adverse effects include nausea, vomiting, myalgia, arthralgia, hyperuricaemia and hepatotoxicity. Hypersensitivity reactions have also been reported.

ETHAMBUTOL

It is tuberculostatic drug effective against many atypical mycobacteria also. It **acts mainly against rapidly multiplying organisms in the cavities walls**.

Ethambutol is well absorbed from the GIT after oral administration, distributed widely and excreted in urine by glomerular filtration and tubular secretion.

Adverse effects include optic neuritis, visual disturbance, colour blindness, hyperuricaemia, skin rash, drug fever, malaise, confusion, disorientation, headache, nausea, anorexia, vomiting and abdominal pain.

SECOND LINE OR RESERVED DRUGS

ETHIONAMIDE

It is chemically related to isoniazid and **inhibit the synthesis of mycolic acids**. It is effective against tubercle bacilli resistant to other drugs and atypical mycobacteria.

After oral administration it is well absorbed from gastrointestinal tract and widely distributed throughout body tissues and CSF. It crosses the placental barrier and is completely metabolised and less than one percent of the drug is excreted in urine.

The common **side effects** are nausea, vomiting and anorexia. Other effects include hepatotoxicity, drowsiness, depression, peripheral neuritis, skin rash, acne, alopecia and hypertension.

PARA-AMINOSALICYLIC ACID (PAS)

It is a tuberculostatic and very less active drug in the treatment of tuberculosis. It is used as sodium salt and its larger dose can cause sodium overload in the body.

Bacteriostatic against *Mycobacterium tuberculosis*. It **inhibits the onset of bacterial resistance to streptomycin and INH**.

Readily absorbed from GI tract. Concentrated in pleural and caseous tissue. Does not enter CSF. 50% metabolised by acetylation.

Adverse effects include nausea, vomiting, diarrhoea, abdominal pain, skin rashes, goitre, fever and blood dyscrasias.

CYCLOSERINE

It is an antibiotic obtained from *S. orchidaceus*. It is a chemical analogue of D-alanine. It is a **second line tuberculostatic antitubercular drug** and **inhibitor of cell wall synthesis**.

After oral administration, it is rapidly absorbed and is distributed in various body tissues including CSF. It is excreted largely unchanged in urine by glomerular filtration. It is used for treatment of multidrug resistant tuberculosis with other primary drugs. It is also used in acute urinary tract infections caused by susceptible microorganisms.

Adverse effects include skin rash, nervousness, dizziness, drowsiness, vertigo, tremors, convulsions and psychotic state.

CAPREOMYCIN

It is a peptide protein synthesis inhibitor antibiotic isolated from *Streptomyces capreolus*. It is second line antimycobacterial drug which exhibits activity against human strains of *Mycobacterium tuberculosis.*

After oral administration, it is insignificantly absorbed. It is administered parenterally and is excreted unchanged by glomerular filtration.

Adverse effects include tinnitus, vertigo, leucopenia, hypokalemia, skin rash, urticaria, fever, pain and induration at injection site, excessive bleeding at injection site and abnormalities in liver function.

KANAMYCIN

It is **used** in the treatment of tuberculosis caused by streptomycin resistant strains but since agents with lesser toxicity e.g. capreomycin and amikacin are available, its use is obsolete.

The pharmacology of quinolones e.g. ciprofloxacin and ofloxacin is discussed in chapter 'Sulfonamides, nitrofurans and quinolones' and the pharmacology of macrolide antibiotics e.g. clarithromycin and azithromycin is discussed in chapter 'Macrolide and polypeptide antibiotics.'

RIFABUTIN

It is similar to rifampicin and shows significant activity against *M. tuberculosis, M. avium* complex and *M. fortuitum.* Rifabutin is both **substrate and cytochrome 450 enzyme inducer**. Because it is less potent inducer, rifabutin is used (in place of rifampicin) for the treatment of tuberculosis in HIV-infected patients, who are on concurrent antiretroviral therapy with a protease inhibitor. It is used alone or in combination with pyrazinamide.

RIFAPENTINE

It is an analog of rifampicin active against *M. tuberculosis* and *M. avium.* It **inhibits bacterial RNA polymerase and it is a potent inducer of cytochrome P450 enzymes.**

It is **indicated** in the treatment of tuberculosis caused by rifampicin susceptible strains.

❑❑❑

CHAPTER 9.12 Chemotherapy of Leprosy

Leprosy is caused by *Mycobacterium leprae*. The various drugs used in the treatment of leprosy are classified as in table 9.12.1.

SULFONES

DAPSONE

It is diamino diphenyl sulfone (DDS), chemically related to sulfonamides, have been used effectively in the long term treatment of leprosy. Its mechanism of action is same as that of sulfonamides i.e. **inhibition of paraamino benzoic acid (PABA) incorporation into folic acid (inhibition of folate synthesis)**. In large proportion of *Mycobacterium leprae* infections e.g. in lepromatous leprosy, resistance can develop, so combination of dapsone, rifampicin and clofazimine is used in initial therapy.

After oral administration, it is completely absorbed and is concentrated in lepromatous skin, liver, kidney and muscles. It is metabolized in liver and excreted in urine as glucuronic acid and sulfate conjugates.

Table 9.12.1: *Classification of drugs used in leprosy.*

I.	**Sulfones**	
	Dapsone (DDS)	100 mg daily
II.	**Phenazine derivative**	
	Clofazimine (CLOFOZINE)	100 mg TDS
III.	**Antitubercular drugs**	
	Rifampicin	600 mg monthly/daily
	Ethionamide	250 mg daily
IV.	**Other antimicrobial agents**	
	Quinolones e.g. ofloxacin;	400 mg/day
	Others include pefloxacin, sparfloxacin	
	Macrolides e.g. clarithromycin	500 mg/day
	Minocycline	100 mg/day

Adverse effects include haemolysis which is most common and dose related. Patients with G-6-PD deficiency are more susceptible. Nausea, vomiting, anorexia, headache, methaemoglobinaemia, drug fever, allergic skin reactions, insomnia and paresthesia. Rarely hepatitis and agranulocytosis.

It is also **used** with pyrimethamine in chloroquine resistant malaria.

Phenazine Derivatives

CLOFAZIMINE

Clofazimine is phenazine dye and used as alternative to dapsone in dapsone intolerant/resistant cases and in combination with dapsone and rifampicin in the multidrug treatment of leprosy. It's probable mechanism of action is its **involvement in DNA binding**, it may **interfere with template function of DNA**.

After oral administration, it is slowly absorbed, stored widely in reticuloendothelial system and fatty tissues. It has long elimination half life.

Adverse effects include discolouration of skin (red brown to black) and skin lesion persists for month after discontinuation of therapy. Other side effects include dry skin, itching, phototoxicity, nausea, abdominal pain, anorexia and diarrhoea.

Antitubercular Drugs

RIFAMPICIN

It is bactericidal and highly effective in leprosy. A single monthly dose of 600 mg may be used in combination with other antileprosy drugs to avoid any probable risk of rifampicin resistant *M. leprae.*

The detailed pharmacology is discussed in chapter 'Chemotherapy of Tuberculosis'.

ETHIONAMIDE

It is antitubercular drug used as an alternative to clofazimine in the treatment of leprosy. But due to its hepatotoxicity, its use in leprosy is very limited.

Other Antimicrobial Agents

Among fluoroquinolones, ofloxacin, pefloxacin and sparfloxacin can be used in alternative regimen, when drugs like rifampicin can not be used. Detailed pharmacology of quinolones is discussed in chapter 'Sulfonamides, nitrofurans and quinolones'.

Among macrolide antibiotics, clarithromycin is effective against *M. leprae* as an alternative multidrug therapy (MDT) regimen (detailed pharmacology is discussed in 'Macrolide antibiotics').

MINOCYCLINE

It is a tetracycline which is active against *M. leprae* and its bactericidal activity is higher than that of clarithromycin. Used in alternative multidrug treatment regimen (MDT).

CLARITHROMYCIN

Only macrolide antibiotic useful in leprosy. It is used in alternative MDT regimen.

Recently, **thalidomide** (50-100 mg capsule form, approved by FDA), an immunomodulatory agent is used in erythema nodosum leprosum (ENL) which is a complication of leprosy occurring in approximately one half of borderline lepromatous and lepromatous leprosy patients.

❑❑❑

CHAPTER

9.13 Chemotherapy of Malignancy

Cancer is a disease of cells characterized by a shift in the control mechanism which govern cell proliferation and differentiation and the anticancer agents either kill cancer cells or modify their growth. The various anticancer agents are classified according to their mode of action as in table 9.13.1.

Table 9.13.1: *Classification of anticancer agents.*

I.	**Alkylating agents**	
	Cyclophosphamide (CYCLOXAN)	2-3 mg/kg/day oral; 10-15 mg/kg IV every 7-10 days
	Mesna (UROMITEXAN)	20% of a dose of anticancer agent IV
	Chlorambucil (LEUKERAN)	0.1-0.2 mg/kg daily for 3-6 weeks then 2 mg daily for maintenance
	Busulfan (MYLERAN)	4-8 mg/day, 1-3 mg/day for maintenance
	Lomustine (LUSTIN)	120-130 mg/m^2 BSA single dose orally every 6 weeks
	Thio-TEPA (THIOTEPA)	0.3-0.4 mg/kg IV every 1-4 week interval
II.	**Antimetabolites**	
	Methotrexate (ONCOTRAX)	15-30 daily for 5 days orally repeat after one week or 20-40 mg/m^2 BSA IM/IV twice weekly.
	6-Mercaptopurine (ZYPURIN)	2.5 mg/kg daily
	5-Fluorouracil (FLURACIL)	12 mg/kg OD for 4 successive days IV, 10-15 mg/kg/week maintenance
	Cytarabine (Cytosine arabinoside; CYTABIN)	1.5-3.0 mg/kg IV BD for 5-10 days
III.	**Cytotoxic antibiotics**	
	Dactinomycin (Actinomycin-D) (COSMEGEN)	15 µg/kg IV daily for 5 days
	Doxorubicin (ONCODRIA)	60-75 mg/m^2 BSA every 3 wks slow IV
	Bleomycin (ONCOBLEO)	30 mg twice weekly IV/IM
	Mitomycin-C (MITODUS)	2-10 mg/m^2 BSA IV twice weekly

Contd....

...Contd.

IV. **Vinca alkaloids**	
Vincristine (Oncovin; BIOCRISTINE)	1.5 mg/m² BSA IV weekly
Vinblastine (CYTOBLASTIN)	0.1-0.15 mg/kg IV weekly (total 3 doses)
Vinorelbine (VINELBINE)	30 mg/m² BSA IV weekly
V. **Taxanes**	
Paclitaxel (MITOTAX)	175 mg/m² BSA IV infusion repeated every 3 weeks
Docetaxel (DOXOTEL)	
VI. **Topoisomerase-I inhibitors**	
Irinotecan (IRINOTECAN)	125 mg/m² BSA weekly IV
Topotecan (TOPOTEL)	1.5 mg/m² BSA IV infusion for five consecutive days
VII. **Hormone & hormone antagonists**	
Fosfestrol (Stilboestrol)	40-80 mg IM every 2-4 weeks
Ethinyl estradiol (LYNORAL)	1-3 mg daily
Tamoxifen (ONCOTAM)	10-20 mg BD
VIII. **Radioactive isotopes**	
Radioactive iodine (^{131}I)	3-6 mci oral/IV
Radioactive phosphorus (^{32}P)	2.5-5.0 mci IV
Radioactive gold (^{198}AU)	35-150 mci IP
IX. **Miscellaneous agents**	
Hydroxyurea (CYTODROX)	20-30 mg/kg daily or 80 mg/kg every 3rd day
Procarbazine	100-300 mg/day
L-Asparaginase (LEUNASE)	50-200 KU/kg daily IV infusion for 2-4 weeks
Cisplatin	50-100 mg/m² BSA single IV dose every 3-4 wks
Interferon alfa (ALFERON)	3-36 million IU daily SC/IM (depending upon the type of cancer)
X. Immunosuppressants	
Azathioprine	
Cyclosporine	

* BSA = Body surface area

ALKYLATING AGENTS

The alkylating agents can transfer an alkyl radical to a suitable receptor site. Alkylation of DNA within the nucleus represent the major interactions which will lead to cell death. These agents react chemically with sulfhydryl, carboxyl, amino and phosphate groups of other cellular nucleophiles in the cells which make them unavailable for the normal metabolic reactions. Alkylating agents **react with nucleic acid and inhibit DNA synthesis and also interfere with cell replication**. Alkylating agents has got cytotoxic action and damage the nuclei of growing and multiplying cells. They have got immunosuppressant action also and suppress antibody production. They also have radiomimetic (like ionizing radiation) actions.

CYCLOPHOSPHAMIDE

It is an alkylating agent given orally or by intravenous route. It **exerts its action by alkylation of DNA**.

After oral administration it is well absorbed. It is a prodrug and converted in the blood and liver to its active form (metabolites) namely hydroxyphosphamide and aldophosphamide. It is excreted in urine.

Adverse effects include nausea, vomiting, visual blurring, facial burning with IV administration, teratogenic effect, **haemorrhagic cystitis**, bone marrow depression, hyponatremia, sterility, inappropriate secretion of ADH, alopecia and increased skin pigmentation.

It is **indicated** in leukaemias, lymphogranulomatosis, lymphosarcoma, reticulum cell sarcoma, Hodgkin's disease, multiple myeloma, retinoblastoma, carcinoma of the breast, adenocarcinoma of the ovary, inoperable solid malignancies. It is used in combination with surgery, radiation and other therapeutic measures.

MESNA

Cyclophosphamide and ifosfamide cause urothelial toxicity (haemorrhagic cystitis) which is caused by metabolite 'acrolein'. Mesna reacts with this metabolites in the urinary tract to prevent toxicity and is **used** in prevention of toxicity to the urinary passage caused by oxazaphosphorins e.g. ifosfamide and cyclophosphamide.

CHLORAMBUCIL

It is a slow acting alkylating agent. After oral administration, it shows adequate and reliable absorption and almost completely metabolised.

It is **indicated** in chronic lymphocytic leukaemia (drug of choice), primary (Waldenstrom's) macroglobulinaemia, advanced ovarian adenocarcinoma, breast cancer, certain forms of nonHodgkin's lymphoma and Hodgkin's disease.

Adverse effects include nausea, vomiting, pulmonary fibrosis, dermatitis, hepatotoxicity, seizures, amenorrhoea, azoospermia, peripheral neuropathy and bone marrow depression.

BUSULFAN

After oral administration, it is well absorbed and excreted in urine as methanesulfonic acid. It is mainly **used** in chronic myeloid leukaemia, polycythemia vera, essential thrombocythemia and myelofibrosis.

Adverse effects include, thrombocytopenia, amenorrhoea, azoospermia, skin pigmentation, nausea, vomiting, cataract, gynaecomastia, pulmonary fibrosis and hyperuricaemia.

LOMUSTINE

It is rapidly absorbed from GIT after oral administration and is completely and rapidly metabolised. It is **indicated** in Hodgkin's disease, brain tumour, lung carcinoma, solid tumours and malignant melanoma.

Adverse effects include nausea, vomiting, delayed bone marrow depression (four to six weeks), leucopenia, thrombocytopenia and pulmonary fibrosis.

THIO-TEPA

Chemically it is ethylenimine and because of high toxicity, it is rarely used.

ANTIMETABOLITES

Antimetabolites are analogues of normal DNA components or of coenzymes involved in nucleic acid synthesis. They get incorporated or competitively inhibit utilization of normal substrate to form dysfunctional nucleic acid molecules.

METHOTREXATE

It is a broad spectrum antineoplastic drug which **act as an antimetabolite of folic acid**.

It **acts by inhibiting dihydrofolate reductase**. It inhibits conversion of dihydrofolic acid to tetrahydrofolic which is essential for purine synthesis and amino acid interconversions. It primarily affects DNA synthesis but also RNA and protein synthesis. It has cell cycle specific action and kills cells in S phase. It is readily absorbed from gastrointestinal tract but larger doses are absorbed incompletely, little drug is metabolised and it is excreted largely unchanged in urine.

Adverse effects include nausea, vomiting, diarrhoea, anaphylaxis, hepatic necrosis, fever, bone marrow depression, osteoporosis, menstrual dysfunction, cirrhosis, pulmonary infiltrates and fibrosis, renal toxicity and depigmentation.

It is **indicated** in lymphoblastic leukemia and choriocarcinoma, psoriasis, adjuvant therapy of non-metastatic osteosarcoma and to reduce corticosteroid requirement in patients with severe steroid dependent asthma.

It is also used as 'disease modifying drug' in rheumatoid arthritis as it reduces lymphocyte proliferation, rheumatoid factor production and interferes with the release of inflammatory cytokines.

6-MERCAPTOPURINE

It is an antimetabolite antineoplastic, which being an analogue of hypoxanthine and adenine inhibits purine metabolism.

After oral administration absorption is incomplete and drug is metabolised in liver. The active metabolites have longer half life than parent drug.

Adverse effects include nausea, vomiting, diarrhoea, cholestasis, bone marrow depression, pancreatitis, oral and intestinal ulcers. Rarely hepatic necrosis.

It is **used** in acute leukaemia, choriocarcinoma and chronic granulocytic leukaemia.

FLUOROURACIL

It is fluorinated analogue of pyrimidine, **act by binding the enzyme thymidylate synthetase and preventing the production of basic component of DNA-thymine**. It is converted into 5-fluorouridine triphosphate and is incorporated into RNA where it interferes with RNA processing and function.

It is **used** in the treatment of carcinoma of breast, colon, urinary bladder, stomach liver, rectum and ovaries.

The major **toxicity** includes myelosuppression and mucositis.

CYTARABINE

Cytarabine or cytosine arabinoside **competitively inhibits DNA polymerase** and **blocks generation of cytidylic acid** and is a drug of choice for acute myeloid leukaemia.

It is **indicated** in acute myelocytic leukaemia, acute lymphocytic leukaemia, chronic myeloid leukaemia (blast phase), non-Hodgkin's lymphoma in children, treatment and maintenance of meningeal neoplasms, erythroleukaemia.

Adverse effects include depression of bone marrow which gives rise to leukopenia, thrombocytopenia, reticulocytopenia. GI disturbances, oral and anal ulceration, hepatic and renal dysfunction and peripheral neurotoxicity with high doses.

CYTOTOXIC ANTIBIOTICS

These drugs are obtained from various microorganisms and have antitumor activity. They act by binding to double stranded DNA and interfere with its functions.

DACTINOMYCIN (ACTINOMYCIN D)

It is a potent antitumor antibiotic isolated from *Streptomyces* organism. It binds tightly to double stranded DNA through intercalation between adjacent guanine cytosine base pair and **inhibit all forms of DNA dependent RNA synthesis**.

It is **used** in choriocarcinoma, Hodgkin's disease and Wilm's tumour in combination with irradiation.

Adverse effects include damage of skin, alopecia, bone marrow depression, vomiting and diarrhoea.

DOXORUBICIN

It is a cytotoxic anthracycline antibiotic isolated from *Streptomyces pneuceticus.* It is DNA intercalator and it generates free radicals.

It is usually administered by intravenous route. It does not cross blood brain barrier.

Adverse effects include nausea, vomiting, diarrhoea, fever, red urine (harmless), ventricular arrhythmia, severe local tissue damage on extravasation, cardiotoxicity, bone marrow depression, anorexia, stomatitis, alopecia, conjunctivitis.

It is **indicated** in GI tract carcinoma, acute myeloblastic leukaemia, bronchogenic, breast and ovarian carcinoma, soft tissue and bone sarcomas, malignant lymphoma; primary management of nonmetastatic bladder carcinoma (intravesical administration), Wilm's tumor and neuroblastoma.

Epirubicin (FARMORUBICIN) is structurally similar to doxorubicin and is similarly effective in the treatment of breast cancer, lung cancer and lymphoma.

BLEOMYCIN

It is a mixture of cytotoxic glycopeptide antibiotic isolated from a strain of *Streptomyces verticillus.*

It exerts its cytotoxic action by **causing fragmentation of DNA** and it generates free radicals.

It is usually administered by parenteral route. It does not cross blood brain barrier.

Adverse effects include nausea, vomiting, allergic reactions, fever, anaphylaxis, skin rash, Raynaud's phenomenon, stomatitis, pulmonary fibrosis, hyperpigmentation, renal and hepatic toxicity.

Bleomycin is **used** as palliative and adjuvant to surgery and radiation therapy in testicular tumour, squamous cell carcinoma of skin, neck and head, genitourinary tract and oesophagus neoplasm, malignancy of cervix, Hodgkin's and non Hodgkin's lymphoma, choriocarcinoma and embryonal cell carcinoma of testis, brain tumour and glioma.

MITOMYCIN-C

It is a highly toxic antibiotic with antitumour activity isolated from *Streptomyces caespitosus*.

It **inhibits DNA synthesis and cross links DNA**.

After oral administration it exhibits inconsistent absorption. Hence it is administered by IV route and is metabolised in liver.

It is **used** in the treatment of adenocarcinoma, lymphosarcoma and seminoma. It is also used in squamous cell carcinoma of cervix.

Adverse effects include nausea, vomiting, alopecia, pulmonary fibrosis, bone marrow depression, sterility, amenorrhoea and renal toxicity.

VINCA ALKALOIDS

The vinca alkaloids are isolated from plant *Vinca rosea*. They are **cell cycle specific** and **mitotic inhibitors**.

VINCRISTINE

It **blocks mitosis and produces metaphase arrest by binding to microtubular protein 'tubulin', preventing its polymerization**.

After oral administration the absorption is unpredictable. It is metabolised in liver.

Adverse effects include local reaction if extravasation occurs, constipation, paralytic ileus, jaw pain, alopecia, bone marrow depression, peripheral neuropathy, inappropriate ADH secretion, shortness of breath and bronchospasm.

It is **indicated** in acute leukaemias, lymphomas, Ewing's sarcoma, neuroblastoma, Wilm's tumour and idiopathic thrombocytopenic purpura.

VINBLASTINE

It **interferes with metabolic pathways of amino acids** leading from glutamic acid to the citric acid (Krebs) cycle and urea.

Vinblastine has an effect on cell energy production required for mitosis and interferes with nucleic acid synthesis. Reversal of antitumour effect by glutamic acid or tryptophan has occurred.

It undergoes rapid distribution and extensive tissue binding following IV injection. It is metabolised in liver.

Adverse effects include hepatic function impairment, leucopenia, aspermia, nausea, vomiting, hypertension and alopecia.

It is **indicated** in Hodgkin's and non Hodgkin's lymphoma, testicular carcinoma, mycosis fungoides and Kaposi's sarcoma.

VINORELBINE

It is semisynthetic vinca alkaloid. It **interferes with microtubules, in miotic spindle fibres leading to cell cycle arrest**

in metaphase.

It is **used** for the treatment of non small cell lung carcinoma, breast carcinoma, Hodgkin's disease, ovarian carcinoma, squamous cell carcinoma of the head and neck, cervical squamous cell carcinoma, renal cell cancer and Kaposi's sarcoma.

TAXANES

PACLITAXEL

It is an alkaloid ester derived from the western yew *Taxus brevifolia*.

It is a diterpenoid compound and is a natural product with antitumour activity.

It **binds specifically to the β-tubulin subunit of microtubule and appears to antagonise the disassembly of this cytoskeletal protein** i.e. enhances polymerization of tubulin. Arrest in mitosis follows. The cell killing is dependent on both drug concentration and duration of cell exposure.

It is **indicated** in metastatic ovarian and breast cancer.

Adverse effects include bone marrow depression, hypersensitivity reactions, chest pain, bradycardia, sensory neuropathy, nausea, vomiting, diarrhoea, alopecia and impaired liver function tests.

Docetaxel (DOXOTEL), a related drug, used in metastatic breast cancer.

TOPOISOMERASE-I INHIBITORS

IRINOTECAN

It **inhibits topoisomerase-I**, the enzyme which is involved in DNA replication.

It is **used** in the treatment of metastatic carcinoma of colon or rectum.

Adverse effects include vomiting, diarrhoea, abdominal discomfort, leukopenia, anemia, neutropenia, haemorrhage, insomnia and dizziness.

TOPOTECAN

Topotecan also **inhibits topoisomerase I**.

Adverse effects include abdominal discomfort, vomiting, diarrhoea, intestinal obstruction, nausea, stomatitis, anorexia, bone marrow suppression (primarily neutropenia, anaemia and thrombocytopenia).

It is **valuable** in control of metastatic ovarian cancer, including cisplatinresistant neoplasms.

HORMONE AND HORMONE ANTAGONISTS

These are not cytotoxic drugs. They act by modifying the growth of hormone dependent tumours.

FOSFESTROL (STILBOESTROL)

Fosfestrol is a synthetic non-steroidal estrogen which is activated by the enzyme acid phosphatase to produce stilboestrol.

Metabolism occurs primarily in the liver. It is **used** as palliative treatment of disseminated mammary or prostatic carcinoma.

Adverse effects include hepatic cutaneous porphyria, perineal pain, erythema and feminising effects in man.

ETHINYL ESTRADIOL

It is also **indicated** in palliative treatment of disseminated mammary or prostatic carcinoma. The detailed pharmacology is discussed in chapter 'Oral Contraceptives.'

MEGESTROL ACETATE

It belongs to group of progesterone which are mainly used as second or third line therapy in breast and endometrial cancer.

Adverse effects include nausea, acne, fluid retention, GI disturbances and weight changes.

TAMOXIFEN

It **exerts its action by binding to estrogen receptors**. Tumours with estrogen receptors respond.

It is given orally, the drug has biphasic half life and is primarily excreted in bile.

Adverse effects include nausea, vomiting, hot flushes, vaginal bleeding, pruritus vulvae and menstrual irregularities.

It is **used** as palliative treatment of estrogen receptor positive advanced or metastatic carcinoma of breast.

MISCELLANEOUS AGENTS

HYDROXYUREA

The primary action is inhibition of enzyme ribonucleoside diphosphate reductase. The drug is specific for S phase of the cell cycle and **causes cell to arrest at the G_1-S interface**.

After oral administration it is readily absorbed from GI tract. Hydroxyurea readily crosses blood brain barrier.

It is **indicated** in treatment of chronic granulocytic leukaemia, polycythemia vera, essential thrombocytosis, melanoma, metastatic or inoperable carcinoma of ovary. In combination with radiotherapy in carcinoma of cervix, head, neck and lung.

Adverse effects include nausea, vomiting, rash. Bone marrow depression is the major toxic effect. Alopecia, stomatitis, dysuria; inflammation and increased pigmentation may occur in areas exposed to radiation. Rarely neurological disturbances occur.

PROCARBAZINE

After metabolic activation, it **depolymerizes DNA and causes chromosomal damage** and **also nucleic acid synthesis inhibition**. It is found to be effective in Hodgkin's disease and carcinoma of lungs.

Adverse effects include drowsiness, restlessness, anaemia, leucopenia, thrombocytopenia, bone marrow toxicity and disulfiram like reaction with alcohol.

L-ASPARAGINASE

It **destroys essential amino acid (asparagine) hence leukaemic cells are deprived of amino acid and leads to cell death.** It is given by parenteral route.

Adverse effects include nausea, vomiting, headache, fever, abdominal pain, hyperglycemia leading to coma, hypersensitivity, renal damage, coagulation defects, thrombosis, CNS depression or hyperexcitability and **acute haemorrhagic pancreatitis**.

It is **used** in the treatment of malignant lymphoma and acute leukaemia.

CISPLATIN

It **acts by cross-linking of DNA.** It also has radiomimetic property. It is bound to plasma proteins and is excreted slowly unchanged in urine. It is **effective** in metastatic testicular and ovarian carcinoma, advanced bladder carcinoma and refractory squamous cell head and neck carcinoma.

Adverse effects include nausea, vomiting, fever, anaphylactic reactions, hypokalemia, hypomagnesaemia, haemolysis, renal damage, sterility, teratogenesis, ototoxicity, peripheral neuropathy, Raynaud's disease and bone marrow depression.

INTERFERON ALFA

It is highly purified protein containing 165 amino acids and is manufactured by recombinant DNA technology.

Mechanism of action is not clearly understood but direct antiproliferative action against tumour cells and modulation of the host immune response may play important roles.

It exhibits half life of 3.7-8.5 hours. Alpha interferons are filtered through the glomeruli and undergo rapid proteolytic degradation during tubular reabsorption.

It is **indicated** in hairy cell leukemia, AIDS related Kaposi's sarcoma (the detailed pharmacology and its use as antiviral agent is discussed in chapter 'Antiviral agents').

Adverse effects include GI haemorrhage, leukopenia and elevation in liver enzyme levels.

Recently introduced interferon a-2b is used in chronic myeloid leukaemia, chronic hepatitis B and C.

IMMUNOSUPPRESSANTS

The drugs like azathioprine and cyclosporine A are used chiefly to prevent transplant rejection and in the treatment of autoimmune diseases. They are used to prevent graft rejection after kidney, liver, lung, pancreas transplant or bone marrow transplantation.

AZATHIOPRINE

It is a purine antimetabolite which has marked effect on T-lymphocytes, suppresses cell mediated immunity (CMI). It selectively affects differentiation and functions of T cells and inhibits cytolytic lymphocytes. It is used primarily as immunosuppressant in organ transplantation, progressive rheumatoid arthritis and some other autoimmune diseases.

CYCLOSPORINE

It is a cyclic polypeptide with 11 amino acids. It selectively inhibits T-lymphocytes proliferation, IL-2 and other cytokine production. It is the most effective drug for prevention and treatment of graft rejection reaction. It is used in cardiac, hepatic, renal, bone marrow transplantation and as second line drug in rheumatoid arthritis, inflammatory bowel disease, dermatomyositis, bronchial asthma and certain other autoimmune diseases.

Mycophenolate mofetil, a semisynthetic derivative of mycophenolic acid, isolated from the mould *Penicillium glaucum* is used in kidney and liver transplant patient. Another newer compound **mizoribine** is used in kidney transplantation.

❑❑❑

Section 10

Vitamins and Trace Elements

CHAPTER 10.1 Vitamins and Trace Elements

Vitamins are exogenous chemical substance required by the body in very small amount for the various metabolic functions of the body and categorized as essential nutrients. They do not yield energy but enable the body to use other nutrients and are primarily used in the prevention and treatment of certain deficiency diseases.

Vitamins are vital for normal metabolism in body. They vary in their chemical structure and are supplied in very small quantity in diet, because they are not synthesized in body or their rate of production is not sufficient for maintenance of health. Vitamin deficiency leads to development of deficiency symptoms. Different vitamin preparations are available for treatment and prophylaxis. Most of the vitamins are non-toxic but on chronic administration can cause toxicity especially vitamin A and D.

Vitamins are classified into two main groups:

I. **Fat soluble vitamins,** includes vitamin A, D, E and K.

II. **Water soluble vitamins,** includes B-complex group and vitamin C.

The fat soluble vitamins are stored in the body and excessive administration of fat soluble vitamins can cause toxicity, while water soluble vitamins are rapidly excreted in the urine and cause very less toxicity.

The different market preparation available for vitamins are given in table 10.1.1 and the deficiency diseases which occur with deficient supply of various vitamins are listed in table 10.1.2.

Table 10.1.1: *Classification of various preparations of vitamins.*

Vitamin A (ROVIGON)
Vitamin D (CALCIROL)
Vitamin E (EVION)
Alfacalcidol (ALCIDOL)
Vitamin B complex group
Vitamin B_1 (Thiamine; BENALGIS)
Vitamin B_2 (Riboflavin; LIPABOL)
Vitamin B_5 (Calcium pantothenate; SIGMA PANTOTHENATE)
Vitamin B_6 (Pyridoxine; PYRICONTIN)
Vitamin B_{12} (Cyanocobalamin/Mecobalamin; METHYCOBAL)
Folic acid (FOLVITE)
Vitamin C (Ascorbic acid; CELIN)
Multivitamins preparations
$B_1 + B_6 + B_{12}$ (NEUROBION)
B complex (B_1, B_2, B_3, B_5, B_6, B_{12} + folic acid; BECOSULE)

Table 10.1.2: *Diseases due to deficient supply of vitamins.*

Vitamins	Deficiency
1. Vitamin A	Night blindness (inability to see in dim light), conjunctival xerosis (dry and non-wettable conjunctiva), corneal xerosis (dry and non-wettable cornea and become opaque), keratomalacia (cornea becomes soft and burst open and vision is lost), Bitot's spots, growth retardation, dry and rough skin, sterility due to faulty spermatogenesis.
2. Vitamin D	Rickets (reduced calcification of growing bones).
3. Vitamin E	Axonal degeneration, ophthalmoplegia (however, vitamin E deficiency does not occur clinically).
4. Vitamin K	Decreased prothrombin content of blood and blood clotting time is prolonged.
5. Vitamin B_1 (Thiamine)	Beriberi (characterized by nerve involvement – peripheral neuritis), Wernicke's encephalopathy (characterized by ophthalmoplegia, polyneuritis and mental disorientation).
6. Vitamin B_2 (Riboflavin)	Angular stomatitis (occurs in malnourished children).
7. Vitamin B_3 (Niacin or Nicotinic acid)	Pellagra (characterized by diarrhoea, dermatitis and dementia).
8. Vitamin B_5 (Pantothenic acid)	Clinical deficiency is not known (has role in biosynthesis of corticosteroids).
9. Vitamin B_6 (Pyridoxine)	Peripheral neuritis, mental confusion, impairs the optimal utilization of pyridoxine [INH (anti TB drug) is a recognised antagonist].
10. Vitamin B_{12} (Cyanocobalamin)	Megaloblastic anaemia (pernicious anaemia), demyelinating neurological lesions in the spinal cord & infertility.
11. Vitamin C (Ascorbic acid)	Scurvy
12. Folic acid	Megaloblastic anaemia and gastrointestinal disturbances such as diarrhoea, distension and flatulence. Severe folate deficiency causes infertility or even sterility.

FAT SOLUBLE VITAMINS

VITAMIN A

Vitamin A is widely distributed in plant and animal foods. In plants, the main source of vitamin A is green leafy vegetables e.g. spinach and amaranth. The darker the green leaves, the higher the carotene present. Vitamin A is also present in green & yellow vegetables and fruits e.g. pumpkin, papaya and mango, and in roots e.g. carrots (richest source among plant source). The most important carotenoid is betacarotene which has the highest vitamin A percentage. Carotenes are converted to vitamin A in the small intestine.

In animal foods, vitamin A is present in liver, eggs, butter, cheese, milk, fish and meat. Fish liver oil are the richest source of retinol.

It is vital for the functioning of retina. Vitamin A is essential for differentiation and growth of epithelial tissue. It enhances function of immune system and protect against development of certain malignancies. Different forms of vitamin A mediate different functions.

Retinoids: They influence a wide variety of biological activities including cellular proliferation, cellular differentiation, immune function, inflammation. e.g. tretinoin, isotretinoin, etretinate.

Isotretinoin is a retinoid, recently approved for use in capsule form (10-20 mg). It decreases the amount of sebum that sebaceous glands produce. Isotretinoin exhibits antiproliferative and antiandrogenic effects on the sebaceous glands. It also interacts with the formation of androgens in sebaceous glands. It is **indicated** in the treatment of severe nodular acne, acne conglobata and recalcitrant acne. It is available in International market under the brand name 'ACCUTANE' by Roche pharmaceuticals.

Deficiency symptoms: Bitot's spots, xerosis, night blindness, keratomalacia, diarrhoea, follicular hyperkeratosis, papular eruptions, drying of epidermis, urinary calculi, degeneration of testis, impaired spermatogenesis, sterility, abortion, impairment of smell and taste.

It is **indicated** in night blindness, vitamin A deficiency (in infants, in pregnancy, lactation, malabsorption syndrome), for prophylaxis of vitamin A deficiency, acne, ichthyosis, psoriasis, xerophthalmia, Bitot's spots (especially children).

Dosage:

Severe deficiency with xerophthalmia: 50,000 IU per day for three days followed by 50,000 IU per day for two weeks.

Severe deficiency: 100,000 IU per day for three days followed by 50,000 IU per day for two weeks.

Children: 5,000 to 10,000 IU per day for two weeks.

VITAMIN D

The term vitamin D is used for a range of compounds which possess the property of preventing or curing rickets. They include ergocalciferol (calciferol, vitamin D_2), cholecalciferol (vitamin D_3), dihydrotachysterol, alfacalcidol (1α-hydroxycholecalciferol) and calcitriol (1,25-dihydroxycholecalciferol).

It plays an important role in calcium metabolism. It regulates calcium homeostasis and maintains normal levels of plasma calcium and phosphate.

Deficiency symptoms: Rickets occurs in patients who are having deficiency of vitamin D. The bones are unusually soft and due to stress and strain of weight bearing produce characteristic deformities.

It is **indicated** in prophylaxis and treatment of rickets, postmenopausal osteoporosis, Fanconi syndrome and hypoparathyroidism.

Adverse effects include headache, weakness, nausea, vomiting, dry mouth, muscle pain, constipation, somnolence, ectopic calcification, hypertension, nephrocalcinosis and weight loss.

ALFACALCIDOL

It regulates calcium metabolism by increasing calcium and phosphate absorption from the intestinal tract and also mobilises minerals from the bone.

After oral administration it is absorbed in the small intestine and undergoes rapid metabolism to 1,25 $(OH)_2$ D_3 in liver and further distribution to bone and intestine is nearly similar to its physiological distribution.

Adverse effects include hypercalcaemia and hyperphosphataemia.

It is **indicated** in osteoporosis, hypoparathyroidism, hyperparathyroidism (with bone disease), renal osteodystrophy, nutritional and malabsorptive rickets, hypophosphataemic vitamin D resistant rickets and osteomalacia.

Dosage:

Adults: Initially 1 mcg daily adjusted according to response. **Elderly:** Initially 0.5 mcg daily adjusted according to response.

Children: Over 20 kg: Initially 1 mcg daily adjusted according to response. Under 20 kg: 0.05 mcg/kg body wt. daily.

VITAMIN E

It is an antioxidant vitamin. It presumably prevents oxidation of coenzyme Q and inhibits generation of peroxidation products from unsaturated fatty acids.

Vitamin E is a family of eight compounds, four tocopherols and four tocotrienols. Tocotrienols appear to affect a key enzyme in the liver (HMG CoA reductase), which plays a key role in the synthesis of cholesterol. As such tocotrienols help maintain good cardiovascular health. Vitamin E is an antioxidant and prevents the oxidation of LDL (the bad cholesterol). Vitamin E functions as anticoagulant, which means it delays the clotting of the blood. It can help prevent thrombosis, the formation of blood clots in the arteries.

Deficiency symptoms: In vitamin E deficiency in experimental animals the manifestations are seen in several systems including cardiovascular, reproductive and haematopoietic.

The clinical manifestations are axonal degeneration, gait disturbances, ophthalmoplegia, hyporeflexia and necrotizing myopathy.

Adverse effects include nausea, fatigue, headache, blurred vision, diarrhoea.

It is **indicated** in premature infants exposed to high concentration of oxygen, correction of established vitamin E deficiency, in patients at risk of developing vitamin E deficiency, nocturnal muscle cramps, intermittent claudication, fibrocystic breast disease, coronary artery disease and as an antioxidant.

Dosage:

Adults:

- *Nocturnal muscle cramps*: 400 mg daily for 8 to 12 weeks.
- *Intermittent claudication*: 400 mg daily for 12 to 18 weeks.
- *Fibrocystic breast disease*: 600 mg daily for 2 to 6 months.

Children: 200 mg daily.

WATER SOLUBLE VITAMINS

VITAMIN B GROUP

Vitamin B_1 (Thiamine)

Vitamin B_1 is the first member of the B complex.

Thiamine pyrophosphate is a coenzyme and the active form of vitamin B_1. It functions as coenzyme in decarboxylation of α-keto acid and in hexose monophosphate shunt.

Deficiency symptoms: In severe vitamin B_1 deficiency beriberi develops.

It is **indicated** in wet beriberi, dry beriberi, Wernicke's encephalopathy, prophylaxis of thiamine deficiency, hyperemesis gravidarum, Korsakoff's syndrome, chronic alcoholics, multiple neuritis, toxic and confusional states, delirium tremens and anorexia nervosa.

Dosage: *Mild chronic deficiency:* 10-25 mg daily; *severe deficiency*, 200-300 mg daily.

VITAMIN B_2 (RIBOFLAVIN)

It carries its physiological function in its active forms, flavin mononucleotide (FMN) and flavin adenine dinucleotide. These coenzymes are involved in various biochemical reactions.

Deficiency symptoms: It is characterized by glossitis, dermatitis of trunk and extremities, angular stomatitis, cheilosis, anaemia, neuropathy, cataract formation and vascularization of cornea.

It is **indicated** in arteriosclerosis, as adjunct in treatment of hypertension, diabetes and obesity.

VITAMIN B_3 (NIACIN)

Niacin was initially called pellagra preventing factor.

It is converted to coenzymes, nicotinamide adenine dinucleotide (NAD) or nicotinamide adenine dinucleotide phosphate (NADP). These coenzymes are bound to hydrogenases, function as oxidants by accepting hydrogen and electrons from substrates and become reduced.

Deficiency symptoms: In niacin deficiency, pellagra develops. The main features of this condition are diarrhoea, dermatitis and dementia. Nausea, vomiting, stomatitis, dizziness, depression, insomnia, headache develops. In severe deficiency hallucinations and dementia occurs.

Adverse effects include flushing, activation of peptic ulcer, vomiting, diarrhoea, pruritus, skin rash and transient headache.

It is **indicated** in pellagra, for prophylaxis, Hartnup disease, hyperlipoproteinaemia.

VITAMIN B_5 (CALCIUM PANTOTHENATE)

Pantothenic acid is traditionally considered to be vitamin B substance. It is widely distributed in meat, legume and whole grain cereals, egg, milk, vegetables and fruit.

It is a component of coenzyme A which is essential in the metabolism of carbohydrate, fat and protein.

Deficiency symptoms: Deficiency of panthothenic acid is unlikely in man because of its widespread distribution in food, though it has been administered by mouth as a nutritional supplement as the calcium salt and usually in conjunction with other vitamins of the B group.

Dosage: 50 to 100 mg per day.

VITAMIN B_6 (PYRIDOXINE)

It is involved as a coenzyme (pyridoxal phosphate) in metabolism of tryptophan, in several metabolic transformations of amino acids including transamination, decarboxylation and racemization.

Deficiency symptoms: Peripheral neuritis, seizures, stomatitis, anaemia, seborrhoea like lesions, mental confusion and growth retardation.

It is **indicated** to prevent and treat isoniazid, hydralazine, penicillamine and cycloserine induced neurological disturbances, mental symptoms in women on oral contraceptives, pyridoxine responsive anaemia and homocystinuria, morning sickness and hyperemesis gravidarum, convulsions in infants and children.

Dosage: ***Adults*:** 100 mg daily. In suppression of lactation: 2 tablets thrice daily followed by one tablet daily.

CYANOCOBALAMIN (METHYLCOBALAMIN)

Methylcobalamin is the coenzyme form of vitamin B_{12}. It is neurologically active, most bioavailable and best utilized. Unlike cyanocobalamin, it does not require any conversion after absorption by the body and is better retained by the liver and other tissues. It has exhibited beneficial effects against brain aging, irregular sleep patterns. It supports immune function and promote normal cell growth. It represents one of the best values in nutritional products, given its comparably low cost and its wide range of potential benefits.

Methyl B_{12} is the superior form of vitamin B_{12}.

Deficiency symptoms are glossitis, GIT disturbances, megaloblastic anaemia, subacute combined degeneration of spinal cord, peripheral neuritis, poor memory, mood changes and hallucinations.

Clinical Applications

Bell's palsy: It increases the recovery time for facial nerve function in Bell's palsy.

Cancer: Experimental studies indicate that it inhibits the proliferation of malignant cells.

Diabetic neuropathy: Oral administration of methylcobalamin (500 mcg three times daily for four months) resulted in subjective improvement in burning sensation, numbness, loss of sensation and muscle cramps.

Immune system regulation: It has been suggested that vitamin B_{12} plays an important role in immune system regulation, but the details are still obscure.

Rheumatoid arthritis: Vitamin B_{12} is a potential agent in management of RA. It mainly acts by correcting abnormalities in RACD8+ T cells in autologous mixed lymphocyte reaction (AMLR).

Eye function: It protects retinal neurons against N-methyl-D-aspartate receptor mediated glutamate neurotoxicity. Deterioration of accommodation following visual work has also been shown to improve in individuals receiving methylcobalamin.

Heart rate variability: Methylcobalamin produces improvement in several components of heart rate variability, suggesting a balancing effect on the nervous system.

HIV: Under experimental conditions, methylcobalamin inhibited HIV-1 infection of normal human blood monocytes and lymphocytes.

Homocysteinemia: Elevated levels of homocysteine can be a metabolic indication of decreased levels of the methylcobalamin form of vitamin B_{12}.

Male impotence: It is known to increase sperm count in male patients with impotence.

Sleep disturbances: The use of methylcobalamin in the treatment of a variety of sleep-wake disorders is very promising.

Vitamin B complex preparations are **indicated** in vitamin deficiency states. Specific vitamin B preparations can be used as per indications mentioned above in the pharmacological write up; as an adjuvant to antibiotic therapy; combination with lactobacillus are indicated in aphthous stomatitis, thrush.

Preparations of **vitamin B_1 + B_6 + B_{12}** are **indicated** to prevent and treat isoniazid, hydralazine and cycloserine induced neurological disturbances, mental symptoms in women on oral contraceptives, pyridoxine responsive anaemia and homocystinuria, neuropathies, subacute combined degeneration, beriberi, anaemia, hepatitis, debility.

FOLIC ACID

It plays a vital role in various intracellular reactions e.g. conversion of serine to glycine, synthesis of thymidylate, synthesis of purines, histidine metabolism etc. Due to folic acid deficiency these reactions are affected.

Deficiency symptoms: The characteristic feature of folic acid deficiency is megaloblastic anaemia. Deficiency also leads to glossitis, enteritis, diarrhoea, general debility, weight loss and sterility.

It is **indicated** in folic acid deficiency states e.g. megaloblastic anaemia, tropical and nontropical sprue, alcoholism; adjunctive therapy in nutritional anaemias and anaemias of pregnancy.

Dosage:

Adults: *Therapeutic*: 5 to 20 mg daily in divided doses.

Children: 5 to 10 mg daily in divided doses.

VITAMIN C (ASCORBIC ACID)

It functions as a cofactor in number of amidation and hydroxylation reactions.

The active form of **vitamin C** is ascorbic acid itself. The main function of ascorbate is as a reducing agent in a number of different reactions. Vitamin C has the potential to reduce cytochrome a and c of the respiratory chain as well as molecular oxygen. The most important reaction requiring ascorbate as a cofactor is the hydroxylation of proline residues in collagen. Vitamin C is, therefore, required for the maintenance of normal connective tissue as well as for wound healing since synthesis of connective tissue is the first event in wound tissue remodeling. Vitamin C is also necessary for bone remodeling due to the presence of collagen in the organic matrix of bones. It is also required for conversion of folic acid to folinic acid, biosynthesis of adrenal steroids, catecholamines, oxytocin and ADH; metabolism of cyclic nucleotides and prostaglandins.

Deficiency symptoms: In vitamin C deficiency **scurvy** develops. It is characterized by ecchymosis, petechiae, swollen and bleeding gums, subperiosteal haemorrhage, bones are painful to touch, impaired wound healing, anaemia, loosening of teeth and gingivitis.

It is **indicated** for treatment of scurvy, for prophylaxis of vitamin C deficiency, to acidify urine, anaemia of vitamin C deficiency, as antioxidant to protect natural colour and flavour of many foods, dental caries and increased capillary fragility.

Dosage:

Adults: *Prophylaxis* : 50-500 mg daily.

Pregnancy and lactation: 100-150 mg daily.

CALCIUM

Calcium is the most abundant body constituent (approx. 2% of body weight). It controls excitability of nerves and muscles and regulates permeability of cell membranes. It act as intracellular messenger for hormones and autacoids and help in coagulation of blood.

Plasma calcium level is precisely regulated by three hormones e.g. parathormone, calcitonin and calciferol (which is a active form of vitamin D). They control its absorption, exchange with bone and excretion.

Calcium is present in three forms e.g., as free calcium ion, bound to plasma protein albumin and in diffusable complexes. The endocrine system, through parathyroid hormone and calcitonin, helps in keeping the concentration of ionized plasma calcium in normal level. Decrease in plasma levels of ionized calcium leads to increased parathyroid hormone secretion. Parathyroid hormone tends to increase plasma calcium level by increasing bone resorption, increasing intestinal absorption and increasing reabsorption of calcium in kidney. Vitamin D acts by stimulating intestinal absorption of calcium and decreasing the renal excretion.

Calcium play vital role in excitation - contraction coupling in myocardium. Calcium mediates contraction in vascular and other smooth muscles. Calcium is required for exocytosis and also involved in neurotransmitters release. Calcium also help in maintaining integrity of mucosal membranes and mediating cell adhesions. Hypercalcemia may occur in hyperthyroidism, vitamin D intoxication and renal insufficiency, which can be treated by administration of calcitonin, edetate sodium, oral phosphate etc. Hypocalcemia may occur in hypothyroidism, malabsorption, osteomalacia secondary to leak of vitamin D or vitamin D resistance, pancreatitis and renal failure. Hypocalcemia can be treated by chloride, gluconate, gluceptate, lactate and carbonate salts of calcium.

TRACE ELEMENTS

NICKEL

It is an essential trace element for mammals, but little is known about its role or requirement in human metabolism. In humans, serum levels of nickel are about 1.1 to 1.6 mcg/l. This level increases in conditions such as stroke and acute myocardial infarction. A dietary requirement for adults is about 30 mcg/day.

Nickel occurs mainly in plant foods, especially grains and vegetables with little in animal food sources or fats.

CHROMIUM

Less than 6 mg of chromium is found in the body, with the highest concentrations occurring in the adrenal glands, brain, skin, muscles and fat.

The total body content of chromium is estimated to be 6 to 10 mg. The recommended safe limit for daily chromium intake by adult is 0.05 to 0.2 mg.

MANGANESE

The body contains only 20 mg of manganese, found mostly in the bones and glands. The plasma level is low, about 2.5 mcg/dl.

The best sources of manganese are wheat bran, dried legumes, seeds, nuts and leafy green vegetables, other good sources are cereal grains, coffee and tea. The adequate range in adult diet is 2.5 to 5.0 mg/day.

Manganese is a cofactor of enzymes involved in energy metabolism and is required for hemoglobin synthesis, thiamin utilization and tendon and bone formation. Unlike nutrients that fulfil unique functions, other minerals sometimes can substitute for manganese.

MOLYBDENUM

Molybdenum is found primarily in the liver, kidneys, bone, skin and adrenal glands.

Organ meats, legumes and grains are good sources. The adequate range of molybdenum intake for adults is 75 to 250 mcg/day. It is equally excreted in the urine and the faeces.

Because molybdenum is a copper antagonist, high levels of copper decrease the absorption of molybdenum. It is equally excreted in the urine and the faeces.

Molybdenum is a cofactor for enzymes involved in protein synthesis.

SELENIUM

Selenium is an essential trace element in the human body. This nutrient is an important part of antioxidant enzymes that protect cells against the effects of free radicals that are produced during normal oxygen metabolism. Selenium is also essential for normal functioning of immune system and thyroid gland.

❑❑❑

Section 11

Chelating Agents and Treatment of Poisoning

CHAPTER 11.1 Chelating Agents & Treatment of Poisoning

Antidotes are used in life threatening situations and are administered for a short treatment course. They can be divided into three main categories:

- Antidotes that remove active poison from its site of action e.g. hydroxylamine used in organophosphate anticholinesterase poisoning.
- Antidotes that act pharmacologically e.g. naloxone used in opioid poisoning.
- Antidotes that antagonised other macromolecules e.g. carbon monoxide produce poisonous condition by binding the haemoglobin and other cellular components.

The antidotes are classified into four main types.

i. **Mechanical antidotes:** These substances interfere with the absorption of poison. They act by forming a coat over mucous membrane of the stomach. e.g. fats, oils, albumin, activated charcoal is specifically used in adsorbing alkaloidal poisons.

ii. **Chemical antidotes:** They react with poison to form harmless insoluble form e.g. acids are neutralised by alkalis, $KMnO_4$ used in opium poisoning.

iii. **Systemic antidotes:** They produce the action which are opposite to that of poison e.g. caffeine for morphine and atropine for pilocarpine.

iv. **Universal antidotes:** These antidotes can be given in all such conditions where nature of poison is not known or where more than one poison is suspected to be taken e.g. charcoal as adsorbent of toxins and alkaloids, tannic acid for precipitating alkaloids, glycoside and many metals.

CHELATING AGENTS

Chelating agents are widely used as specific antidotes for heavy metals. They form stable, soluble, nontoxic complexes and in easily excreted form. They promote dissociation of bound metal from tissue enzymes and other functional macromolecules. These metal chelates are water soluble. e.g. EDTA, BAL, desferrioxamine etc.

DIMERCAPROL (BRITISH ANTI LEWISITE, BAL)

It **acts by forming chelation complexes between its sulphydryl groups and metals**. Its effectiveness is much more, if given immediately after exposure to the metal.

It is given by parenteral route (deep IM injection) and has short plasma half life.

Adverse effects include increased blood pressure, burning sensation in lips, mouth and throat; nausea, vomiting, sweating, pain in chest, throat or hands; painful sterile abscess at site of injection; haemolytic anaemia in patients with G-6-PD enzyme deficiency; hypertension, tachycardia, salivation, lacrimation and conjunctivitis.

It is **indicated** in metallic intoxication due to arsenic, mercury, gold, bismuth, lead, nickel, thallium and antimony; in conjunction with sodium calcium edetate for lead poisoning. It is also useful in hepatolenticular degeneration (Wilson's disease). It is **contraindicated** in iron and cadmium poisoning.

Dose: BAL; 2.5 to 5.0 mg/kg QID depending upon the severity of the poisoning.

D-PENICILLAMINE

It is a monothiol, prepared by alkaline hydrolysis of benzyl penicillin and chemically it is beta-dimethylcysteine.

It acts as a chelating agent which helps in elimination of heavy metal ions by forming stable soluble complexes which can be easily excreted by the kidneys.

It is **used** in poisoning due to copper, mercury and lead; Wilson's disease, cystinuria, scleroderma and rheumatoid arthritis.

Adverse effects include skin rash, proteinuria, bone marrow depression, nausea and loss of taste sensation.

Dose: CILAMIN; 0.5-1 g/day in divided dose.

DESFERRIOXAMINE

It is a iron chelating agent, available for intramuscular, subcutaneous and intravenous administration.

When injected, it **forms a stable water-soluble iron complex (ferrioxamine) that prevents the iron from entering into further chemical reactions** and is readily excreted in the urine giving the urine a characteristic reddish colour. Some of it is also excreted in the faeces via the bile. It can also chelate aluminium and thus is useful in aluminium overload. It is primarily a chelator used in acute iron poisoning and chronic iron overload as in thalassemia patients needing multiple transfusions.

Adverse effects include flushing, urticaria, hypotension, shock, tachypnoea, hypoxaemia, tachycardia, cardiac arrhythmias, convulsions, erythema, swelling, GIT disturbances, dysuria, fever, allergic skin rashes. Leg cramps on long term therapy and reversible ocular and auditory disturbances have also been reported.

DESFERAL

Acute iron intoxication: Initially 1 g IM followed by 500 mg every four hours for two doses. Subsequent doses of 500 mg are given 4 to 12 hourly depending on response, maximum 6 g in 24 hours.

Patients with cardiovascular collapse: IV infusion 50 mg/kg/hour up to a maximum of 80 mg/kg in 24 hours.

Chronic iron overload: 0.5 to 1 g IM daily. In addition 2 g IV infusion given separately with each unit of blood transfused.

CALCIUM DISODIUM EDETATE

It is the calcium chelate of disodium edetate having high affinity for metals like lead, zinc, cadmium, copper, manganese and some radioactive metals. Given by IV route, it is distributed extracellularly and excreted unchanged in urine by glomerular filtration carrying the toxic metal along.

It is primarily **indicated** in lead poisoning. It is also useful in iron, zinc, copper, manganese and radioactive metal but not mercury poisoning.

Adverse effects include nephrotoxicity, anaphylactoid reaction, chills, bodyache and malaise.

DEFERIPRONE

It is an orally active iron chelator. It is **useful** in acute iron poisoning, iron overload in cirrhosis, transfusion siderosis in thalassemia patients. **Adverse effects** are anorexia, vomiting, altered taste, joint pain and neutropenia.

DISULFIRAM (ESPERAL)

It is relatively nontoxic, used as an adjunct in the treatment of chronic alcoholism.

It exerts its action by **inhibiting aldehyde dehydrogenase enzyme**. Disulfiram thus increases the concentration of acetaldehyde in body when ethanol is ingested by an individual pretreated with disulfiram. The symptoms and signs produced are flushing, pulsating headache, nausea, vomiting, thirst, marked uneasiness, vertigo, weakness, confusion, hypotension and circulatory collapse.

After oral administration it is rapidly absorbed from gastrointestinal tract.

Adverse effects include urticaria, allergic dermatitis, restlessness, tremor, dizziness, metallic taste, fatigue, decrease in sexual [illegible] lassitude.

It is **indicated** in chronic alcoholism in a dose range of 1 g on 1st day, 0.75 g on 2nd day, 0.5 on 3rd day, decreasing to 0.125-0.25 g/day. Sensitization to alcohol develops after two to three hours of first dose and lasts for 7 to 14 days after stopping it.

LEUCOVORIN

It is used as leucovorin calcium (calcium folinate). It is 5-formyl derivative of tetrahydrofolic acid and it acts as an antidote to folic acid antagonists like methotrexate or pyrimethamine which **inhibit the enzyme dihydrofolate reductase**.

Well absorbed by the oral or IM route and is rapidly converted to biologically active folate. Distribution occurs to all body tissues and it is concentrated in the CSF. It is excreted in the urine.

Adverse effects include pyrexia which occurs rarely.

It is **indicated** in overdose of methotrexate, folic acid antagonists and as adjuvant treatment of colorectal carcinoma.

Dose: NYRIN; 120 mg per day by IM or IV infusion.

PRALIDOXIME

It **causes reactivation of the phosphorylated acetylcholinesterase enzyme**. After administration, it is metabolised in liver.

Adverse effects include blurred vision, dizziness, diplopia, headache, tachycardia, mild weakness and nausea. In high dose it can cause neuromuscular blockage.

It is **indicated** as antidote for organophosphorus poisoning like malathion, TEPP, parathion etc.

NICOTINE

Nicotine is a tertiary amine compound composed of a pyridine and a pyrrolidine ring. It **binds selectively to acetylcholine receptors at the autonomic ganglia in the adrenal medulla at neuro-muscular junction and in the brain**. It exerts a stimulating effect in the cortex and a 'reward' effect via the 'pleasure system' in the limbic system.

Adverse effects include erythema, pruritus or burning at the site of application, headache, somnolence, dizziness, arthralgia, myalgia, dyspepsia, dry mouth, diarrhoea, sweating, BP changes, angioneurotic edema, urticaria and dyspnea.

It is **used** in the treatment of nicotine dependence and as an aid to stop smoking.

BUPROPION

The mechanism by which bupropion acts as an aid in smoking cessation is unknown. Bupropion **weakly inhibits neuronal reuptake of noradrenaline and serotonin and inhibits the reuptake of dopamine**. In tissues from rat brain, bupropion produced greater inhibition of dopamine reuptake than noradrenaline reuptake; however in, *in vivo* models, bupropion is a stronger inhibitor of noradrenaline than dopamine reuptake. The metabolites hydroxybupropion and threohydrobupropion are pharmacologically active *in vitro* and in animal models of depression and are expected to contribute to the therapeutic effects of bupropion.

Adverse effects include abdominal pain, chest pain, facial edema, nausea, dry mouth, constipation, diarrhoea, anorexia, mouth ulcer, thirst, myalgia, arthralgia, anxiety, disturbed concentration, dizziness, nervousness, tremor, dysphoria, rhinitis, increased cough, pharyngitis, sinusitis, dyspnea, epistaxis, agitation, insomnia and headache.

It is **indicated** in smoking cessation in the dose of 150 to 300 mg twice daily.

TREATMENT OF POISONING

The treatment of different drug poisoning is discussed in individual chapters. In this section, general treatment is discussed.

The general principles of treatment are:

1. Support ventilation.
2. Maintain cardiovascular function.
3. Reverse hypothermia if present.
4. Treat convulsions.
5. Correct fluid, acid-base and electrolyte imbalance.
6. Relieve pain.
7. Good nursing care.

Prevention of Poison Absorption

The aim is to reduce the absorption of poison.

1. Gastric lavage may be useful for six hours after ingestion of poison. The lavage should be done as early as possible but only if vital functions are adequate.
2. It is inappropriate to employ gastric lavage unless the lungs can be protected, either by virtue of patient having an adequate cough reflex or by means of a cuffed endotracheal tube.
3. Gastric lavage is **contraindicated** if corrosive or caustic substances have been taken, because oesophageal and gastric erosion and perforation may occur.
4. Activated charcoal is probably more effective than either emesis or lavage.

Accelerating Poison Elimination

Alkalinisation of urine (alkaline diuresis) is effective for salicylates and phenoxyacetate herbicides.

Repeated dose of activated charcoal administered by oral route have been shown to enhance the non-renal elimination of carbamazepine, salicylates, phenobarbitone, phenytoin, digoxin, theophylline and meprobamate. In severe cases activated charcoal is to be administered via a nasogastric tube.

Haemoperfusion, using a cartridge containing charcoal or an uncharged resin is effective in enhancing drug excretion in few selected cases of poisoning e.g. theophylline, barbiturates, non-barbiturate hypnotics, etc. (Also see Section I for the management of poisoning).

Frequent administration of activated charcoal is effective for the following substances:

1. *Substances which form masses:* Aspirin, iron, lithium, enteric-coated tablets, meprobamate.
2. *Substance which remain in the stomach for a long time:* Barbital, aspirin, iron, alcohol, cholinergic blockers, narcotic drugs, phenytoin, antidepressants.
3. *Substances which have a long half-life when present in large amounts:* Theophylline, aspirin, alcohol, phenytoin, chloral hydrate, acetaminophen.
4. *Substances which have active metabolites:* Benzodiazepines, chloral hydrate, acetaminophen, antidepressants, procainamide.
5. *Substances whose poisonous metabolites are eliminated slowly:* Ethylene glycol, methanol, primidone, isopropyl alcohol, carbon tetrachloride, levothyroxine.
6. *Substances which are reabsorbed from the urinary tubules in a pH dependent manner:* Phenobarbital, aspirin, amphetamine.
7. *Substances with persistent tissue accumulation:* Iron, lithium.
8. *Substances which enter the enterohepatic circulation:* Carbamazepine, digoxin, phenobarbital.

The specific antidotes for various poisons are listed in table 11.1.1

ORGANOPHOSPHORUS POISONING

These compounds are mainly used as agricultural and household insecticides. The poisoning may be occupational (for those who are involved professionally with these agents), accidental (accidental consumption) or suicidal due to intentional ingestion of these compounds.

Table 11.1.1 *List of specific antidotes for various poisons.*

Poison	Antidote
1. Arsenic	Dimercaprol, BAL, D-penicillamine
2. Cyanide	Oxygen (100%), dicobalt edetate, Amyl nitrite, sod. nitrite
3. Ethylene glycol, methanol	Ethanol
4. Opioids	Naloxone
5. Organophosphorus insecticides	Atropine and pralidoxime mesylate
6. Iron	Desferrioxamine
7. Beta-blockers	Atropine for bradycardia, glucagon
8. Digoxin	Digoxin specific antibody fragments (DIGIBIND)
9. Carbon monoxide	Oxygen (100%)
10. Oral anticoagulants	Vitamin K (phytomenadione)
11. Heparin	Protamine sulfate
12. Lead (inorganic)	Sodium calcium edetate, D-penicillamine
13. Mercury (inorganic)	Dimercaprol, D-penicillamine, BAL
14. Methanol	Ethanol
15. Paracetamol, gold	N-acetylcysteine
16. Benzodiazepines	Flumazenil
17. Atropine	Physostigmine
18. Isoniazid	Pyridoxine
19. Folic acid antagonists	Folinic acid
20. Acetaminophen (Paracetamol)	N-acetylcysteine
21. Copper	BAL, EDTA D-penicillamine
22. Methotrexate	Folic acid, Leucovorin
23. Snake bite	Antisnake venom polyvalent
24. Hydroxzines	Pyridoxine
25. Theophylline	Esmolol
26. Curare compounds	Neostigmine
27. Insulin	Glucose

a. Local exposure produces miosis, spasm of accommodation, headache, irritation of eye, lacrimation and blurring of vision.

b. On ingestion fall in blood pressure, tachycardia, cardiac arrhythmias, ataxia, convulsion, respiratory paralysis and vasomotor collapse occurs. The death is generally due to respiratory failure.

Treatment

1. Gastric lavage, fresh air for termination of further exposure to compound.
2. Maintenance of a patent airway. Use oropharyngeal or nasopharyngeal airway or endotracheal intubation if airway obstruction persists.
3. Washing of skin, mucous membrane and eye.
4. Supportive therapy: Maintenance of blood pressure, artificial respiration, rehydration (fluid/electrolyte therapy) and control of convulsions.
5. Antidote/Reactivators.

a. Atropine is highly effective in counteracting the muscarinic symptoms. It is given in a dose of 2 mg IV every 10 min till muscarinic effects are controlled.

b. The cholinesterase reactivators are used to restore neuromuscular transmission. **Pralidoxime** (pyridine-2-aldoxime methiodide; 2-PAM) is an antidote and cholinesterase reactivator. It breaks the bond between the organophosphate poison and the molecular surface of acetylcholinesterase and the enzyme is freed and reactivated to hydrolyse the excess of acetylcholine at the receptor sites. It is to be given in the dose of 1-2 g IV infusion along with 100-200 mg of atropine.

Other cholinesterase reactivators are diacetylmonoxime (DAM) which combines with free organophosphate molecule in the body fluids. It is administered 1-2 g IV slowly.

CHRONIC ALCOHOLISM

It is associated with development of psychic dependence, tolerance and physical dependence and sudden withdrawal of alcohol may lead to withdrawal syndrome.

In addition, the alcohol addicts are liable to other neuropsychiatric syndrome (Korsakoff's psychosis) which is associated with hallucination, suicidal tendencies and encephalopathy. They may also suffer from hyperlipidemia, hyperuricemia, pancreatitis and hepatitis.

Drug Treatment of Chronic Alcoholism (Aldehyde Dehydrogenase Inhibitors)

DISULFIRAM

Chemically it is tetraethyl thiuram disulphide, commonly known as antabuse and available in 200 mg tablet. The treatment is initiated with 800 mg single dose which is gradually reduced over 5 days to a maintenance dose of 100 to 200 mg daily and treatment may be continued up to one year.

After a week's therapy, if a small quantity of alcohol is consumed by the patient, it produced unpleasant toxic reactions such as flushing, palpitation, nausea, vomiting throbbing headache, uneasiness, dizziness, visual disturbances, fall in blood pressure and even collapse. The patient thus realizes that during the treatment he can not tolerate even a small amount of alcohol and would abstain from alcohol drinking.

The drug disulfiram interferes with the oxidation of acetaldehyde formed during the metabolism of alcohol. This increases the blood level of acetaldehyde which acts directly on cardiovascular system and produce these toxic reactions. Disulfiram also inhibits dopamine beta oxidase and thus interferes with the synthesis of noradrenaline, which causes depletion of catecholamines.

Disulfiram is slowly absorbed incompletely from the gut and is metabolised slowly.

METHYL ALCOHOL (METHANOL)

Methyl alcohol is only used to denature ethyl alcohol in 5 percent concentration. It is metabolised to formaldehyde and formic acid by alcohol and aldehyde dehydrogenases. Its absorption and distribution are similar to ethyl alcohol.

Ingestion of methyl alcohol produces the following signs and symptoms:

- Nausea and vomiting.
- Blurring of vision, hyperemia of optic disc and blindness.
- Pancreatitis.
- Albuminuria.
- Coma followed by death.

Treatment of Methanol Poisoning

- Gastric lavage, activated charcoal.
- Hospitalization: Correction of acidosis.
- IV/oral ethyl alcohol.
- Maintenance of nutrition.
- Administration of folinic acid (1 mg/ kg, IV) together with folic acid (1 mg/ kg IV) to accelerate the metabolic degradation of formate.
- Administration of 4-methylpyrazole (inhibitor of alcohol dehydrogenase).
- In severe case: Haemodialysis.

TREATMENT OF SNAKE BITE

Vipers, Cobras and Kraits are the common poisonous snakes and in India 40,000 to 50,000 deaths recorded per year due to snake bite.

Local Signs & Symptoms in the Bitten Part

- Fang marks.
- Local pain & bleeding.
- Bruising.
- Lymphangitis.
- Inflammation (swelling, redness, heat).
- Blistering.
- Lymph node enlargement.
- Local infection, abscess formation & necrosis.

Generalised (Systemic) Symptoms & Signs

- Nausea, vomiting, malaise, abdominal pain weakness.
- Visual disturbances, faintness, collapse, shock, hypotension, pulmonary edema & conjunctival edema.
- Bleeding & clotting disorders.
- Skeletal muscle breakdown.
- Acute pituitary/adrenal insufficiency.

First-aid Treatment

- First aid treatment is carried out immediately before hospitalisation.
- Immobilise the bitten limb with a splint or sling.
- Consider pressure-immobilisation for some elapid bites.
- Avoid any interference with the bite wound as this may introduce infection, increase absorption of the venom and increase local bleeding.
- Tight (arterial) tourniquets are not recommended.

Treatment in hospital

- Rapid clinical assessment and resuscitation.
- History (especially the snake identification).
- Physical examination.
- Investigation/laboratory tests:
  - 20 minute whole blood clotting test (20 WBCT).
  - Haemoglobin concentration/ haematocrit.
  - Platelet count.
  - WBC count.
  - Biochemical abnormalities.
  - Urine examination etc.

Supportive Therapy

Blood pressure, ECG, blood gas analysis, urine output and respiration are to be monitored. To correct coagulation parameters, blood transfusion may be needed.

ANTISNAKE VENOM

Antivenom is the only specific antidote to snake venom. Antivenom is immunoglobulin purified from the serum or plasma of a horse or sheep that has been immunised with the venoms of one or more species of snake. Antivenom should be given by the intravenous route. Freeze dried (lyophilised) antivenoms are reconstituted, usually with 10 ml of sterile water for injection per ampoule. Adrenaline should always be drawn up in readiness before antivenom is administered for any possible anaphylactic reactions.

❑❑❑

Section 12

Dental Pharmacology

CHAPTER 12.1

Antiseptics & Disinfectants

These are the agents which inhibit or kill microbes on contact. Conventionally

- **Antiseptics** are used on living surfaces.
- **Disinfectants** are used for inanimate objects.

The practical distinction of these two agents is on the basis of a growth inhibiting or direct lethal action. There are concentration dependent. Germicide covers these two category. Potency of germicide is generally expressed by its **"phenol coefficient or Rideal Walker (RW) coefficient"** – "which is the ratio of the minimum concentration of the test drug required to kill a 24 hour culture of *B. typhosa* in 7.5 minutes at 37.5°C to that of phenol (as standard) under similar conditions."

In dentistry, they are used for sterilization of certain instruments and prevention and treatment of dental plaque and peridental diseases. They are also used in root canal therapy (RCT), treatment of acute necrotizing gingivitis and other infective oral conditions. Antiseptics and disinfectants are also used as ingredient in various dentifrices.

Factors which Modify the Activity of Germicides

1. Temperature & pH.
2. Period of contact with the microorganisms.
3. Nature of microbes involved.
   - Spectrum of activity of majority of antiseptic disinfectants is wide reflecting non selectivity of action. However, some are selective e.g. hexachlorophene, chlorhexidine, quarternary ammonium antiseptics, gentian violet, acriflavine are more active for gram +ve than gram –ve. Silver nitrate is highly active against gonococci and benzoyl peroxide against *P. acnes*.
4. Size of inoculum.
5. Presence of blood, pus & other organic matter.

Mechanism of Action (Cidal or Inhibiting Action)

i. Oxidation of bacterial protoplasm.
ii. Denaturation of bacterial proteins including enzymes.

iii. Detergent like action increasing permeability of bacterial membrane.

Classification

i. Phenol derivatives.
ii. Oxidizing agent.
iii. Halogens.
iv. Biguanides.
v. Quarternary ammonium compounds.
vi. Acids.
vii. Metallic salts.
viii. Dyes.
ix. Furan derivatives.
x. Alcohol.
xi. Aldehydes.
xii. Soaps.

Phenol Derivatives

Used as disinfectants

- ***Phenol (carbolic acid):*** Acts by denaturing bacterial proteins.
- ***Methylphenol (cresol; LYSOL):*** 3-10 times more active.
- ***Resorcinol:*** 1/3 as potent as phenol (used both as an antiseptic/ disinfectant). **Used as antiseptic.**
- ***Hexyl-resorcinol:*** More potent. Used as mouth wash, lozenges & as antifungal.
- ***Chloroxylenol:***
  - 4.8% sol. (DETTOL): Used for surgical antisepsis.
  - 1.0% sol. (DETTOLIN) used as mouth washes, 0.8% cream & soap; 1.4% lubricating obstetric cream (for vaginal examination).
- ***Hexachlorophene:***
  - Act by inhibiting bacterial enzyme and in high concentration cause bacterial lysis.
  - Incorporated in soap & other cleansing antiseptics. Also acts as deodorant.
  - Highly active against gram +ve microorganisms.

Phenol is used to disinfect urine, faeces, pus, sputum of patients and sometime included in antipruritic preparation because of its mild anaesthetic action.

Oxidizing Agents

1. **Potassium permanganate ($KMnO_4$):**

lWater soluble purple crystals.

- Liberates oxygen which oxidizes bacterial protoplasm.
- Potassium permanganate ($KMnO_4$) is used as Condy's lotion (1 : 4,000 to 1 : 10,000 solution).
- **As antiseptic:**
  - Used for gargels, irrigating cavities, urethra & wounds.
  - Higher concentration cause burns & blistering.
- **As disinfectants:**
  - To disinfect water (well, ponds) & for stomach wash in alkaloidal poisoning (except atropine & cocaine which are not efficiently oxidized).
  - Not suitable for surgical instruments (promotes rusting).

2. **Hydrogen peroxide (H_2O_2):**
   - Used as antiseptic.
   - Removes slough, ear wax etc.

- Used in cosmetic preparation.
- As gargels.
- Potency loses on keeping and not much used.

3. **Benzoyl peroxide** (PERSOL 2.5, 5.0% gel, 10% cream):
   - Used in acne.
   - Gradually liberates oxygen (in the presence of water) which kills bacteria, specially anaerobic.
   - Mild irritant to skin.
   - Can cause dryness of skin, edema etc.

HALOGENS

1. **Used as disinfectants:**

- ***Chlorine:***
  - Highly reactive element & potent germicide.
  - 0.1-0.25 ppm kills most pathogens in 30 secs.
  - Used to disinfect urban water supplies.
  - More active in acidic & neutral medium.

2. **Used as antiseptic:**

- ***Iodine:***
  - Act by iodinating and oxidizing microbial protoplasm.
  - 1:20,000 solution kills most vegetative forms within 1 min.
  - **Tr. iodine (2%) in alcohol:** Used on cuts, for degerming skin before surgery.
  - **Mandel's paint (1.25%):** Used in sore throat.
  - **Non-staining iodine ointment (4%** – IODEX) used as counter irritant & antiseptic.
  - **More than 5%** can cause burning & blistering of skin.
- ***Iodophores:***
  - Are soluble complexes of iodine with large molecular organic compounds that serve as carrier – release free iodine slowly.

  Povidone (polyvinyl pyrrolidone):
  - BETADINE (5% sol.; 5% ointment; 200 mg vag. pessaries).
  - 1% mouth wash.
  - 10% solution.
  - 10% cream.
  - 5% spray (aerosol) (RANVIDONE AEROSOL): Used in boils, burns, ulcers, non-specific vaginitis & all surgical dressings. Also for disinfections of endoscopes and instruments.
- **Chlorophores:**
  - Compounds that slowly release hypochlorous acid (HOCl).
  - Used in preference of gaseous chlorine due to ease of handling.
- **Chlorinated lime** (bleaching powder):
  - Used as disinfectant for drinking water, swimming pools & sanitizer for privies etc.
- **Sodium hypochlorite solution** (4-6% sod. hypochlorite):
  - Used as disinfectant in dairies for milk.
  - Used for root canal therapy in dentistry as antiseptic.
- **Chlorinated lime (1.25%) with boric acid** (1.25%) (EUSOL):
  - Used to clean infected wounds.

- **Chloramine-T** and **halazone:**
  - Used as sanitizer.

BIGUANIDES

- **Chlorhexidine:**
  - Having high antiplaque activity.
  - Used as antiseptic.
  - Nonirritating antiseptic that disrupts bacterial cell membrane.
  - More active against gram +ve bacteria
  - Used for surgical scrub, mouthwash, neonatal bath & general skin antiseptic.

QUARTERNARY AMMONIUM ANTISEPTICS (CATIONIC)

- Act by altering permeability of cell membranes.
- Soaps (being anionic) neutralise their action while alcohol potentiates.
- Non-irritating & mild keratolytic.

- **Cetrimide:**
  - 20% sol. (CETAVLON).
  - Chlorhexidine gluconate (1.5%) + cetrimide (3%) [SAVLON LIQUID].
  - SAVLON CREAM: Chlorhexidine (0.1%) + cetrimide (0.5%).
  - SAVLON HOSPITAL CONCENTRATE: Chlorhexidine (7.5%) + cetrimide (15%).
  - Also used in soaps, shaving creams.
  - Used for cleansing action.
  - Used as antiseptic & disinfectant for surgical, instruments, utensils, baths etc.
- **Cetylpyridinium chloride** (similar to cetrimide)**:** Used in mouth wash & in lozenges.
- **Benzalkonium chloride:** 1 : 5000-1 : 10,000 sol. used for douches, irrigation etc.
  - Used as preservative for eye/ear/nasal drops.
- **Dequalinium chloride:**
  - As an antiseptic used in gum paints & lozenges.

ACIDS

- **Boric acid:**
  - Bacteriostatic & weak antiseptic.
  - **4% sol.:** Used for irrigating eyes, mouth washes, douche etc.
  - **Boroglycerine paint (30%):** Used for stomatitis & glossitis.
  - **10% ointment** (BOROCIDE)**:** Used for cuts & abrasion.
- **Acetic acid:**
  - Weak antiseptic.
  - Bactericidal (>5%).
  - Occasionally used for burn dressing.

METALLIC SALTS

a. **Mercury compounds:** Act by inactivating SH enzymes and acts as bacteriostatic.

- **Ammoniated mercury:**
  - ***5-10% ointment:*** Used for dermatophytosis & anal pruritus.
  - Phenyl meruric nitrate: EPHYTOL PAINT used for tinea. MEDITHANE – anorectal use.
  - Merbromin 1-2% solution (MERCUROCHROME): Used in first aid kit.

b. **Silver compounds:**
  - Astringent action.
  - React with SH, COOH, PO_4 & NH_2 groups of proteins.

- **Silver nitrate:**
  - Rapidly kills microbes, action persisting for long periods because of slow release of Ag^+ ions from silver proteinate formed by interaction with tissue proteins.
  - Silver nitrate touch is used for hypertrophied tonsillitis and aphthous ulcers.
  - Highly active against gonococci (10% sol.).
- **Silver sulphadiazine** (SILVEREX 1%):
  - Highly active against *Pseudomonas*.
  - Used in burns.

c. **Zinc salts:** Astringent & mild antiseptic.

- **Zinc sulphate:**
  - 0.1-1.0% solution used for eye wash and eye/ear drop (ZINCOSULFA eye drops).
  - Lotion containing zinc sulfate & saturated potash (THIOSOL 2.5% 24%): Used in acne.
  - Zinc oxide and calamine: Used as dermal protectives & adsorbants.

Dyes

- Rosaniline dye:
  - **Gentian violet** (0.5-1% alcoholic solution): Effective against staphylococci, gram +ve bacteria & fungi.
  - **Brilliant green:** Rosaniline dye, similar to gentian violet.
  - **Acriflavine & proflavine:** Orange-yellow acridine dye. ACRINOL 0.1% cream. Effective against gram +ve bacteria & gonococci. Activity enhanced in alkaline medium. Used in chronic ulcers & wounds
  - Combination of gentian violet (0.25%) + brilliant green (0.25%) + acriflavine (0.1%) (TRIPLE DYE): Used for burns & for dressing umbilical stump in neonates.

Furan Derivatives

- **Nitrofurazone** (FURACIN 0.2% cream, ointment, powder):
  - Bactericidal to both gram +ve & –ve, aerobic & anaerobic bacteria.
  - Highly effective in burns & for skin grafting.
  - Act by inhibiting enzymes necessary for carbohydrate metabolism in bacteria.

Alcohols (Ethanol)

- Act by precipitating bacterial proteins.
- Effective antiseptic & cleansing agent at 40-90% concentration (above 70% antiseptic & up to 90%).
- Used for hypodermic inj. & on minor cuts.
- In open wounds it produces burning sensation
- Poor disinfectant for instruments (does not kill spores & promotes rusting).
  - **Isopropanol:** Used as substitute of ethanol.

Aldehydes (Formaldehyde)

- It denatures proteins, general protoplasmic poison (but acts slowly).
- Broad spectrum germicide.
- Use as antiseptic is restricted because of its irritating nature & pungent odor.
- 4% solution is used for hardening & preserving dead tissues.

- 37% sol. is called FORMALIN.
- Occasionally used to disinfect instruments & excreta.

- **Glutaraldehyde:**
  - Less volatile, less pungent, less irritating. 2% solution is used to disinfect surgical instruments & endoscopes.

SOAPS

- Anionic detergent.
- Weak antiseptic, mainly used for cleansing action.
- Affect only gram +ve bacteria.
- Medicated by other antiseptic & herbal origin compounds (DETTOL, SAVLON, NEEM, MEDIMEX etc).

❑❑❑

CHAPTER 12.2 Astringent and Obtundents

ASTRINGENTS

Astringents act by precipitating proteins in superficial layers of cells and are used to diminish the excretion or exudation of superficial cells. They are also used as local haemostatics and mummifying agents (discussed elsewhere). The different types of astringents used in dentistry are:

TANNIC ACID

It is vegetable astringent obtained from nutgalls. It acts by precipitating protein and gelatin as tannates owing to its acid radical. While hardening the superficial cells it forms pellicle on them. Tannic acid glycerine (30% tannic acid) and mouth-washes/gumpaints containing 1-5% of tannic acid are used to strengthen gums and check bleeding. Its preparations are used as astringent mouth wash, astringent dentrifices, local haemostatics, mummifying agent and obtundent.

Another astringent of vegetable origin i.e. catechu is also used as an astringent mouthwash.

ZINC CHLORIDE

It is a caustic astringent, used as 5-10% solution in ulcerative gingivitis, pyorrhoeal pockets and apthous ulcers.

ZINC SULPHATE

It is used as astringent in 0.5-1% concentration in the form of mouthwash and lotion in mastoiditis, stomatitis and chronic alveolar abscess

COPPER SULPHATE

It is used as astringent mouth in 0.5-2% concentration in indolent ulcer of gums.

ALUM

It has an astringent, antiseptic and haemostatic properties and used in 1-2% concentration to harden the gum or for inflamed and ulcerated gums.

Certain other metallic astringents e.g. ferric chloride solution, lead acetate, silver nitrate, mercuric chloride etc. are used as astringents in dentistry.

OBTUNDENTS

Obtundents are the agents which are used to either diminish or eliminate the dentine sensitivity to make the excavation painless. But due to the availability of local anaesthetics e.g. xylocaine for painless excavation, the use of obtundents is very limited.

An ideal obtundent should possess the following characteristics

(i) It should remove dentive sensitivity and penetrate the dentine sufficiently.

(ii) It should not stain the dentine.

(iii) It should be free from any local irritation or pain.

Obtundents may be classified into three main categories according to their mechanism of action.

I Act by destroying the nervous tissue
- Absolute alcohol

II Act by paralysing the sensory nerve endings
- Phenol creosote
- Benzyl alcohol
- Camphor
- Thymol
- Menthol
- Eugenol (clove oil)

III Act by precipitating proteins
- Silver nitrate
- Zinc chloride

ETHYL ALCOHOL

Ethyl alcohol (70%) is painless and nontoxic to the pulp and penetrates rapidly. It does not cause staining of the dentive. It is to be applied locally, allow the alcohol to evaporate and carry out the excavation.

PHENOL

On local application, it causes irritation followed by numbness. It is used alone and in combination with chloroform and olive oil in a 2:4:10 ratio. It acts rapidly but does not penetrate deeply and due to its protoplasmic poisonous nature it produces its obtundent action.

CREOSOTE

Its characteristics and action is same as that of phenol, in addition its penetrability is relatively more.

BENZYL ALCOHOL

Due to its local anaesthetic property it is used as obtundent agent. It can be used either alone or in combination of chloroform and ethyl alcohol in a 5:3:2 ratio.

CAMPHOR, THYMOL, MENTHOL

All three are volatile oils and are used in a mixture in a ratio of 1:2:1 for rapid action. The mixture acts initially stimulating and then paralysing the sensory nerve endings.

EUGENOL (CLOVE OIL)

Clove oil is used due to the presence of eugenol as its main constituent. It acts by paralysing the sensory never endings. It is non-irritating but stains the dentine yellow.

SILVER NITRATE

It is an astringent and caues pain on application followed by desensitization. It acts by precipitating dentine proteins and liberating acid and stains the dentine black.

ZINC CHLORIDE

Its action is similar to that of silver nitrate but it causes sharp pain and does not stain the dentine.

❑❑❑

CHAPTER 12.3 Mummifying and Bleaching Agents

MUMMIFYING AGENTS

In dentistry, when astringents and antiseptics are used to harden and dry tissues of the pulp and root canal so that the tissues are resistant to infection, they are termed as mummifying agents. It is used in certain dental procedures when it is not possible to completely remove the pulp and contents of root canal. For this, generally a combination of various mummifying agents are used in the form of paste or semi-liquid preparation like tannic acid glycerine.

The following are mummifying agents used in dentistry.

TANNIC ACID

It is an astringent which is yellowish white to light brown amorphous powder obtained from nutgalls (excrescences produced on the young twigs to *Quercus infectoria* which gradually darkens on exposure to air and light. It is used along with glycerine and it hardens the tissues and precipitates proteins and thereby avoids bacterial action.

PARAFORM (PARAFORMALDEHYDE):

It is a prodrug used in combination of zinc oxide or zinc sulphate glycerine and creosote and act by slow liberation of fomaldehyde. It is also used alone as obtundents. Its main disadvantage is that formaldehyde may penetrate the pulp and can cause inflammation.

Liquid formaldehyde is also used in the form of paste with zinc oxide, glycerine along with local anaesthetic and it hardens the tissue without causing the shrinkage.

IODOFORM

It acts by slow liberation of iodine and has both antiseptic and local anodyne properties. It is used in the form of paste which contains tannic acid, phenol, eugenol (clove oil), cinnamon oil and glycerine.

TOOTHACHE DROPS

These are the preparations used for temporary relief of toothache by application of a small pledget of cotton soaked with the product into the tooth cavity. Certain local anaesthetic compounds. e.g. benzocaine, eugenol or clove oil, camphor, menthol, creosote and alcohol has been considered safe and effective for toothache but restricted its use only for first aid type or temporary relief.

BLEACHING AGENTS

Bleaching agents are used to remove pigmentation of teeth. They are classified as

(i) Oxidizing agents e.g. perhydrol, pyrozone, sodium peroxide
(ii) Reducing agents e.g sodium thio sulphate
(iii) Chlorinated lime
(iv) Ultraviolet rays

OXIDIZING AGENTS

Hyrdrogen peroxide in various percentages e.g. perhydrol (30% H_2O_2 in water) and sodium peroxide (50% aqueous solution) are used as oxidizing agents to remove pigmentation of teeth.

REDUCING AGENTS

Saturated solution of sodium thio sulphate is used to remove superficial stains with silver, iodine or permanganate.

CHLORINATED LIME

It is a chlorine compound, which acts by evolution of chlorine to remove the pigmentation of teeth. It is also used clinically by packing into the cavity as a dry powder.

ULTRAVIOLET RAYS

To bleach the dentine from a carbon or mercury, arc lamp UV rays have been used.

Other agents are also available, which are used to remove pigmentation of teeth e.g. weak ammonia solution is used to remove iodine stains, hypochlorite or iodine solution are used to remove silver stains, hypochlorites are used to remove iron stains of teeth and for dye stains, chlorinated lime and acetic acid are used.

❑❑❑

CHAPTER 12.4

Styptics (Local Haemostatics) and Disclosing Agents

STYPTICS (LOCAL HAEMOSTATICS)

After tooth extraction and many dental procedures, bleeding occurs due to disruption of arterioles and minute blood vessels which can not be surgically repaired or sutured. Styptics or local haemostatics are the agents used to arrest bleeding, or to control oozing of blood form minute blood vessel, by the formation of an artificial clot, or by providing a matrix which facilitates bleeding. After extraction of tooth, bleeding from the tooth socket is generally controlled by a cotton guaze pressure pack which may be aided by use of local haemostatics.

They can be categorized as

(i) **Gelatin sponge-** It is used for packing wounds after moistening with normal saline or thrombin solution which is completely absorbed in 2 to 4 weeks and generally cause no foreign body reaction. Gelatin sponge is also available with 5% colloid silver (GELATAMP). It facilitates optimum wound treatment when applied to a surgical cavity and can be cut to the required size to fit smaller wound cavities or tooth socket after tooth extraction. The evenly porous foam structure absorbs its own weight in blood several time over, promotes thrombocyte aggregation due to large surface and fills the wound cavity. It remains in the wound and is completely absorbed within four weeks. The addition of colloid silver has an antimicrobial effect whilst being nontoxic and these type of preparations can be easily gamma sterilised.

(ii) **Fibrin foam-** Fibrin foam or sheets are prepared from human plasma and these dried sheets are used to cover or pack the bleeding surfaces where it gets absorbed in the body. It is applied directly to the bleeding area and it is also combined with thrombin.

(iii) **Human or bovine thrombin-** Dry powder or freshly prepared solution of human or bovine thrombin can be applied on the oozing surfaces and it is employed in haemophilia, skin grafting and in neurosurgery. Thrombin solution with fibrinogen is also used locally to induce clotting.

(iv) **Oxidized cellulose-** It is a surgical gauze, specially treated to promote clotting by reaction between haemoglobin and cellulosic acid. Since it is not well absorbed it is used only for surface haemostatics.

(v) **Russel's Viper venom-** It has a strong thromboplastin activity and used in haemophilia cases by applying locally.

(vi) **Vasoconstrictors -** Adnenaline (1% solution) is used in the form of cotton-gauze pack in the bleeding socket. It stops bleeding by causing local vaso-constriction and useful in epistaxis.

(vii) **Astringents-** Tannic acid (20% in glycerine) is used for bleeding gums and bleeding piles.

Certain systemic haemostatics e.g. tranexamic acid, ethamsylate etc. are also used in the prevention and treatment of capillary bleeding in epistaxis, haematuria and after tooth extraction.

DISCLOSING AGENTS

A dye used in dentistry as a diagnostic acid, applied to the teeth to reveal the presence of dental plague.

❑❑❑

CHAPTER 12.5 Dentifrices and Mouth Washes

DENTIFRICES

These are the agents or mechanical aids which are available as tooth powder, paste, or gel and used with tooth brush to cleanse and polish natural teeth. They are prepared in the form of bulk powder and containing soap or detergent and mild abrasive agent which should have maximum cleansing efficiency with minimum tooth abrasion.

Properties of an Ideal Dentifrice

1. An ideal dentifrice should assist the toothbrush to mechanically remove debris, soft deposits and stains from the teeth.
2. It should be non-decalcifying and non-overabrasive to the teeth.
3. It should impart a polished surface to the teeth.
4. It swallowed, it should be non-poisonous to the body as a whole and also to the mucous membrane.
5. Should have pleasant taste and odour and having sufficient cleansing property.
6. Should help to reduce caries, maintain healthy gingiva, improve aesthetics and reduce mouth odours.

For getting all these properties in one single oral preparation, the following ingredients/agents are used together.

1. **Abrasive agents**

   These are fine dental preparations used to help the scouring action to toothbrush mechanically. And, abrasion is defined as the wearing away of a substance or structure through a mechanical process, such as grinding, rubbing or scrapping. The abrasives is made into a paste and supplied in a tube.

Abrasives used in dentistry can be classified into three categories.

(i) **Finishing abrasives-** They are hard, coarse abrasives which are used initially to develop contour and remove gross irregularities e.g. coarse stones.

(ii) **Polishing abrasives-** They have fine particle size and less hard than abrasive used for finishing. They are used for smoothening the surfaces that have been roughened by coarse stones e.g. pumice, polishing cakes etc.

(iii) **Cleansing abrasives-** They are soft materials with small particle size and are used to remove soft deposits that adhere to enamel or restorative material.

Commonly used abrasives are:

(i) **Pumice-** It is a highly siliceous material of volcanic origin and is used either as an abrasive or polishing agent depending upon particle size. It consists of aluminium, potassium and sodium chiefly. It is available as pumice with glycerine and its use ranges from smoothening dentures to polishing teeth in the mouth.

(ii) **Emery-** It consists of a natural oxide of aluminium called corundum. The different impurities e.g. iron oxide present in it also act as an abrasive.

(iii) **Aluminium oxide-** It can be replaced by emery for abrasive purpose. Pure alumina which is manufactured from bauxite (an impure aluminium oxide) is also used as a polishing agent.

(iv) **Chalk/precipitated calcium carbonate-** Chalk is a calcium carbonate prepared by precipitation method. Various grades of precipitated calcium carbonate is available depending upon its fineness, weight and colour. It is mild abrasive and used to give final polish to silver amalgam fillings.

The other abrasive agents used are tin oxide, chromic oxide, sand, carbides (silicon carbide and boron carbide), zirconium silicate, zinc oxide, garnet, rouge (fine red powder of iron oxide), kieselgurh, tripoli, magnesium oxide, hydrated silica etc.

2. **Humectants**

   These are the agents which are used to keep paste from drying out e.g. glycerine, sorbitol, propylene glycol etc.

3. **Detergents and foaming agents**

   These are cleansing agents and decreases surface tension of dentrifrice. Most common detergent used in dentistry is sodium lauryl sulfate. They cause loosening of debris which adhere to teeth and also dissolving fatty substances and mucous plaques. They also act as an lubricant when scrubbed over the teeth.

4. **Binders**

   Carboxy methyl cellulose is the most commonly used binder in the dental preparation.

5. **Sweetening agents**

   Artificial sweeteners such as sorbitol saccharin is used as synthetic sweetening agent which is more palatable having no food value and can be used by diabetic patients.

6. **Antiseptics/therapeutic agents**

   Certain antiseptic and therapeutic agents (such as sodium fluoride, stannous fluoride, strontium chloride, urea, dibasic ammonium phosphate, are used in dentrifrices for their anticarcinogenic, bacteriostatic and bactericidal actions.

7. **Coloring and flavoring agents**

   Certain coloring agents (methylene blue (0.001%), magenta (0.05%) and flavoring agents (peppermint, clove etc.) are also used to make the preparation more attractive, palatable and acceptable.

8. **Preservatives**

   To preserve the quality and stability, certain preservative e.g. methyl paraben etc. are also used in dental preparations.

MOUTH WASHES

Mouthwashes are aqueous concentrated solutions containing one or more active ingredients and excipients. They are used by swishing the liquid in the oral cavity. Approximately 15–30 ml. of mouthwash are used for single mouthful of rinse for about a minute. Mouthwashes can be used for therapeutic and cosmetic purpose. Therapeutic mouthwashes are used to reduce plaque, dental caries, gingivitis and stomatitis while cosmetic mouthwashes are used to reduce bad breath and it contains used antimicrobial and/or flavoring agent. Mouthwashes other than used for cosmetic purpose, should only be used under the direction of physician/dentist since it contains certain medicines.

Mouthwashes contain the following ingredients and excipients:

Alcohols—It is used in the range of 10-20%. Alcohol enhances the flavor, aids in masking the unpleasant taste of certain ingredients and also serve as solubilizing agent and preservative.

Humectants—Humectants such as glycerine and sorbitol (5-20% of the mouthwashes) increase the viscosity of the preparation and enhance the sweetness of the final product. It also enhances the preservative property of the product along with alcohol.

Surfactants—Non-anionic surfactant e.g. polyoxyethylene derivative of sorbitol, fatty acid esters may be used over anionic surfactant e.g. sodium lauryl sulfate. They aid in the solubilization of flavours and in the removal of debris by its foaming action. Certain other agents e.g. cetylpyridinium chloride (cationic surfactant) is used for its antimicrobial property.

Flavouring agents— Flavouring agents e.g. peppermint, spearmint, menthol, cinnamon, oil of wintergreen (methyl salicylate) are used in conjunction with alcohol and humectants to overcome disagreeable taste.

Colouring agents— Certain colouring agents (e.g. methylene blue, magenta etc.) are used in mouthwashes for pleasing colour.

Medicated mouthwashes—Mouthwashes are also being used as a dosage form in certain specific conditions in oral cavity e.g.

(i) Mouthwashes containing a combination of antihistaminics, corticosteroids, antimicrobial agent (nystatin, tetracycline etc.) have been prepared from commercially available syrups, suspensions, solutions, powders for the treatment of stomatitis.

(ii) Mouthwashers containing allopurinol for the treatment of stomatitis.

(iii) Pilocarpine for dry mouth.

(iv) Amphotericin B for oral candidiasis.

(v) Tranexamic acid for prevention of bleeding after oral surgery.

(vi) Chlorhexidine gluconate for control of plaque.

(vii) Hexetidine for its antibacterial and antifungal property.

❑❑❑

CHAPTER 12.6 Caries and Fluorides

DENTAL CARIES

It is a degenerative condition which is characterized by decay of the hard and soft tissues of the teeth. Infection and decaying food are the main causative factors of dental caries. Carbohydrates mainly act as decaying food and acids are formed in the oral cavity due to fermentation of carbohydrates. The acid thus formed then react with the insoluble calcium salts of the teeth and convert them into soluble salts. Proteolytic enzyme (produced by the bacteria present in the mouth) digest the organic enamel matrix and also enhances the action of acids and digest the organic matter of dentine, and organic acids of the oral cavity destroy the inorganic matter. In a later stage, pulp also affected with the advancing decay and infection may progress in the body.

For dental caries, the preventive phase is probably the most important which include regular brushing, flossing and periodic dental checkup. Regular brushing has been shown to be very effective at controlling caries as well as gum problems. Caries involves the actual demineralization and destruction of tooth structure.

Treatment

Dental caries can be treated by using the following chemical agents.

Ammonium ions—To reduce the incidence of dental caries, ammonium ions are applied locally in the oral cavity. Certain dentifrices which contain ammonia or ammonium compounds e.g. dibasic ammonium phosphate and urea carbamide which liberates ammonia in the mouth are used. They decrease the number of acid producing pathogen, decrease the acidity of the oral cavity and dissolve the dental plaques.

Urea—It is used to treat dental caries and is one of the oldest chemical used. In some dentifrices, urease is present. Urea is broken down to ammonia by urease.

FLUORIDES

The role of fluoride in the control of dental caries has been known for a long time.

Fluoride therapy and fluoridation of drinking water has played a significant role in deccreasing the dental caries. The incidence of dental caries can be significantly decreased by adding fluorides into the drinking water supply. Fluorides prevent decalcification of the structure of tooth by inhibiting bacterial enzymes which produce lactic acid. Fluorides also increase the tooth resistance to acid decalcification.

Fluorides can be used prophylactically as well as therapeutically. Prophylactically, fluoride (in the form of sodium fluoride) can be used in drinking water and one part of fluoride to one million part of drinking water is sufficient for reducing the incidence of dental caries by 50%. Therapeutically, 2% sodium fluoride solution is applied locally to the teeth after cleaning. The local application of fluoride leads to the absorption of fluorine on the enamel surface as calcium fluoride. But, sodium fluoride must be used with caution as it may cause nausea, vomiting and abdominal pain and on chronic ingestion it may lead to chronic fluoride poisoning and also affects enamel and dentine of developing teeth.

Antimicrobial agents— Certain antimicrobial agents e.g. penicillin, bacitracin, aeuromycin etc. are being used to reduce the bacterial count which may be beneficial in reducing the incidence of dental caries.

Certain other agents such as hexachlorophene, silver nitrate, chlorophyll are also used to clean debris and decaying material and incidence of dental caries.

❑❑❑

CHAPTER 12.7

Pharmacotherapy of Common Oral Conditions & Dental Emergencies

The most common oral condition and dental emergency is dental caries, which is a destructive disease of the hard tissues of the teeth due to bacterial infection with *Streptococcus mutans* and other bacteria. It is characterized by destruction of enamel and dentine. Dental decay presents as opaque white areas of enamel with grey undertones and in more advanced cases, brownish discoloured cavitations. Dental caries is initially asymptomatic and pain does not occur until the decay impinges on the pulp, and an inflammation develops. Treatment of caries involves removal of the softened and infected hard tissues, sealing of exposed dentines and restoration of the lost tooth structure with porcelain, silver, amalgam, composite plastic, gold etc.

The common dental emergencies are:

Pulpitis- If the caries lesion progresses, infection of the dental pulp may occur, causing acute pulpitis (Pulpal inflammation). The tooth become sensitive to hot or cold, and then severe continuous throbbing pain ensues. In reversible pulpitis, filling is an option but in case of irreversible pulpitis, root canal therapy (RCT) becomes necessary. The contents of the pulp chamber and root canals are removed, followed by thorough cleaning, antisepsis and filling. Alternatively, extraction may be indicated.

Apical peridontitis- A severely inflammed pulp will eventually necrose, causing apical peridontitis, which is the inflammation around the apex of the tooth. It is characterised by severe spontaneous and persistent pain and regional lymphadenopathy can be present. Management is root canal treatment or extraction. Antibiotics are generally not necessary but patients should be advised to report back to dentist/physician, if swelling or other evidence of infection occurs.

Periapical abscess- It is pulpal inflammation characterized by localized pain and swelling. If the pulpitis is not treated successfully, infection may spread beyond the tooth apex into the peridontal ligament. This infection causes acute inflammation with pain on chewing or on percussion is present. The treatment of abscess is incision and drainage or RCT or extraction supported by antimicrobial and NSAlD's.

Cellulitis- Proliferation of epithelial cell cysts may convert the granuloma into a periapical cyst. The pus in the periapical abscess may track through the alveolar bone into soft tissues, causing cellulitis and bacteremia, or may discharge into the oral cavity, into the maxillary sinus, or through the skin of the face or submandibular area. Maxillary infection also may spread to the periorbital area, increasing the risk of other serious complications including loss of vision, carvernous sinus thrombosis and CNS involvement.

Outpatient with localized cellulitis should be treated by the physician with antistreptococcal oral antibiotics e.g. oral penicillin and in case of penicillin allergy, macrolide antibiotics may be substituted with appropriate pain medication. Definitive theraphy is root canal treatment or extraction.

In severe infection, patients be hospitalized under the direct supervision of physician and treatment should be started immediately with intravenous broad- spectrum antibiotics and surgical drainage if abscess formation is detected.

Peridontal disease- It is an inflammatory destruction of the periodontal ligament and supporting alveolar bone and the main etiologic agent is bacterial plaque. Multiple bacteria are implicated but after progressing the disease, gram negative anaerobes predominate. It is characterized by throbbing pain with erythema and swelling over the affected tissue. At this stage, if left untreated, the abscess may rupture or less commonly, progress to cellulitis.

The treatment is drainage and debridement of the infected perdontal area supported with antibiotics.

Pericoronitis- It is the inflammation of soft tissues surrounding the crown of a partially erupted tooth and most commonly, a wisdom tooth. It generally occurs when bacterial plaque and food debris accumulate beneath the flap of gum covering the partially erupted tooth. It is characterized by inflammation, often complicated by trauma from the opposing tooth, leads to swelling of the flap, tenderness, pain and a bad taste due to pus oozing from beneath the flap.

In localized pericoronitis, hot saline mouthwashes and irrigation under the flap can resolve symptoms in most of the cases. Severe disseminated cases with spreading cellulitis should be treated with penicillin and appropriate medication for pain.

Dental trauma- Dental trauma is extremely common in children with injuries to their primary or permanent teeth. Examination of any injury should focus on related soft tissue injuries and the need for suturing, signs of tooth loosening, displacement or fracture or any other disturbance in the bite or other signs of alveolar fracture. The complete diagnosis require dental radiograph (x-rays) and need follow up with the dentist for complete diagnosis, treatment and long-term care.

Tooth fracture may involve the crown, root or both and with or without the exposure of the pulp. Fracture exposing the pulp are often painful and immediately require referral to a dentist and definitive treatment may involve root canal treatment or extraction depending on the exact nature of the root fracture.

Injuries to teeth and their supporting structures can be classified as fractures.

(i) **Lateral or extrusive (loosening and displacement of the tooth)-** It requires immediate referral to dentist. Luxated permanent teeth require repositioning, splinting or root canal treatment and long term follow up. Any luxated tooth that interferes with normal occlusion requires immediate dental evaluation and treatment for pain and other complications.

(ii) **Instrusion (displacement of the tooth vertically into the alveolar bone)-** Teeth subject to intrusive luxation have been intruded into the alveolar bone, which may occur at the point that the teeth are not visible. Dental referral is required for monitoring to determine if the teeth will re-erupt. For permanent teeth, monitoring and treatment is required to promote re-eruption (surgical or orthodontic) and often coupled with root canal treatment.

(iii) **Avulsion (complete displacement of the tooth out of its socket-** It is a true dental emergency. Primary teeth are never implanted. Permanent teeth that are avulsed should be reimplanted as soon as possible and care should be taken not to touch or clean the root, which could remove periodontal ligament fibres and which ultimately reduce the chance of successful re-implantation. The patient should be immediately referred to dentist for splinting and antibiotic prophylaxis. Antibiotic prophylaxis with penicillin should be given and tetanus toxoid vaccine should be administered

Dental caries and peridontal disease which can lead to certain dental emergencies can be minimised by regular dental care i.e. regular tooth brushing, appropriate fluoride use, decreasing ingestion of sugar containing confectionery items and regular dental examination. Dental trauma especially in children and sport persons can be avoided by using certain mouth guards and face shields.

❑❑❑

Section 13

Miscellaneous

CHAPTER 13.1 Vaccines, Sera and Other Immunological Agents

The **immunological agents** are the agents which produce active or passive immunity and are used to prevent or to modify certain infectious disease. **Immunity** can be defined as the ability of the body to neutralize and eliminate the pathogens and their toxic products.

The immunity can be divided into two sub-groups:

I. **Active immunity:**
   Humoral immunity.
   Cellular immunity.
   Combination of these two.

II. **Passive immunity:**
   Normal human Ig.
   Specific human Ig.
   Animal antitoxins or antisera.

Active Immunity

Active immunity depends upon the humoral and cellular responses of the host. It is the immunity which an individual develops as a result of infection and production of antibodies or cells having a specific action on the microorganisms concerned with a particular infectious disease or on its toxin.

The active immunity may be acquired following clinical infection (chicken pox, rubella, measles), following subclinical infection (polio and diphtheria) and following immunization with an antigen which may be killed vaccine, live attenuated vaccine or a toxoid.

When an antigen is administered for the first time in human body, the antibodies that is elicited first is entirely of the IgM type. The IgM antibody titres rise steadily during the next three to four days, reaches a peak and then declines. Meanwhile if the antigenic stimulus was sufficient, IgG antibody appears in a few days, reaches a peak in a week time and gradually falls over a period of weeks or months, this is called as **primary response**.

The **secondary response** is also known as booster response. It differs from primary response and has a shorter latent period, production of antibodies is more rapid, antibodies are more abundant, antibody response is maintained at a higher level for a longer period and antibodies elicited tend to have a greater capacity to bind to the antigen.

Passive Immunity

When antibodies produced in one body are transferred to another to induce protection against disease, it is known as passive immunity. It can be acquired naturally i.e. in foetus receiving mother's antibodies through placenta or artificially by administration from outside in the form of antisera containing antibodies.

Types of Immunizing Agents

The various preparations employed for conferring immunity are:

VACCINES

It is an immunobiological substance for producing specific protection against a given disease. It stimulates the production of protective antibodies and other immune mechanisms. Vaccines may be prepared from attenuated live organisms, inactivated or killed microorganisms, toxoids or combination of these and more recent one are recombinant vaccines.

Live Vaccines

These are prepared from live organisms e.g. BCG, measles and polio oral vaccine. The live vaccines are more potent immunizing agent because live organisms multiply in the host and the resulting antigenic dose is larger than what is injected and live vaccines have all the major and minor antigenic components. Besides that live vaccines engage certain tissues of the body e.g. intestinal mucosa by polio oral vaccine.

But there are some limitations with live vaccines, such as live vaccines should not be administered in a person with immune deficiency disease or a person with leukemia, lymphoma or are on cytotoxic chemotherapy, radiation or corticosteroid therapy because of malignancy.

The examples of live vaccines are:

- **Live (bacterial)**: BCG, typhoid oral.
- **Live (viral)**: Polio oral vaccine, yellow fever, measles, rubella, mumps, influenza.
- **Live (rickettsial)**: Epidemic typhus.

Killed or Inactivated Vaccines

These consist of microorganisms killed by heat or chemicals. Killed vaccines usually require a primary series of two-three doses of vaccine to produce an adequate antibody response and generally booster dose is required. The duration of immunity varies from months to years. (e.g. in case of polio vaccine) The examples are:

- **Killed (bacterial) vaccine**: Typhoid, cholera, pertussis, plague, meningitis.
- **Killed (viral) vaccine**: Rabies, influenza, hepatitis B, encephalitis (Japanese), polio.

Toxoids

These are produced by addition of formalin to the toxin of microorganisms and incubating them at 37°C for three to four weeks. Certain microorganisms produce endotoxins e.g. tetanus and diphtheria. The toxins produced by these organism are detoxicated and used for the preparation of vaccine. The toxoids have lost their toxicity but antigenicity is retained.

Polysaccharides

Certain vaccines are prepared from extracted cellular fractions e.g. meningococcal vaccine from polysaccharide antigen of the cell wall, pneumococcal vaccine from polysaccharides contained in the capsule of the organism and hepatitis B polysaccharide vaccine.

Combined Vaccines

When more than one kind of immunizing agents are included in the vaccines, it is known as mixed or combined vaccine. For example, DPT (diphtheriapertussistetanus), MMR (measlesmumpsrubella), DT (diphtheriatetanus), DP (diphtheriapertussis) etc.

The various types of vaccines and the immunization schedule are listed in table 13.1.1.

IMMUNOGLOBULINS

There are five major classes IgG, IgM, IgA, IgD and IgE, which form human immunoglobulin system. The various classes and sub-classes of immunoglobulin represent different functional groups that are required to meet different types of antigenic challenges (Table 13.1.2).

Normal human Ig: Normal human Ig is an antibody rich fraction and used to prevent measles in highly susceptible individuals and also provide protection against hepatitis A & B, mumps, poliomyelitis and chicken pox.

Specific human Ig: These preparation are made from the plasma of the patients who have recently recovered from infection. The specific human Ig are used for the prophylaxis of chicken pox and hepatitis B, rabies and tetanus.

The various immunoglobulins used for passive immunization are listed in table 13.1.3.

VACCINATION PROGRAMMES

The result of vaccination programmes have been very impressive. The treatment of certain infectious diseases have been drastically reduced, with their virtual elimination from some countries where they formerly caused considerable disability and many deaths. Vaccination has also opened up the possibility of completely eradicating some diseases from the face of the earth e.g. small pox and polio.

The general schedule of vaccination age-wise is listed below in table 13.1.4.

VACCINE PREPARATIONS

TB (BCG VACCINE)

This vaccine is routinely given to infants and small children in countries where TB is common. This vaccine contains a live attenuated (weakened) strain of *Mycobacterium tuberculosis*, the bacterium which causes tuberculosis. The bacterium has been modified to produce a strain known as Bacille Calmette-Guerin, named after its discoverer. Killed vaccines (strain) can not be used to protect against tuberculosis infection since they do not produce the necessary cellular immune response.

A single dose of vaccine is administered intradermal into the skin over the upper shoulder area. Protection lasts for several years.

POLIO (OPV)

Poliomyelitis is caused by a highly infectious virus known to affect only

Table 13.1.1. *Vaccines for active immunization.*

Type of vaccine	Agent type	Route of administration	Immunization dose (primary & booster)
LIVE VIRUS			
Measles	Live virus	Subcutaneous	Two doses at least 1 months apart and no booster.
Measles-mumps-rubella (MMR)	Live virus	Subcutaneous	2 doses, first at 12-15 months & then 4-6 years.
Varicella	Live virus	Subcutaneous	Two doses, 4-8 weeks apart.
Yellow fever	Live virus	Subcutaneous	One dose 10 days to 10 years before travel and booster at every 10 yrs.
Rubella	Live virus	Subcutaneous	One dose & no booster.
Mumps	Live virus	Subcutaneous	One dose & no booster.
Polio virus vaccine, oral (OPV)	Live viruses of all 3 serotypes	Oral	3 doses, 4-8 weeks apart and booster dosage at 18 months and 5 yrs.
INACTIVATED VIRUS			
Polio virus vaccine inactivated (IPV)	Inactivated viruses of all 3 serotypes	Subcutaneous	Two doses, 4 to 8 weeks apart and a third dose 6 to 12 months after the second and one-time booster dose for travellers.
Rabies	Inactivated virus	Intramuscular or intradermal	Preexposure: 3 doses (IM or ID) at days 0, 7, and 21 or 28. Postexposure: 5 doses (IM only) at days 0, 3, 7, 14, and 28 and serologic testing every 6 months to 2 years in persons at high risk.
Influenza	Inactivated virus or viral components	Intramuscular	One dose (children ≤12 years of age should receive split virus vaccine only; children < 9 yrs who are receiving influenza vaccine for the first time should receive 2 doses, administered at least 1 month apart) and booster yearly with current vaccine.
Hepatitis A	Inactivated virus	Intramuscular	One dose (administer at least 2 to 4 weeks before travel to endemic areas) and booster at 6 to 12 months for long-term immunity.
Hepatitis B	Inactive viral antigen	Intramuscular	Three doses at 0, 1, and 6 months.
BACTERIA			
Typhoid, Ty 21a oral	Live bacteria	Oral	Four doses given 2 days apart and booster 4 doses every 5 years.
Typhoid, heat-phenol inactivated	Inactivated bacteria	Subcutaneous or intradermal	Two doses ≥ 4 weeks apart & booster every 3 years.
Cholera	Inactivated bacteria	Subcutaneous, intramuscular, or intradermal	Two doses given at least 1 week apart, preferably 1 month apart & booster every 6 months.

Contd....

...Contd.

BACTERIAL POLYSACCHARIDES			
Typhoid, Vi-capsular polysaccharide	Bacterial polysaccharide	Intramuscular	One dose and booster at every 2 years.
Haemophilus, influenzae type b conjugate (Hib)	Bacterial polysaccharide conjugated to protein	Intramuscular	One dose
Pneumococcal	Bacterial polysaccharides of 23 serotypes	Intramuscular or subcutaneous	One dose & booster after 6 years in patients at high risk.
Meningococcal	Bacterial polysaccharides of serotypes A/C/Y/W-135	Subcutaneous	One dose
TOXOIDS			
Tetanus-diphtheria (Td or DT)	Toxoid	Intramuscular	Two doses at least 4 weeks apart and a third dose 6 to 12 months after the second and booster at every 10 years or at age 50.
Diphtheria-tetanus-pertussis (DTP)	Toxoids and inactivated whole bacteria	Intramuscular	DTP at 2 months, 4 months, 6 months and at 12 to 18 months then at 4 to 6 years.
Diphtheria-tetanus-acellular pertussis (DTaP)	Toxoids and inactivated bacterial components	Intramuscular	Same as DTP vaccine.
DTP-*Haemophilus influenzae* type b conjugate (DTP-Hib)	Toxoids, inactivated whole bacteria and bacterial polysaccharide conjugated to protein.	Intramuscular	Same as DTP vaccine.

Table 13.1.2: *Types of immunoglobulin.*

Type of immunoglobulin	Characteristics
IgG	75 percent of the total serum immunoglobulin, small molecular wt. (1,60,000), diffuse into the intestinal mucosa.
IgA	15 percent of the total serum immunoglobulin, found in all body secretions (internal & external).
IgM	10 percent of total serum immunoglobulins.
IgD	Normal serum contains 0.3-40 mg/100 ml of IgD.
IgE	Normal serum level is 10 to 130 μg/100 ml.

humans. The virus usually spreads by contact with infected individuals via the water borne route, though mouth-to-mouth transmission is also possible. The disease typically affects very young children, with 80 to 90 percent of cases occurring in children under three years of age.

Polio is a highly contagious disease. By the time first case is detected in a family, all family members may have probably been infected due to the rapidity of viral spread. Viral spread is enhanced by crowding and poor sanitation.

The most prominent example of the effectiveness of OPV is the success of the

Table 13.1.3: *Immunoglobulins for passive immunization.*

Product	Dosage	Use
Immune globulin (intramuscular)	Preexposure prophylaxis: 0.02 mL/kg IM for anticipated risk of ≤3 months, 0.06 mL/kg for anticipated risk of >3 months, repeated every 4 to 6 months for continued exposure. Postexposure: 0.02 mL/kg IM immediately after exposure up to 2 weeks.	Hepatitis A
Hepatitis B immune globulin (HBIG)	0.06 mL/kg IM immediately after exposure up to 1 week for percutaneous exposure or 2 weeks for sexual exposure. 0.5 mL IM within 12 hours after birth for perinatal exposure.	Hepatitis B
Immune globulin (intravenous)	400 mg/kg IV daily for 2 to 5 consecutive days, depending on platelet count and clinical response or 1 g/kg once daily for 1 day or 2 consecutive days.	Idiopathic thrombocytopenic purpura
Immune globulin (intravenous)	400 mg/kg IV daily for 4 consecutive days within 4 days after the onset of illness. A single dose of 2 g/kg IV over 10 hours is also effective.	Kawasaki disease
Immune globulin (intramuscular)	Normal hosts: 0.25 mL/kg IM Immunocompromised hosts: 0.5 mL/kg IM (maximum dose of 15 mL).	Measles
Immune globulin (intravenous)	Minimum effective dosage is 150 mg/kg every 3 to 4 weeks (serum IgG concentration ≥ 400 mg/dL).	Primary immunodeficiency disorders
Rabies immune globulin	20 IU/kg.	Rabies
Rh_o (D) immune globulin	The usual dose (1 vial) administered IM within 72 hours after delivery or termination of pregnancy.	Rh isoimmunization
Immune globulin (intramuscular)	0.55 mL/kg IM	Rubella
Antivenin (*Micrurus fulvius*), equine	At least 3 to 5 vials (30-50 mL) IV initially within 4 hours after the bite. Additional doses may be required.	Snake bite (coral snake)
Antivenin (Crotalidae) polyvalent, equine	The entire dose should be given within 4 hours after the bite by the IV or IM route (1 vial = 10 mL); upto 15 vials can be used depending upon the degree of envenomation.	Snake bite (pit vipers)

Contd....

...Contd.

Tetanus immune globulin	Postexposure prophylaxis: 250 units IM. Treatment: 3,000 to 6,000 units IM.	Tetanus
Varicella-zoster immune globulin	125 units/10 kg IM, up to 625 units. Higher doses may be required.	Varicella
Immune globulin (intravenous)	Initial dose of 400 mg/kg IV every 3 weeks. Dosage should be adjusted upward if bacterial infections occur.	Chronic lymphocytic leukemia
Cytomegalovirus immune globulin (intravenous)	Bone marrow transplantation: 1 g/kg weekly. Kidney transplantation: 150 mg/kg then 50 to 100 mg/kg every 2 weeks.	Cytomegalovirus
Diphtheria antitoxin, equine	20,000 to 120,000 units IV or IM depending on the severity and duration of illness.	Diphtheria
Anti gas gangrene serum	Prophylactic: 10, 000 IU; Therapeutic: 30-75,000 IV SC/IM/IV	Gas gangrene

Table 13.1.4: *General schedule of vaccination.*

Age	Immunization
Birth to 2 months	Hepatitis B vaccine, BCG vaccine.
2 months	Diphtheria and tetanus toxoid and pertussis vaccine (DTP), oral polio virus vaccine (OPV), *Haemophilus influenzae* type b conjugate vaccine (Hib).
2-4 months	HBV and second dose after one month of first dose.
4 months	DTP, Hib, OPV.
6 months	DTP, Hib, OPV.
6-18 months	HBV, OPV, oral polio vaccine at 6 months of age is more preferred.
12-15 months	Measles-mumps-rubella vaccine (MMR), Hib.
12-18 months	DTP or diphtheria and tetanus toxoids and acellular pertussis vaccine (DTaP) at 15 months, varicella vaccine.
4-6 yrs	DTP or DTaP, OPV.
4-6 yrs or 11-12 yrs	MMR.
11-12 yrs	Diphtheria and tetanus toxoids (Td).

worldwide polio eradication programme. Oral polio vaccine (OPV) is used for active immunisation against poliomyelitis. It stimulates the formation of antibodies both in the blood and the mucosal tissues of the GI tract.

DTP (DIPHTHERIA, TETANUS, PERTUSSIS; TRIPLE ANTIGEN, TRIPVAC)

Combined DTP vaccines have been in use worldwide since the 1940s and have contributed substantially to the reduction in clinical pertussis.

Children given three doses of this remarkable vaccine get good protection against three diseases namely diphtheria, tetanus and pertussis.

Diphtheria is an infection that attacks the throat, mouth and nose. It is a highly contagious disease (easy to get), but has become rare ever since the vaccine was introduced.

Tetanus is an infection caused by a bacteria found in dirt, gravel and rusty metal. It usually enters the body through a cut. Tetanus bacteria causes the muscles to spasm (move suddenly). If tetanus attacks the jaw muscles it causes lockjaw, the inability to open the mouth. Tetanus can also cause spasm of the respiratory muscles, which can be fatal.

Pertussis also called whooping cough which is caused by a bacteria that clogs the lungs with mucus (a thick, slimy substance). This can cause a severe cough that sounds like a 'whoop.' The cough can last for two months and allows the infection by other bacteria which can cause pneumonia and bronchitis (infection of lungs).

Diphtheria Antitoxin

It is used for passive immunisation in suspected cases of diphtheria and should be given without waiting for bacteriological confirmation of the infection and antibacterial agent is usually given concomitantly. A test dose of diphtheria antitoxin should always be given to test hypersensitivity.

COMBINATION VACCINE

A combination vaccine consists of two or more separate immunogens physically combined in a single preparation. A combination vaccine gives protection from more than one disease.

Advantages of Combination Vaccines

- It is more convenient for parents and medical staff since number of visits to the hospital are reduced.
- It is less traumatic for children since lesser number of injections have to be given.
- Combined vaccines invariably cost less than the sum of their component individual vaccines.
- The overall number of adverse reactions is lower.
- The chance of compliance is increased benefitting the individual and the community.
- There is more cost-effective use of health-care manpower and resources.
- The cost of purchase, transportation and storage of vaccines are substantially reduced.
- The administration of medical records and vaccine scheduling is simplified.

Some examples of combination vaccines include DTP, MMR etc. Now, newer combination vaccines are available that provide prevention against four diseases (DTP + HB) or even five diseases (DTP + HB/Hib) making it pentavalent vaccine.

COMBINATION VACCINES WITH HAEMOPHILUS B CONJUGATE VACCINE (HIB TITER)

Each lyophilisate for one immunising dose of diphtheria, tetanus toxoids and pertussis with Haemophilus b conjugate vaccine contains *Haemophilus influenzae* type b polysaccharide conjugated to tetanus protein 10 mcg, purified diphtheria toxoid 1 immunising dose, purified tetanus toxoid 1 immunising dose, *Bordetella pertussis* minimum of 4.1 IU.

It is **indicated** in all children from age of two months onwards for the combined prevention of invasive infections such as meningitis, septicaemia, epiglottitis etc. caused by *Haemophilus influenzae* type b, diphtheria, tetanus and pertussis.

Dosage: Three injections of 0.5 ml at one or two months interval followed by a booster injection administered one year after the primary vaccination.

DUAL ANTIGEN

It is a uniform suspension of diphtheria and tetanus toxoid adsorbed on aluminium phosphate and suspended in isotonic saline solution.

Adverse effects include mild local reactions like pain, redness, tenderness at the site of injection. Mild to moderate transient fever and irritability.

It is **used** for active immunisation of children against diphtheria and tetanus in cases where it is decided not to immunize against pertussis also.

Dosage: 3 IM injections of 0.5 ml to be administered with an interval of four to eight weeks between doses. A fourth injection of 0.5 ml should be administered one year after initial injection.

HEPATITIS B (BEVAC)

Hepatitis B is a worldwide disease caused by the hepatitis B virus (HBV). HBV primarily affects the liver inducing an inflammatory reaction that destroys liver cells and often hinders liver function. The consequences of infection are variable and unpredictable. They depend on the age and immunity status of the patient.

The hepatitis B virus is highly infectious. It is estimated to be 100 times more infectious than HIV which causes AIDS. Hepatitis B kills more people in a day than AIDS kills in a whole year.

Blood is the most important vehicle for transmission but other body fluids have also been implicated including semen, vaginal secretions and saliva.

HBV can spread in three ways: From mother to child (MTC), at birth and from person to person.

Hepatitis B vaccine is used for active immunisation against hepatitis B infection. Immunisation should be considered in persons at high risk of contracting hepatitis B.

Adverse effects include mild transient soreness and induration at injection site. Occasionally low grade fever, malaise, fatigue, headache, nausea and dizziness.

It is **used** for active immunization against hepatitis B virus infection.

Dosage:

- *Adults:* 1 ml by IM injection into the deltoid muscle; repeated one month and six months later.
- *Children:* 0.5 ml by IM injection into the anterolateral aspect of thigh; repeated one month and six months later.

Administration: This is for IM use only. In adults the injection should be given in the deltoid region; in neonates and infants the injection should be given in anterolateral thigh. Dose for adults and children above 10 years is 20 mcg and for neonates, infants and children below 10 years the dose is 10 mcg. Three doses are given as above. For rapid immunization the third dose can be given two months after the first dose and a fourth booster dose at 12 months.

HEPATITIS A (AVAXIM)

Hepatitis A is one of the most widespread infectious diseases worldwide. It is caused by the hepatitis A virus and is common in places with poor standards of hygiene and sanitation. The virus attacks the liver and causes varying degrees of illness in patients.

The hepatitis A virus is excreted in the faeces. Direct contact with an infected person's faeces or indirect contamination of food, water, hands and cooking utensils may result in the virus being ingested, causing infection.

Symptoms include nausea, vomiting, jaundice (yellowness of eyes, skin and urine), diarrhoea, pale stools, abdominal pain, malaise, fatigue, fever, chills, lack of appetite, sore throat, etc.

Hepatitis A is often confused with hepatitis B. What is important to remember is that hepatitis A is the single largest cause of jaundice. Also vaccination against hepatitis B does not protect from hepatitis A.

A vaccine is now available and is the most practical means of protection against hepatitis A. A complete course of vaccine should be taken to get long term protection.

Hepatitis A vaccination is indicated for active immunisation against hepatitis A virus (HAV) infection in subjects at risk of exposure to HAV such as travellers to high prevalence areas, armed force personnel travelling to high endemic areas, person in whom hepatitis A is an occupational hazard or in whom there is an increased risk of transmission (persons working in a day care centre, nursing, medical and paramedical personnel especially gastroenterology and paediatric unit, sewage workers, homosexuals, haemophilia patients, abusers of injectable drug and persons with multiple sexual partners.

Adverse effects include injection site soreness, redness and swelling; mild headache, malaise, fatigue, fever, nausea and loss of appetite.

Dosage:

- *Adults* (19 years onwards): A single dose of hepatitis A adults vaccine (1 ml suspension containing not less than 1,440 ELISA units of viral antigen) is used for primary immunization.
- *Children and adolescents* (from 1 year up to 18 years of age): A single dose of hepatitis A junior vaccine (0.5 ml suspension containing not less than 720 ELISA units of viral antigen) is used for primary immunization.

In both a booster dose is recommended any time between 6 to 12 months later to ensure long time protection from hepatitis A.

Administration: By IM route only, in deltoid muscle.

TYPHOID (TYPHIVAX)

Typhoid fever is a disease which starts as an infection of the gastrointestinal tract. It is caused by the bacterium *Salmonella typhi.* It spreads by ingestion of contaminated food or drink. Normally *Salmonella typhi* bacterium is inactivated by acid in stomach. However, if a large number of bacteria are ingested, a substantial number may reach the small intestine. Symptoms include periodic fever, headache, tiredness and weakness, changes in behaviour and abdominal discomfort with constipation in the early stages of the disease followed by diarrhoea later.

Typhoid vaccines are used for active immunisation against typhoid fever. Two types of vaccine, one injectable and other oral are available.

Polysaccharide Typhoid Vaccine

It is prepared from Vi capsular polysaccharide of *Salmonella typhi*. Immunity develops 7 to 15 days after injection and protection lasts for three years.

Adverse effects include slight local pain, fever and rash.

It is **indicated** for prevention of typhoid fever in adults and children over five years.

Dosage: Single dose of 0.5 ml SC or IM.

Oral Typhoid Vaccine

It contains the attenuated strain Ty21a of *Salmonella typhi*. The attenuation is due to the absence of enzyme uridine diphosphate galactose-4-epimerase which is essential for the production of the lipopolysaccharide 'O' antigen. The absence of this enzyme makes Ty21a highly immunogenic.

Adverse effects include fever and/or mild GI effects.

It is **indicated** for prophylactic immunization of adults and children over six years against typhoid fever.

Dosage: One capsule on day 1, 3 & 5 irrespective of age and weight.

HIB (*H. INFLUENZAE* TYPE B; VAXIGRIP)

Haemophilus influenzae is a bacteria which exists in many forms. The type B form called Hib, commonly produces disease in humans by colonizing the upper respiratory tract of up to 80 percent of the population and is major cause of infection and mortality in children.

Almost all Hib disease occurs in children younger than five years and mostly in children younger than one year.

Transmission of Hib from one individual to another primarily occurs via respiratory secretions from carriers. However, Hib can also be spread through direct contact with a person with Hib disease but this accounts for only two percent of cases in children younger than four years old.

The manifestations of Hib disease are varied with the most serious being meningitis and epiglottitis.

Adverse effects include mild and transient local erythema, swelling, fever, irritability, sleepiness, GIT disturbances, rashes and anorexia.

It is **indicated** for immunisation of children against invasive disease caused by *Haemophilus influenzae* type b (meningitis, septicemia, cellulitis, arthritis, epiglottitis).

The safety and efficacy of Hib vaccines have clearly been demonstrated in developed countries and their introduction into the national vaccination programme of developing countries in the future can markedly reduce the incidence of Hib-related disease worldwide.

MMR (MEASLES, MUMPS & RUBELLA; TRESIVAC)

Measles

In developing countries, measles can be a very severe disease, with mortality rates as high as 10 percent. Hence, vaccination is recommended for all children at the earliest possible age. Currently, the WHO recommended nine months as the age for measles vaccination, taking into account maternal antibody levels and vaccine intake, as well as disease incidence.

The signs and symptoms of measles include fever, common cold-like symptoms, conjunctivitis, cough, spots inside the mouth and a skin rash. Diarrhoea, stomach pain and loss of appetite may also be present.

The severity of the symptoms of measles is greater in adolescents and adults than in children. The incubation period is 10 to 12 days and during this period there is virtually no outward sign of illness. During this period the virus first causes a local infection of the upper respiratory tract then spreads to other parts of the body. The virus is then disseminated throughout by bloodstream causing a primary disease.

Mumps

Mumps or infective parotitis is an acute infectious disease usually marked by a painful enlargement of one or both salivary glands around the jaw. In addition, dryness of the mouth may often occur.

Rubella

Rubella or German measles, is a highly infectious disease, which mostly affects children, adolescents and young adults. Rubella soon after birth is a disease which is usually trivial and of short duration. Its most obvious sign is a mild rash. Rubella virus infection during pregnancy can disrupt fetal growth and cause birth defects.

Approximately 25 to 50% of rubella infections may go undetected. When symptoms do present, they are usually quite mild.

Adults who contract rubella present with fever and loss of appetite for two days prior to the onset of the rash.

MMR Vaccination

Live attenuated virus vaccines for measles, mumps and rubella (MMR) have been combined into a single vaccine known as MMR vaccine. The MMR vaccine is effective as the single-virus vaccine composed of the respective strains and has been shown to be highly effective. The immunity induced by MMR is long lasting and may be lifelong.

Adverse effects include hyperthermia, rhinopharyngeal or respiratory symptoms of short duration. Hyperthermia convulsions are rarely observed. Lymphadenopathies or parotitis may be observed.

It is **indicated** for joint prevention of measles, mumps and rubella, normally, given from the age of 12 months, in infants of both sexes.

CHICKENPOX (VARICELLA; OKAVAX)

Chickenpox or varicella is caused by the varicella zoster virus (VZV). Varicella vaccine is indicated for active immunisation against varicella in healthy subjects and their susceptible healthy close contacts from the age of 12 months onwards.

Varicella vaccine is a lyophilized preparation of the Oka strain of live attenuated varicella virus obtained by propagation of the virus in MRC_5 human diploid cell culture.

Varicella vaccine produces an attenuated clinically inapparent varicella infection in susceptible subjects.

Adverse effects include mild and transient reaction at the site of injection, headache, fever, paraesthesia and fatigue.

It is **indicated** for active immunisation against varicella in healthy subjects from the age of 12 months onwards. Susceptible healthy close contacts (parents and siblings of high-risk patients, medical, paramedical personnel and other people who are in close contact with varicella patients) should be immunised in order to reduce the risk of transmission of virus to high-risk patients.

FLU VACCINE (HIBERIX)

Influenza vaccine contains antigens from two or three of the currently circulating types of flu virus.

Vaccination is recommended for elderly people particularly those with heart, lung or kidney disease. Flu vaccination has to be repeated before each winter because of the possible changes in virus types.

MENINGOCOCCAL VACCINE (MENCEVAX A & C)

This vaccine is recommended for both adults and children to protect them from *Meningococcal meningitis*.

A single dose of vaccine provides good protection against infection caused by meningococci. Regular revaccinations are required for long-term protection.

Adverse effects include low grade fever and pain at injection site.

It is **indicated** for prophylaxis against cerebrospinal meningitis due to meningococci A & C groups by SC or IM route in single 0.5 ml dose.

PNEUMOCOCCAL VACCINE (PNEUMO 23)

This vaccine is recommended for those who are at risk of pneumococcal pneumonia. A single dose of vaccine gives protection against infection. Revaccination is required at a later date.

It is prepared from purified pneumococcal capsular antigens and includes 23 serotypes which are responsible for at least 85% of pneumococcal infections and has greater than 90% coverage against serotypes that are penicillin resistant.

Adverse effects include hypersensitivity, redness, slight pain and induration at the site of injection. Rarely fever may occur.

It is **indicated** in prevention of pneumococcal infections, particularly those of respiratory origin in all subjects over the age of two years who are at risk of serious pneumococcal infection.

RABIES VACCINE (RABIPUR)

Commonly known as treatment for dog bite. Rabies is usually caused by the bite of infected dog, monkey, cat, etc. and can lead to hydrophobia (feeling of fear of water) and death. A series of five injections need to be given. Usually rabies vaccine is given once the dog bite has already taken place.

Rabies vaccines which are used for active immunisation against rabies may be used as part of postexposure treatment. It may also be used as preexposure prophylaxis against rabies in high risk persons like dog handlers etc.

Rabies vaccines may be

i. Purified chick embryo cell rabies vaccine.
ii. Inactivated rabies vaccine prepared on vero cells. This vaccine for the pre or postexposure immunization against rabies is obtained by culture on vero continuous cell lines.
iii. Human diploid cell rabies vaccine.
iv. Highly purified duck embryo rabies vaccine.

Adverse effects include pain, reddening and swelling at injection site, swollen lymph nodes, joint pains and GI complaints.

It is **indicated** for immunization against rabies after exposure and for prophylactic vaccination against rabies before exposure.

Dosage: Vaccine should be given intramuscular in the deltoid region only.

a. ***Preexposure***: 3 dose IM injections on day 0, 7 and 28. A booster dose after one year and one dose after every five years. In case of subsequent exposure, only two doses at day 0 and day 3 provide protection, if proper previous vaccination status is available.
b. ***Postexposure***: After exposure start immediately a full course of treatment for both adults and children consists of 5 injections on days 0 (day of exposure), 3, 7, 14 and 30. A booster dose on day 90 is optional.

MEASLES VACCINE

It contains live attenuated Edmonston-Zagreb strain of measles virus propagated on human diploid cells.

Adverse effects include fever which may be accompanied by skin rash, malaise, cough, headache and rarely febrile convulsions.

It is **indicated** for active immunization of children and susceptible adults by SC route in a dose of 0.5 ml.

TETANUS TOXOID

It is a sterile uniform suspension of tetanus toxoid adsorbed on aluminium phosphate and suspended in isotonic saline used for active immunization against tetanus.

Adverse effects include mild local reactions, tenderness and induration at the site of injection.

Dosage:

For active primary immunization: Two doses of 0.5 ml each by IM route at an interval of four to six weeks. Reinforcing dose should be given, six to eight months later, to increase the level of immunity.

Booster dose: In previously immunized persons, a booster dose of 0.5 ml IM should be given every five years to maintain adequate level of immunity. The need for tetanus vaccine in wound management depends both on the condition of the wound and immunisation history of the patient. For tetanus prone wound, tetanus immunoglobulin may also be required.

RUBELLA VACCINE (R-VAC)

It is used for active immunisation against rubella. It is administered to girls aged 10 to 14 years. It is also recommended for women of child bearing age if they are seronegative, women who are found to seronegative during pregnancy should be vaccinated in the early postpartum period. Pregnancy should be avoided for at least one month after vaccination.

ANTISNAKE VENOM

The venom of snake is a complex mixture of protein which has enzymatic activity and may also provoke local inflammatory reaction. The venom may have effect on tissue, blood vessels, blood cell coagulation or neurotoxic effect with sensory, motor and respiratory involvement. Management of snake bite involves general supportive care and monitoring of vital functions but in a systemic snake bite poisoning, specific antivenom is the most effective therapy. It is highly recommended to wait for clear clinical evidence of systemic poisoning before giving antivenom. Monospecific antivenoms are more effective and are less likely to cause side effects than polyvalent antivenoms.

IMMUNOGLOBULINS

These are preparations containing antibodies against infectious microorganisms and are usually prepared from human plasma or serum.

Normal immunoglobulins are prepared from material from blood donors and contain several antibodies against infectious diseases prevalent in the general population. Specific immunoglobulins contain minimum specified levels of one antibody.

Anti-D immunoglobulins are given to prevent the formation of rhesus antibodies in rhesus-negative (Rh –ve) persons on exposure to rhesus positive red blood cells.

TETANUS IMMUNOGLOBULIN (TIG; TETGLOB)

It is a sterile solution of hyperimmunoglobulin prepared from the placenta of healthy volunteers specifically immunised against tetanus.

Adverse effects include local pain, fever, flushing, headache and chills.

It is **indicated** in subjects already sensitised with serums of animal origin, existence of prior or present allergic manifestations (asthma, eczema, etc.), burns, injuries, open and compound fractures; unimmunized or inadequately immunised mothers.

Dosage:

Prophylaxis: 250-500 IU intramuscular.

Therapeutic: Tetanus neonatorum 500 to 10,000 IU intramuscular or 250 IU intrathecal. In adults and children 500 to 10,000 IU intramuscular and/or 250 to 500 IU intrathecally.

RABIES IMMUNOGLOBULIN (BERIRAB-P)

It provides passive protection when given immediately to individuals exposed to rabies virus. This provides maximum circulating antibody with minimum interference of active immunisation with human diploid cell vaccine.

Adverse effects include local tenderness, muscle soreness or stiffness at the injection site, low grade fever, sensitisation to repeated injections of human globulin in immunoglobulin deficient patients.

It is **indicated** in all injuries, even licks, on mucous membranes by wild animals (or even pet animals) suspected to be suffering from rabies.

HEPATITIS B IMMUNOGLOBULIN (HEPABIG)

HBIG provides immediate passive immunity for those individuals with acute exposure to HBsAg positive blood/blood derivatives. Clinical trials have demonstrated reduction in attack rate of clinical hepatitis B following its use. After administration of the usual recommended dose of the HBIG there is a detectable level of circulating anti-HBsAg antibody which persist for three months. No case of transmission of hepatitis B has been associated with the use of this product.

HBIG does not interfere with generation of antibody response to hepatitis B vaccine. Ideally, persons exposed to blood which contains hepatitis B virus should be given combined passive active immunization.

Adverse effects include transient, mild pain at the site of injection and itching.

It is **indicated** for prophylaxis of hepatitis B after exposure to HBsAg e.g. by accidental 'needle-stick', contact by accidental splash or oral ingestion (pipetting accident) involving HBsAg positive material such as blood, plasma or serum.

For prophylaxis of hepatitis B in neonates born to HBsAg positive mothers.

Dosage: Following exposure to HBsAg.

Adults: 1,000 to 2,000 IU IM.

Children: 32 to 48 IU/kg body weight This should be administered within seven days (preferably within 48 hrs) after exposure to HBsAg.

Neonates: Initial dose is 100 to 200 IU. The first dose should be administered within five days after birth. The booster dose should be 32 to 48 IU/kg of body wt. between two to three months after initial dose.

HUMAN NORMAL IMMUNOGLOBULIN (BHARGLOB)

It is **indicated** for prophylaxis of infectious diseases and immunotherapy.

Adverse effects include flushing with chills, nausea and headache.

GAMMAGLOBULIN (HISTOGLOB)

Intravenous gamma globulin preparations are available for replacement therapy for patients with congenital agammaglobulinaemia and hypogammaglobulinaemia, idiopathic thrombocytopenic purpura and Kawasaki syndrome. It is also used for prophylaxis of infection following bone marrow transplantation.

HUMAN ANTI-D IMMUNOGLOBULIN (RHOCLONE)

It is **indicated** for prevention of development of anti-D antibodies in Rh negative mothers after child birth, abortion beyond 13 weeks gestation, antepartum prophylaxis at 26 to 28 weeks gestation.

Dosage:

Adults: Prophylaxis after delivery, abortion, amniocentesis: 300 mcg IM within 72 hours. Massive transplacental haemorrhage: 25 mcg/ml of foetal erythrocytes.

HISTAGLOBULIN

Histaglobulin is a lyophilised preparation of histamine (as histamine dihydrochloride) coupled with human normal immunoglobulin.

Histaglobulin is thoroughly screened for hepatitis B surface antigen and anti HIV using third generation technique RIA and ELISA and is found to be non-reactive.

As histamine by itself is not an antigenic molecule, it is conjugated with globular protein to form a complete antigen wherein histamine acts as hapten when injected into a living body, forming antibodies to the hapten histamine complex. Antibodies thus formed increase the histamine binding capacity of serum. It has been demonstrated that the histamine binding capacity of normal plasma is 20 percent to 30 percent, whereas it is only zero to five percent in allergic patients.

Adverse effects include nausea, vomiting and vasodilatation in the facial area.

It is **indicated** in bronchial asthma, migraine, urticaria, eczema, allergic rhinitis, pruritus, neurodermatitis, atopic dermatitis and other allergic disorders.

IMMUNOSUPPRESSANTS

These are the agents used to suppress the immunity. The drugs like azathioprine and cyclosporin A are used chiefly to prevent rejection in organ transplantation. They are also used for treatment of autoimmune disease.

AZATHIOPRINE (IMURAN)

It is a purine antagonist, immunosuppressant drug which suppresses cell mediated immunity. It acts by inhibiting DNA synthesis and hence prevents proliferation of T-lymphocytes.

After administration in body it is converted to mercaptopurine.

Adverse effects include skin rash, bone marrow depression, GI disturbances and hepatotoxicity.

It is **indicated** in renal transplantation, severe active rheumatoid arthritis unresponsive to other therapy, certain autoimmune diseases, chronic active hepatitis, idiopathic thrombocytopenic purpura and acquired haemolytic anaemia.

Dosage:

Renal transplantation: Initially 3 to 5 mg/kg/day followed by 1 to 3 mg/kg/day as maintenance dose.

Rheumatoid arthritis: Initially 1 mg/kg as a single dose; if required increase after six to eight weeks by 0.5 mg/kg/day at four weeks intervals up to a maximum of 2.5 mg/kg/day.

CYCLOSPORINE A (SANDIMMUN)

It inhibits early cellular response to antigenic and regulatory stimuli, mainly in helper T-cells. At molecular level it affects cyclophilin proteins.

After oral administration it is absorbed and is highly concentrated in erythrocytes. After metabolism in liver most of the drug is excreted in bile. Some metabolites are active and show immunosuppressive activity.

Adverse effects include nephrotoxicity, hypertension, tremor, seizures, increased incidence of infections, gingival hyperplasia, hirsutism, flushing, paraesthesias, tinnitus, headache, gynaecomastia and conjunctivitis. It has no toxic effects on bone marrow and RE system.

It is **used** to prevent graft rejection after kidney, liver, heart, lung, pancreas transplant or bone marrow transplantation and psoriasis not responding to conventional therapy.

Dosage:

Solid organ transplantation: Oral dose should be initiated within 12 hours before surgery at a dose of 10 to 15 mg/kg in two divided doses, then continued for one to two weeks postoperatively followed by maintenance dose of 2 to 6 mg/kg.

Bone marrow transplantation: Start a day before transplantation. IV infusion: 3 to 5 mg/kg/day, continue two weeks postoperatively, then continue with oral preparation in dose of 12.5 mg/kg in two divided doses for six months to one year.

Psoriasis: Initial 2.5 mg/kg/day orally in two divided doses. Maximum dose is 5 mg/kg/day.

❑❑❑

CHAPTER 13.2 Drugs Used in Skin Disorders

For the treatment of various skin disorders, local application of drugs in the form of cream, ointment, gel etc., appears to be the ideal and convenient form of management. However, in severe conditions different drugs can also be given by oral routes. The different agents used in various skin disorders are classified as in table 13.2.1.

The detailed pharmacology of various agents listed in table are discussed in different chapters and only remaining agents are covered in this section.

ANTIBACTERIAL AGENTS

Topical antibacterial agents are used to prevent infection and in the early treatment of infected dermatoses and wounds. Various preparations contain corticosteroids in addition to antibacterial agents.

Detailed pharmacology of various antibacterial agents is discussed in chapter 'Chemotherapeutic agents'.

MUPIROCIN

It is structurally unrelated to other topical anti-bacterial agents. Most of the gram positive aerobic bacteria including methicillin resistant *S. aureus* are sensitive to mupirocin. It inhibits *in-vivo* synthesis of bacterial proteins by specific and reversible binding to isoleucyl transfer-RNA synthetase bacterial enzyme. It is **indicated** in the treatment of impetigo (which is a common skin disease, characterized by superficial bacterial infection caused by *S. aureus* or streptococci. The primary lesion is a superficial pustule crust, which may occur on normal skin or superimposed upon another skin disease).

Topical Antibiotics Used in Acne

Clindamycin is active against *Propionibacterium acnes*. Erythromycin alone and in combination with benzoyl peroxide is used in the treatment of acne vulgaris. Topical metronidazole is effective in the treatment of acne rosacea.

Tetracycline hydrochloride and minocycline sulfosalicylate are used in the treatment of acne vulgaris.

Topical sodium sulfacetamide is used in the form of lotion and in combination of

Table 13.2.1: *Classification of drugs used in different skin disorders.*

I	**Antibacterial agents (used topically)** Bacitracin, polymyxin B sulphate, neomycin, gentamicin, gramicidin, mupirocin (T-BACT)
II.	**Antibiotics used in acne (topically)** Erythromycin (ACNESOL), clindamycin (CLINDAC-A), tetracycline and minocycline sulfosalicylate, metronidazole, sodium sulfacetamide
III.	**Antifungal agents (used orally)** Griseofulvin, ketoconazole, fluconazole, itraconazole **Used topically** Miconazole, oxiconazole, ketoconazole, sulconazole, clotrimazole (along with betamethasone dipropionate), terbinafine (SEBIFIN), naftifine, butenafine, tolnaftate, nystatin, amphotericin B, cyclopirox olamine
IV.	**Antiviral agents (used topically)** Acyclovir, valacyclovir, penciclovir, famciclovir, imiquimod
V.	**Steroid preparations (used topically as antiinflammatory agents)** Beclomethasone dipropionate (BECLATE) Betamethasone valerate (BETNOVATE) with neomycin also Clobetasol valerate (TENOVATE) Dexamethasone sodium acetate (DECADRON) with neomycin Fluocortolone (ULTRALAN) Triamcinolone acetonide (LEDERCORT) Hydrocortisone acetate (WYCORT)
VI.	**Ectoparasiticides** Lindane, crotamiton, permethrin, sulphur, benzyl benzoate
VII.	**Melanizing/demelanizing agents (agents affecting pigmentation)** Hydroquinone, monobenzone (BENOQUIN), trioxsalen (NEOSORALEN), methoxsalen (MACSORALEN), azelaic acid
VIII.	**Sunscreens** Para-aminobenzoic acid (PABA) and its esters, benzophenones
IX	**Acne preparations** Retinoic acid, adapalene, isotretinoin (ADAFERIN), benzoyl peroxide, azelaic acid
X.	**Agents for psoriasis** Acitretin, tazarotene, calcipotriene
XI.	**Keratolytic agents** Salicylic acid, propylene glycol, podophyllum resin & podofilox, urea, cantharidin, fluorouracil, benzoic acid
XII.	**Antipruritic agents** Doxepin, pramoxine
XIII.	**Drugs for alopecia (trichogenic agents)** Minoxidil, finasteride, dutasteride
XIV.	**Antiseborrheic agents** Coal tar compound, chloroxine, selenium sulfide (SELSUN)
XV.	**Miscellaneous compounds** Tacrolimus, sirolimus, antimetabolites e.g. methotrexate, antihistaminics for pruritus dermatitis, prednicarbate (DERMATOP), becaplermin, dapsone, thalidomide, cyclosporine, interferon

sulfur for the treatment of acne vulgaris and acne rosacea.

ANTIFUNGAL AGENTS

Detailed pharmacology of antifungal agents (oral & topical) is discussed in detail in chapter 'Chemotherapeutic agents-Antifungal agents'.

ANTIVIRAL AGENTS

Detailed pharmacology of acyclovir, valacyclovir, penciclovir and famciclovir is discussed in detail in chapter 'Chemotherapeutic agents- Antiviral agents'.

IMIQUIMOD

It is an immunomodulator agent used locally in the treatment of external genital perianal warts in adults.

Adverse effects include local inflammatory reaction, erythema, pruritus etc.

STEROIDAL PREPARATIONS

Topical corticosteroids are used in the treatment of inflammatory dermatoses. The general pharmacology are discussed in chapter 'Glucocorticoids'.

ECTOPARASITICIDES

LINDANE

It is a gamma isomer of hexachlorocyclohexane used as pediculicide and scabicide in the form of lotion, shampoo and cream.

Adverse effects include neurotoxicity, haematotoxicity and local irritation when it comes in contact with eye and mucous membrane.

CROTAMITON

It is scabicide, pediculocide and antipruritic used in the form of lotion and cream.

PERMETHRIN

It is neurotoxic to *Pediculus humanus, Pthirus pubis* and *Sarcoptes scabiei.*

It is **used** in the form of cream. **Adverse effects** include transient burning and stinging.

Sulphur is **used** as scabicide and benzyl benzoate is effective as pediculicide and scabicide.

DEMELANIZING AGENTS

Hyperpigmentation is an aberration in which dark spots on the skin, which often make it cosmetically undesirable. This benign condition is attributed to an overproduction of melanin, a dark-coloured pigment in the skin. The relative amount of melanin as well as other skin pigments, genetically determine an individual's skin colour. Thus, people with innately dark skin have more melanin than people with lighter skin colour. The production of melanin is dependent upon the activity of the enzyme tyrosinase. This enzyme is essential in catalyzing the reaction that produces melanin. Thus drugs that block tyrosinase, inhibit the overproduction of melanin.

Post-inflammatory hyperpigmentation is the most common cause of hyperpigmentation, which occurs after irritation or inflammation of the skin for example after an episode of acne. This type of hyperpigmentation occurs more often in darker skinned people as a result of the increased level of melanin pigment in the skin. If the affected area only extends into the skin epidermis, this makes it easier to treat because the affliction only involves the superficial layers of the skin. Therefore, patients will respond faster to treatment. However, if the condition affects deep layers of the skin, such as dermis, treatment may need to be prolonged or may require other alternatives.

Hydroquinone and **monobenzone** are used to reduce hyperpigmentation of the skin. **Trioxsalen** and **methoxsalen** used for repigmentation of depigmented macules of vitiligo.

Azelaic acid is a newer treatment for hyperpigmentation, primarily for post-inflammatory hyperpigmentation. It works by blocking the activity of tyrosinase and does not cause photosensitivity of the skin or residual changes in the skin. There is decreased incidence of allergic reactions associated with azelaic acid. Corticosteroids also block the activity of tyrosinase. Corticosteroids are used in combination with other drugs to minimize the side effects. The combination of azelaic acid and hydrocortisone acetate (10%) may also be useful in the treatment of post-inflammatory hyperpigmentation of skin

SUNSCREENS

These are the agents which protect the skin from harmful effects of exposure to sunlight by absorbing ultraviolet light. The most commonly used compounds are paraamino benzoic acid (PABA) and its esters and benzophenones include oxybenzone, dioxybenzone and sulisobenzone. These benzophenones provide a broader spectrum of absorption from 250 to 360 nm.

Various physical sunscreens such as heavy petroleum jelly, zinc oxide, titanium oxide, calamine are also used, which can stop and scatter ultraviolet rays

ACNE PREPARATIONS

Acne is a common skin condition, which consists of blackheads, white heads, and sometimes deeper boil-like lesions called nodules or cysts. It occurs during the teenage years in boys and girls.

Acne vulgaris affects the pilosebaceous units to the skin, leading to their eventual blockade and development of acne lesions. Abnormal desquamation, defective keratinisation, blockade of the follicular orifice and collection and colonization of sebum lead to proliferation of *Propionibacterium acnes.*

RETINOIC ACID

Retinoic acid is an effective treatment of acne vulgaris and is used topically. It stabilizes lysosomes, increases ribonucleic acid polymerase activity, increases prostaglandin E_2, cAMP and cGMP level.

Adapalene is a napthoic acid derivative with retinoid-like activity used for the topical treatment of acne vulgaris. **Adverse effects** include erythema, dryness of skin and skin irritation.

Isotretinoin is a synthetic retinoid which acts by inhibiting sebaceous gland size and function.

Azelaic acid is also used in the treatment of acne.

PSORIASIS

It is an autoimmune disease which is characterized by marked increase in undifferentiated epidermal cell proliferation and can increase the number of superficial cells having abnormal keratinization.

ACITRETIN

It is a metabolite of the aromatic retinoid, etretinate used in the treatment of psoriasis.

Adverse effects include elevation of cholesterol and triglycerides levels; hepatotoxicity and raised liver enzyme levels has also been reported.

TAZAROTENE

It is an acetylenic retinoid prodrug which is hydrolysed to active metabolite tazarotenic acid, binds to retinoic acid receptors resulting in modified gene expression.

CALCIPOTRIENE

It is a synthetic vitamin D_3 derivative effective in the treatment of plaque type psoriasis vulgaris. **Adverse effects** include itching and mild irritation.

KERATOLYTIC AGENTS

These are the agents used in the treatment of disorders of keratin which cause mild peeling of superficial layers of the skin.

Salicylic acid is used to treat various hyperkeratotic lesions like corns, warts, ring- worm, athlete's foot, chronic dermatitis etc.

Propylene glycol is an effective keratolytic agent for the removal of hyperkeratotic debris. It is also used in combination with salicylic acid in the treatment of ichthyosis, psoriasis, keratosis pilaris and hypertrophic lichen planus.

Podophyllum resin, an alcoholic extract of *Podophyllum palatum* is used in the treatment of *condyloma acuminatum* and other verrucae.

Urea is used in cream or ointment to make it less greasy, it increases the water content of stratum corneum which may be because of its hygroscopic property. It also possesses keratolytic property.

Cantharidin is the active irritant isolated from cantharides. It is mainly used in the treatment of *molluscum contagiosum* and *verruca vulgaris*, particularly periungual warts.

Fluorouracil, a fluorinated pyrimidine antimetabolite is used topically for the treatment of multiple actinic keratoses and intralesionally for keratoacanthomas.

Benzoic acid is a antifungal with mild keratolytic action.

ANTIPRURITIC AGENTS

Pruritus is a common symptom in skin along with itching. Antihistaminics and hydrocortisone are very effective in pruritus due to inflammation.

DOXEPIN

Topical doxepin in the form of cream is used in the treatment of pruritus associated with atopic dermatitis or lichen chronicus. **Adverse effects** include marked burning and stinging at the treatment site.

PRAMOXINE

It is a topical anaesthetic which can provide temporary relief from pruritus with mild eczematous dermatoses.

Trichogenic Agents

MINOXIDIL

Topical minoxidil is effective in reversing the progressive miniaturization of scalp hairs associated with **androgenic alopecia** (male pattern baldness). It is a hereditary disorder due to excessive conversion of testosterone to dehydrocorticosterone in the scalp skin in genetically susceptible men.

FINASTERIDE

It is a inhibitor of 5-alpha reductase and blocks the conversion of testosterone to dehydrotesto-sterone. It prevents further hair loss in the significant proportion of men in the androgenic alopecia.

Adverse effects include decreased libido, ejaculation disorders and erectile dysfunction.

It is **used** in the treatment of benign prostatic hypertrophy in the dose of 5 mg daily. In 1 mg dose it is used in the treatment of androgenic alopecia.

Dutasteride is newer compound similar to finasteride.

Antiseborrheic Agents

These agents are effective in seborrheic dermatitis which is characterized by erythematous scaling lesions.

The various agents, e.g. selenium sulfide and imidazole antifungals lotion or shampoo are used in dandruff which is most common problem. Selenium sulfide also has antikeratolytic and fungicidal properties.

Miscellaneous Compounds

These are the agents which can be used in various skin disorders e.g., atopic dermatitis, seborrheic dermatitis and certain types of psoriasis and other related disorders.

TACROLIMUS

It is an immunosuppressant macrolide antibiotic produced by *Streptomyces tsukubaensis*. Like cyclosporine, tacrolimus binds to a cytoplasmic immunophylin and the complex inhibits the activity of the calcium dependent phosphatase known as calcineurin. This in turn, inhibits the translocation of the transcription factor NF-AT into the cell nucleus, blocking the initiation of NF-AT dependent T-cell responses. It is **indicated** in atopic dermatitis.

It is recently approved for immunosuppression in liver and kidney transplant patients.

SIROLIMUS

It is a newer agent derived from *Streptomyces hygroscopicus* that binds immunophylin (same as in tacrolimus and cyclosporine). It is **indicated** in the management of psoriasis and uveoretinitis.

PREDNICARBATE

It is a halogen free steroid and highly active corticosteroid for topical application.

It has pronounced antiinflammatory, antiallergic, anti-exudative and antipruritic properties. It is **indicated** in atopic dermatitis, seborrheic dermatitis and certain types of psoriasis.

Certain other agents are also used in other skin disorders like antimalarials in lupus erythematosus, antimetabolites in psoriasis, dapsone in dermatitis herpetiformis and erythema elevatum diutinum, interferon in viral warts and thalidomide in erythema nodosum leprosum.

❑❑❑

Appendices

APPENDIX I

List of Recently Approved New Drugs and Combinations in India

(During 1999-July 2006)

Name of the drugs	Pharmacological classification
1. Glimepiride	Antidiabetic agent
2. Mycophenolate mofetil	Immunosuppressant
3. Meloxicam	NSAID
4. Tetrabenazine	Pre-synaptic monoamine depleting agent
5. Doxazosin mesylate	Antihypertensive agent
6. Nafarelin acetate	Antiendometriotic agent; gonadotropin inhibitor
7. Milrinone lactate inj	Cardiotonic
8. Brimonidine tartrate	Alpha 2-adrenoreceptor agonist, adjunct in glaucoma
9. Nabumetone	NSAID
10. Zolpidem	Sedative-Hypnotic
11. Basiliximab inj	Immunosuppressant
12. Topotecan hydrochloride	Antineoplastic
13. Fludarabine phosphate IV inj	Antineoplastic
14. Zuclopenthixol acetate	Antimaniac and antischizophrenic
15. Piperacilin-Tazobactam inj	Antibiotic
16. Topiramate	Antiepileptic
17. Eptifibatide	Platlet aggregation inhibitor
18. Atorvastatin	Antihyperlipidemic; HMG-CoA reductase inhibitor
19. Sulpiride	Antipsychotic
20. Bambuterol	Bronchodilator
21. Bulaquine	Antimalarial
22. Fenofibrate	Lipid lowering agent
23. Sibutramine hydrochloride	Appetite suppressant
24. Oxiconazole	Antifungal
25. Temozolomide	Antineoplastic
26. Olanzapine	Antipsychotic

Contd....

...Contd.

27. Fluvoxamine maleate	Antidepressant
28. Celecoxib	NSAID
29. Nevirapine	Anti HIV
30. Repaglinide	Antidiabetic
31. Ganciclovir	Antiviral
32. Trapidil	Adjunct in angioplasty
33. Cerivastatin	Lipid lowering agent
34. Rofecoxib	NSAID
35. Irbesartan	Antihypertensive
36. Rosiglitazone maleate	Antidiabetic
37. Granisetron	Antiemetic
38. Rituximab	Antineoplastic
39. Trastuzumab	Antineoplastic
40. Rosiglitazone	Antidiabetic
41. Moclobemide	Antidepressant
42. Candesartan	Antihypertensive
43. Venlafaxine hydrochloride	Antidepressant
44. Paroxetine hydrochloride	Antidepressant
45. Iomeprol	Contrast medium
46. Capecitabine	Antineoplastic
47. Daclizumab	Immunosuppressive agent
48. Pioglitazone hydrochloride	Antidiabetic
49. Didanosine	Anti-HIV
50. Octylonium bromide	For irritable bowel syndrome
51. Pravastatin	Lipid lowering agent
52. Sildenafil citrate	Male erectile dysfunction
53. Triflusal	Platelet aggregation inhibitor
54. Thymosin Alfa-1 inj	Immunomodulator (for chronic hepatitis-B)
55. Vinorelbin tartrate inj	Antineoplastic aggregation inhibitor
56. Broncho-Vaxom	Antiasthmatic, immune boosting drug
57. Indinavir sulphate	Antiviral (Anti-HIV)
58. Butenafine hydrochloride cream	Antifungal
59. Mirtazapine	Antidepressant
60. Clopidogrel	Antithrombotic; platelet aggregation inhibitor
61. Mosapride	Prokinetic agent
62. Donepezil hydrochloride	For Alzheimer's dementia
63. Bupropion SR	Smoking cessation adjunct
64. Raloxifene hydrochloride	Menopausal osteoporosis
65. Efavirenz	Anti-HIV
66. Moxifloxacin	Antibacterial
67. Misoprostol	Antiulcer agent

Contd....

...Contd.

68. Human Recombinant Granulocyte Colony Stimulating Factor inj	Haemopoietic stimulant, antineutropenic
69. Nelfinavir mesylate	Anti-HIV
70. Ciprofloxacin 1g SR	Antibacterial
71. Toiterodine-L-tartrate	For overactive bladder
72. Ebastine	Antiallergic
73. Leflunomide	Anti-rheumatoid arthritis
74. Citalopram hydrobromide	Antidepressant
75. Gatifloxacin	Antibacterial
76. Linezolid	Antibacterial
77. Genirelix	Antigonadotropin releasing hormone (fertility drug)
78. Racecadotril	Antidiarrhoeal
79. Cefdinir	Antibacterial
80. Iobitridol	Contrast medium
81. Estemestane	Antineoplastic
82. Decapeptide	For vitiligo
83. Oxcarbazepine	Antiepileptic
84. Desloratidine	Antiallergic
85. Zolendronic acid	For hypercalcaemia
86. Zafirlukast	Antiasthmatic (leukotriene receptor antagonist)
87. Ropinirole	Dopamine agonist (for parkinson's disease)
88. Esomeprazole	Antiulcer
89. Etanercept-Recombination	Antirheumatic, tumor necrosis factor receptor
90. Imatinib mesylate	Anticancer
91. Valsartan	Antihypertensive
92. Rabeprazole	Antiulcer; proton pump inhibitor
93. Bimatoprost (ophthalmic sol)	Anti-glaucoma
94. Meropenem inj	Beta-lactum antibiotic
95. Fosinopril sodium	Antihypertensive
96. Divalproax sodium	Antiepileptic
97. Zaleplon	Sedative-hypnotic
98. Tizanidine SR	Multiple sclerosis
99. Thymogen inj	Anticancer
100. Montelukast sodium	Antiasthmatic (leukotriene receptor antagonist)
101. Mifepristone	Progesterone antagonist
102. Dexarazoxane inj	Cardioprotective agent
103. Tranexamic acid	Antifibrinolytic
104. Bicalutamide	Anticancer
105. Loteprednol etabonate (ophthalmic sol)	Corticosteroid, ophthalmic anti-inflammatory
106. Apraclonidine (ophthalmic sol)	Alpha 2-adrenoreceptor agonist
107. Mizolastine	Antiallergic

Contd....

...Contd.

108. Miltefosine	For Kalaazar
109. Ziprasidone hydrochloride	For Schizophrenia
110. Abacavir	Anti-HIV
111. Nadifloxacin cream	Antibacterial; antiacne
112. Meloxicam inj (vet)	NSAID
113. Mesalazine SR	For bowel disease (inflammatory)
114. Tamsulosin hydrochloride	For BPH (benign prostate hypertrophy)
115. Famciclovir	Antiviral
116. Nateglinide	Antidiabetic
117. Lercanidine hydrochloride	Antihypertensive
118. Itopiride capsule	Gastroprokinetic agent
119. Alprostadil inj	For erectile dysfunction
120. Vimpocetine	Vasodilator
121. Quetiapine fumarate	Antipsychotic
122. Isotretinoin soft gel cap	For Acne vulgaris
123. Nebivolol hydrochloride	Antihypertensive
124. Sirolimus	Immunosuppressant
125. Drotrecogin alpha	For severe sepsis
126. Pygenum africum	For BPH (benign prostate hypertrophy)
127. Valdecoxib	NSAID
128. Thalidomide	For leprosy
129. S (–) Amlodipine besylate	Antihypertensive
130. Cabergoline	For hyperproloactemia
131. Butarphenol tartarate	Opoid analgesic
132. Gemtuzumab	For myeloid leukemia
133. Quinapril	antihypertensive
134. Valacyclovir	Antiviral
135. Fosphenytoin sodium	Anti-Epileptic
136. Ceftiofur sodium and hydrochloride	Antibiotic (For veterinary use)
137. Metaxalone	Muscle relaxant
138. Meglumine gadoteric	Contrast media
139. Cafepine hydrochloride	Antibiotic
140. Acamprosate calcium	For alcohol dependency
141. Aztreonam	Antibacterial
142. Tegasserod maleate	For irritable bowel syndrome
143. Parecoxib inj	NSAID
144. Balsalezide disodium	For ulcerative colitis
145. Cefetemet-piroxil	Antibacterial
146. Telmisartan	Antihypertensive
147. Levocetrizine	Antihistaminic
148. Poractant α	For respiratory distress in preterm babies

Contd....

...Contd.

149. Reboxetine	Antidepressant
150. Cefprozil	Antibiotic
151. Cilostazol	For intermittent claudication
152. Escitalopram oxalate	Antidepressant
153. Anastrazole	Anticancer
154. Rizapriptan	Antimigraine
155. Gadobenate (Dimeglumine IV injection)	MRI contrast medium
156. Tacrolimus ointment	Immunomodulator
157. Metolazone	Diuretic
158. Tiotropium bromide	Antiasthmatic
159. Gadoversetamide inj	MRI contrast medium
160. Torsamide	Diuretic
161. Cyproterone	For prostatic cancer
162. Aripiprazole	Anti schizophrenia
163. Azelaic acid	Antiacne
164. Bendrofluazide	Diuretic
165. Vinpocetin	Antipsychotic
166. Tirofiban hydrochloride IV	Antiplatelet
167. Teriparatide	For Osteoporosis
168. Cladribine	Anticancer
169. Tadalafil	For erectile dysfunction
170. S-Atenolol	Antihypertensive
171. Rosuvastatin	Lipid lowering agent
172. Tazarotene	Antiacne
173. Aceclofenac	NSAID
174. Ibopamine hydrochloride	Ophthalmic
175. Trandolapril	Antihypertensive
176. Dorzolamide	Ophthalmic
177. Fenoverine	Antispasmodic
178. Risedronate sodium	For osteoporosis
179. Fondaparinax sodium	LMWH (Low Molecular Weight Heparin)
180. Metadoxine	For hepatic disorder
181. Valgancyclovir	For CMV (Cyto Megalo virus)
182. Isopropyl Unoprostone	Ophthalmic
183. Amorolfine	Antifungal
184. Fluvastatin sodium	Lipid lowering agent
185. Modafinil	For sleeping disorder
186. Sufentanil citrate	Anaesthetic agent
187. Ezetimibe	Lipid lowering agent
188. Dutasteride	For BPH
189. Gefitinib	Anti-cancer

Contd....

...Contd.

190. Imidapril	Anti-hypertensive
191. Adefovir Dipivoxil	Anti-viral (Hepatitis-B)
192. Etoricoxib	NSAID
193. Dicerein	For osteoarthritis
194. Nitazoxanide	Anti-diarrhoeal
195. Trolamine cream (0.67%)	For topical use
196. Neotame	Sweetening Agent
197. Oxybutynine	For neurogenic bladder disorder
198. Cabergoline	For parkinson's disease
199. Rabeprazole Sodium Injection	For gastric and Deudonal Ulcers & GERD
200. Alfuzosin E.R.	For BPH
201. Tiagabine HCl	Anti-epileptic
202. Racecadotril Sachet	Anti-diarrhoeal
203. Ibandronic Acid Inj	Anti-cancer
204. Tacrolimus Capsule	For organ rejection
205. Cefdinir Dispersible	Antibiotic
206. Linezolid	For osteomyelitis in adults
207. Cefprozil Dispersible tablet	Antibiotic
208. Divalproex Sodium E.R. tablets	Anti-epileptic
209. Lithium Carbonate ER tablet	Anti-depressant
210. Nimesulide Injection	For short-term treatment of post-operative pain
211. Levosalbutamol Tablet & Syrup	For obstructive airway disease
212. Memantine HCl	For dementia of Alzheimer's type
213. Pimcrolimus cream	For atopic dermatitis
214. Rebamipide	For gastric ulcer
215. Cefetamet Pivoxil Suspension	Antibiotic
216. Diclofenac Transdermal patch	For osteoarthritis & soft tissue injury
217. Fluconazole Gel	Anti-fungal
218. Miglitol	Anti-diabetic
219. Citicholine Tablet & Injection	Membrane permeability enhancer
220. Lamotrigine S.R. tablet	Anti-epileptic
221. Moxifloxacin Eye drops	For bacterial conjunctivitis
222. Risperidone long-acting suspension for injection	For schizophrenia
223. Everolimus	Immunosuppressant
224. Gemcitabine	Anti-cancer
225. b-arteether Injection	Anti-malaria
226. Ziprasidone powder for injection	Anti-psychotic
227. Voriconazole Tablet & Infusion	Anti-fungal
228. Cefuroxime Axetil ER tablets	Antibiotic

Contd....

...Contd.

229. Diclofenac Transdermal Patch	For pain relief
230. Gatifloxacin Eye Ointment	Ophthalmic use
231. Nimesulide Injection	Veterinary use
232. Isotretinoin Gel	For acne
233. Levosalbutamol rotacaps & inhaler	For obstructive airway disease
234. Celecoxib Injection	For acute pain
235. Orlistat	Anti-obesity
236. Duloxetine HCl	Anti-depressant
237. Delfazacort	Anti-asthma, anti-arthritis
238. Atomoxetine HCl	For ADHD
239. Ursodeoxycholic acid S.R. Capsule	For dissolution of gall stones
240. Methylphenidate Hcl E.R. tablet	For ADHD
241. Calcium Polycarbophil	For constipation
242. Imiquimod Cream	For warts in adults
243. Entacapone	For Parkinson's disease
244. Levocetirizine Syrup	For allergic rhinitis & urticaria
245. Pitavastatin	Lipid lowering agent
246. Bacillus calusii spores suspension	For alteration of intestinal bacterial flora
247. Diflorasone Diacetate Cream	For corticosteroid responsive dermatoses
248. Azelaic acid Cream	For the treatment of inflammatory papules and pustules of mild to moderate rosacea
249. Levodropropizine oral suspension	For non-productive cough in adults
250. Duloxetine HCl	Anti-depressant
251. Levofloxacin Ophthalmic Solution	For susceptible bacterial conjunctivitis
252. Metformin Oral Solution	For type-II diabetes mellitus
253. Tirofiban injection	For acute coronary syndrome including patients undergoing PTCA or atherectomy
254. Stavudine powder for suspention	For HIV-1 infusion
255. Erdosteine	For chronic obstructive brochilits
256. Levetiracetam	As adjunctive therapy in treatment of partial onset seizures in adults with epilepsy.
257. Esomeprazole Sodium for Injection	For GERD in patients with esophagitis and/or severe symptoms of reflux as an alternative to oral therapy when oral intake is not appropriate
258. Rupatadine	For perinial allergic rhinitis
259. Acesulfame Potassium	As sweetener in pharmaceutical preparation
260. S(–) Metoprolol Succinate S.R.	For hypertension
261. R(–) Ondansetron	For chemotherapeutic induced nausea and vomiting
262. Balanced salt intraocular irrigating solution enriched with glutathione dextrose, bicarbonate	For intraocular irrigating during intraocular surgical procedures

Contd....

...Contd.

263. Intralipid	For patients with essential fatty acid deficiencies
264. Montelukast Granules	For prophylaxis and chronic treatment of asthma in adult and pediatric patients of 12 months age and older
265. Bortezomib for injection	For the treatment of myeloma patients
266. Nelfinavir	For HIV patients
267. Sevelamer	For control of serum phosphorus in patients with chronic kidney disease and hemodialysis
268. S(–) Pantoprazole	For gastric ulcer, duodenal ulcer & GERD
269. R(–) Ondansetron oral Solution	For chemotherapy, induced nausea and vomiting
270. Emtricitabine	For HIV infection in adults
271. Eplerenone	For hypertension
272. Strontium Ranelate Granules	For post-menopausal women with osteoporosis
273. Midazolam Maleate Bulk	Anesthetic
274. Calcium Polycarbophil	For IBS
275. Testosterone Gel	For replacement therapy in male with testosterone deficiencies and hypogonadotropic hypoganadism
276. Erlotinib Hydrochloride	For metastatic non-small cell lung cancer
277. Chloroquine Phosphate eye drops	For dry eye syndrome
278. Mecobalamine E.R. tablet	For neuropathic pain
279. Olmesartan Medoxomil	Anti-hypertension
280. Ursodeoxycholic Acid S.R Tablet	Addl. strength
281. Feropenem Sodium	Anti-bacterial
282. Saquinavir (as mesylate) 500 mg. tablet	Addl. strength
283. Pramipexole Di-hydrochloride	For Parkinson's disease
284. Phenytoin Sodium 300 mg. tablet	Addl. strength
285. Tenofovir Disproxil Fumarate	Anti-HIV
286. Bivalirudin Injection	Anti-coagulant in PTCA
287. Efavirenz oral solution	Anti-AIDS
288. Didanosine Powder for oral solution	Anti-AIDS
289. Sodium Valproate C.R. Tablet (750/1000 mg)	Addl. strength
290. Oxcarbazepine S.R. Tablet	Anti-epileptic
291. Acitretin	For sever psoriasis in adults
292. Dried IVY Leaf Extract (7.5 gm/100ml)	Cough syrup
293. Ketorolac Tromethamine Eye drops	Ophthalmic
294. Levetiracetam oral Solution	Anti-epileptic
295. Zinc (Gluconate) oral solution	For acute diarrhoea
296. Trimebutine Maleate	For IBS
297. Oseltamivir (as phosphate) Capsule & oral suspension	For influenzae
298. Cetrizine HCl drops	Anti-histaminic

Contd....

...Contd.

299. Lanthanum Carbonate Chewable tablet	For the treatment of hyperphosphatemia
300. Sodium Hyaluronate eye drops	Ophthalmic use.
301. Voglibose	anti-diabetic
302. Lactitol Sachet	For the treatment of consipation.
303. Aspirin Bolus	For Veterinary use
304. Pregabalin	For neuropathic pain
305. Methotrexate Topical gel	Psoriasis
306. Testosterone Spray	For replacement therapy in males with testosterone deficiency
307. Omeprazole Powder for suspension	Anti-ulcer
308. Doxazosin (as Mesylate) E.R. Tablet	For hypertension
309. Phenylephrine Eye drops	For ophthalmic use
310. Entecavir Tablet & oral solution	For chronic Hepatitis-B infection
311. Travoprost Eye drops	For glaucoma & ocular hypertension.
312. Atomoxetine (as HCl) Sachet	For ADHD
313. Levofloxacin oph. solu.	Ophthalmic
314. Zonisamide	Anti-epileptic
315. Methimazole	For hyperthyroidism
316. Caspofungin Acetate injection	For invasive candidiasis fungal infection
317. Cefprozil Powder for oral suspension	Antibiotic
318. Ciclesonide Inhaler	For persistent Asthma
319. Pegaptinib Sodium Injection	For neovascular (wet) age related macular degeneration
320. Dexibuprofen	For OA, RA & ankylosing spondylitis
321. Moxifloxacin Eye Ointment	For ophthalmic use
322. Erdosteine Powder for oral suspension	For chronic obstructive bronchitis
323. Doxofylline	For bronchila asthma & COPD
324. Zanamavir inhalation powder	For influenzae
325. Testosterone Transdermal Spray	For replacement therapy in males with testosterone deficiency.
326. Cefetamet Pivoxil HCl oral suspension	Antibiotic
327. Voriconazole Powder for oral solution	Anti-fungal
328. Aceclofenac S.R. tablet	NSAID
329. Desflurane liquid for inhalation	For induction & maintenance of anaesthesia
330. Levetiracetam Oral Solution	Anti-epileptic
331. Atomoxetine	For ADHD
332. Fluorescein Sodium Solution for Injection	Ophthalmological diagnostic agent
333. Cefditeron (as pivoxil)	Antibiotic
334. Sodium Hyaluronate Cream	For leg ulcer, diabetic ulcer etc.
335. Saquinavir	Anti-AIDS

Contd....

...Contd.

336. Tobramycin Inhalation solution	For chronic pulmonary infection cystic fibrosis.
337. Propionyl-L-Carnitine HCl Tablet & injection	Chronic congestive heart failure
338. Eflornithine HCl Cream	For reduction of unwanted facial hair in women.
339. Lactulose Enema	For constipation & hepatic encephalopathy
340. Doxofylline Syrup	For bronchial asthma & COPD.
341. Cholestyramine Powder for oral suspension	For hypercholesterolaemia
342. Haloperidol	As approved earlier (Antipsychotic)
343. Resperidone Tablet & Syrup	Acute mania & mixed episode in bipolar-I disorder.
344. D-trans Fentantyl Transdermal patches	For pain
345. Oseltamivir formulation (additional indication)	For Prophylaxis of influenzae in adult and children > 14 years of age
346. Atazanavir	Anti-HIV in adults.
347. Nicorandil E.R. Tablet	Angina Pectoris
348. Nadifloxacin Gel 1%	Acne vulgaris
349. Midazolam (as maleate)	For insomnia
350. Olmesartan (as Medoxomil) 10 mg (Addl. Strength)	Anti-hypertensive
351. Pregabalin capsule 25/50/100/200 mg (Addl. Strength)	Same as approved
352. Oxcarbazepine S.R 450 mg/900 mg (Addl. Strength)	Anti-epileptic
353. Ciclesonide rotacaps	For Asthma
354. Itopride capsule (S.R)	For GERD
355. Ibandronic Acid Tablet (150 mg) (Addl. Strength)	Same as approved.
356. Zonisamide capsule 25/50 mg (Addl. Strength)	Same as approved
357. Perflutren liquid microsphere injectable suspension	For diagnostic use
358. Cyclosporin Eye drops (0.1%) (Addl. Strength)	For Ophthalmic use
359. Bemiparin Sodium Solution	For deep vein thrombosis
360. Icodextrin peritoneal dialysis solution	For peritoneal dialysis
361. Lamotrigin 200 mg tablet (Addl. Strength) dispersible tablet	Anti-epileptic
362. Olopathadine Ophthalmic solution	For allergic conjunctivitis
363. Methyl Prednisolone Aceponate Cream	For atopic dermatitis
364. Levofloxacin Ear drops	For otitis media
365. Buclizine HCl tablet & syrup	As appetite stimulant
366. Solifenacin Succinate Tablet	For overactive bladder with urge urinary incontinence urgency & urinary frequency
367. Zolpidem Tartrate E.R. tablet	For insomnia
368. Deferasirox dispersible tablet	For chronic iron overload due to blood transfusion
369. Sodium Hyaluronate Injection	For OA
370. Forskolin Eye drop	For open angle glaucoma

Fixed dose combinations

1. Mometasone furoate + Terbinafine
2. Rosiglitazone + Metformin
3. Mosapride + MPS (Methyl polysiloxane)
4. Formeterol + Budesonide
5. Butenafine+ Betamethasone
6. Amlodipine + Benazapril
7. Sucralfate + Metronidazole
8. Glycopyrrolate + Neostigmine
9. Betamethasone + Salicylic acid
10. Mefenamic acid + Tizanidine
11. Latanoprost + Timolol
12. Tobramycin + Fluromethalone
13. Betamethasone + Gentamicin
14. S-Amlodipine + Losartan
15. S-Amlodipine + Atenolol
16. Pioglitazone + Glimeperide
17. Glimeperide + Metformin
18. Rosiglitazone + Glimeperide
19. Tramadol + Paracetamol
20. Ramipril + s(-) Amlodipine
21. Olanzapine + Fluoxetine
22. Ciprofloxacin + Ornidazole
23. Quinapril + HCTZ (Hydrochlorothiazide)
24. Aspirin + Dipyridamole
25. Cyproterone + Ethinyl estradiol
26. S-Amlodipine + Lisinopril
27. Valsartan + HCTZ
28. Montelukast + Bambuterol
29. Adapeline + Clindamycin
30. Ramipril + Candisartan
31. Telmisartan + HCTZ
32. Rofecoxib + Tizanidine
33. Losartan + Ramipril
34. Rofecoxib + Paracetamol
35. Lamivudine + Zidovudine + Abacavir
36. Nadifloxacin + Clobetasol
37. Lercanidipine + Atenolol
38. S-Amlodipine + Valsartan
39. S-Atenolol + S-Amlodipine
40. Imipenem + Cilastatin

Contd....

...Contd.

41. Gatifloxacin + Dexamethasone Phos. Eye drops
42. Esomeprazole + Domperidone SR Capsule
43. Aceclofenac + Paracetamol
44. Lamivudine (E.R) + Zidovudine (E.R) + Nevirapine tablets
45. Rabeprazole + Masopride S.R. Tablet
46. Atorvastatin + Ezetimibe
47. Buprenorphin + Naloxone
48. Sucralfate + Metronidazole + Lignocaine cream
49. Glibenclamide + Metformin SR tablet
50. Escitalopram + Clonazepam
51. Dorzolamide + Timolol Eye drops
52. Nebivolol + S(–) Amlodipine
53. Valdecoxib + Paracetamol
54. Amlodipine + Ramipril
55. Rabeprazole Sodium + Domperidone S.R. Capsule
56. Epi-Growth Factor + Silversulphadiazine Cream
57. Amlodipine + Atorvastatin
58. Lovastatin + Nicacin ER tablet
59. Gatifloxacin + Ambroxol HCl
60. Nebivolol HCl + Hydrochlorothiazide
61. Atorvastatin Calcium + Finofibrate
62. Pantoprazole + Domeridone
63. Centbucridine + Feracrylem
64. Atenolol + HCTZ
65. Ofloxacin + Ornidazole
66. Lamivudine + Nevirapine + Stavudine powder for suspension
67. Etonogestrel + Ethinylestradiol Contraceptive rings
68. Metaxalone + Diclofenac Potassium
69. Tranexamic acid + Mefenamic acid
70. Fluconazole + Zinc Pyrethione suspension
71. Desloratadine + Ambroxol + Guiphenasine + Menthol Syrup
72. Omeprazole Enteric coated + Domeperidone (S.R.) capsule
73. Buprenorphine + Naloxone S/L tablet
74. Lamivudine +Stavudine reconstituted solution
75. Gliclazide M.R. + Metformin HCl ER tablets
76. Drosperinone + Ethinylestradiol
77. Simvastatin + Ezetimibe
78. Ramipril + Telmisartan
79. Tazarotene + Mometasone Furoate Cream
80. Gatifloxacin + Ornidazole

Contd....

...Contd.

81. Combikit of 2 tablet of Stavudine + Lamivudine each & 1 tablet of Efavirenz
82. Aceclofenac gel 1.5% alongwith linseed oil, menthol, Salicylate, Capsaicin
83. Lamivudine + Stavudine + Nevirapine dispersible tablet
84. Nitazoxanide + Olfoxacin
85. Papain + Urea Ointment
86. Amlodipine + Bisoprolol
87. Ceftriaxone + Tazobatum Injection
88. Levodopa + Carbidopa + Entacapone
89. Atorvastatin + Niacin E.R. Capsule
90. Levocetirizine + Ambroxol S.R. Capsule
91. Gabapentin + Methylcobalamin
92. Calciprtriol + Betamethasone Dipro Ointment
93. Glimepiride + Pioglitazone + Metformin E.R. Tablet
94. Sucralfate + Povidone lodine Ointment
95. Nimesulide + Methyl Salicylate Aerosol
96. Feracrylum + Metronidazole
97. Methylobalamin + Pyridoxine + Folic Acid
98. Enalapril + HCTZ
99. Ambroxol HCl + Desloratadine
100. S-Metoprolol Succinate Tartrate + HCTZ
101. Stavudine + Lamivudine + Nevirapine dispersible tablet
102. Domperidone + Activated dimethicone chewable tablet
103. Moxifloxacin + Dexamethasone Phosphate Eye drops
104. Brimonidine Tartrate + Timolol
105. Amlodipine (as besylate) + Bisoprolol
106. Olmesartan Medoxomil + HCTZ
107. Ketorolac Tromethamine + Ofloxacin Eye drops
108. Hyoscine-N-Butylbromide + Paracetamol
109. Amlodipine (as besylate) + Losartan Pot
110. Ceftriaxone (as sodium) + Sulbactam (as sodium) powder
111. Nebivolol (as HCl) + Valsartan
112. Combikit of Tamsulosin HCl & Dutasteride Soft Gelatin Capsule
113. Alendronate Sodium + Cholecalciferol
114. Atenolol + HCTZ
115. Tamsulosin HCl + Dutasteride
116. Metoprolol Succinate + Amlodipine
117. Aspirin + Clopidogrel (as bisulphate)
118. Tenofovir Disoproxil fumarate + Emtricitabine
119. Diclofenac Sodium + Misoprostol
120. Pantoprazole (as Sodium) (E.C) + Itopride S.R.

Contd....

...Contd.

121. Amlodipine (as besylate) + HCTZ
122. Formoterol Fumarate + Fluticasone Propionate dry powder inhaler
123. Nevibolol (as HCl) + Amlodipine (as besylate)
124. Levocetrizine + Ambroxol Hydrochloride SR
125. Gatifloxacin + Prednisolne Acetate eye drops
126. Amlodipine (as besylate) + Metoprolol Succinate equivalent to Metoprolol Tartrate 50 mg.
127. Nadifloxacin + Miconazole Nitrate + Mometasone Furoate Cream
128. Amoxycillin + Clavulanate Potassium E.R. tablet
129. Lopinavir 200 mg + Ritonavir 50 mg Tablet (Addl. Strength)
130. Ferrous ascorbate + Folic acid
131. Aspirin + Clopidogrel (as bisulphate)
132. Olmesartan 40 mg + HCTZ 25 mg tablet (Addl. Strength)
133. Ceftriaxone (as sodium) 25 mg + Tazobactam 31.25 mg for injection (Addl. Strength)
134. Bimatoprost + Timolol (as maleate) eye drops
135. Mebeverine HCl + Isabgula husk sachet.
136. Vitamin C + Zinc Citrate + Selenium tablet.
137. Lamivudine + Stavudine dispersible tablet
138. Levocetrizine + Ambroxol syrup
139. Cefixime + Pot. Clavulanate tablet
140. ISMN SR 30 mg + Aspirin 75/150 mg tablet (Addl. Strength)
141. Clobestasol Propionate + Calcipotriol ointment

List of recently approved new drugs and combinations in Indian Market by *Directorate General of Health Services, Min. of Health & Family Welfare,* Govt. of India.

APPENDIX II

List of Banned Drugs and Fixed Dose Combinations in India (Updated till January 2007)

1. Amidopyrine
2. Fixed dose combinations of vitamins with antiinflammatory agents and tranquilizers.
3. Fixed dose combinations of atropine and analgesics and antipyretics.
4. Fixed dose combinations of strychnine and caffeine in tonics.
5. Fixed dose combinations of yohimbine and strychnine with testosterone and vitamins.
6. Fixed dose combinations of iron with strychnine, arsenic and yohimbine.
7. Fixed dose combinations of sodium bromide/chloral-hydrate with other drugs.
8. Phenacetin.
9. Fixed dose combinations of antihistaminics with antidiarrhoeals.
10. Fixed dose combinations of penicillin with sulphonamides.
11. Fixed dose combinations of vitamins with analgesics.
12. Fixed dose combinations of tetracyclines with vitamin C.
13. Fixed dose combinations of hydroxyquinoline group of drugs with any other drug except for preparations meant for external use only.
14. Fixed dose combinations of corticosteroids with any other drug for internal use.
15. Fixed dose combinations of chloramphenicol with any other drug for internal use.
16. Fixed dose combinations of crude ergot preparations except those containing ergotamine, caffeine, analgesics, antihistamines for the treatment of migraine, headache.
17. Fixed dose combinations of vitamins with anti TB drugs except combination of isoniazid with pyridoxine hydrochloride (vitamin B_6).
18. Penicillin skin/eye ointment.
19. Tetracycline liquid oral preparations.
20. Nialamide.
21. Practolol.
22. Methapyrilene, its salts.
23. Methaqualone.
24. Oxytetracycline liquid oral preparations.
25. Demeclocycline liquid oral preparations.

Contd....

...Contd.

26. Combinations of anabolic steroids with other drugs.
27. Fixed dose combinations of estrogen and progestin (other than oral contraceptive) containing per tablet estrogen content of more than 50 mcg (equivalent to ethinyl estradiol) and of progestin content of more than 3 mg (equivalent to norethisterone acetate) and all fixed dose combination injectable preparations containing synthetic estrogen and progesterone.
28. Fixed dose combination of sedatives/hypnotics/ anxiolytics with analgesics-antipyretics.
29. Fixed dose combination of pyrazinamide with other antitubercular drugs except combination of pyrazinamide with rifampicin and INH as per recommended daily dose given below:

Drugs	Minimum	Maximum
Rifampicin	450 mg	600 mg
INH	300 mg	400 mg
Pyrazinamide	1000 mg	1500 mg

30. Fixed dose combination of histamine H_2-receptor antagonists with antacids except for those combinations approved by the Drugs Controller, India.
31. The patent and proprietary medicines of fixed dose combinations of essential oils with alcohol having percentage higher than 20% proof except preparations given in the Indian Pharmacopoeia.
32. All pharmaceutical preparations containing chloroform exceeding 0.5%, w/w or v/v whichever is appropriate.
33. Fixed dose combination of ethambutol with INH other than the following:

INH	Ethambutol
200 mg	600 mg
300 mg	800 mg

34. Fixed dose combination containing more than one antihistaminic.
35. Fixed dose combination of any anthelmintic with cathartic/purgative except piperazine.
36. Fixed dose combination of salbutamol or any other bronchodialator with centrally acting antitussive and/or antihistaminics.
37. Fixed dose combination of laxatives and/or anti-spasmodic drugs in enzyme preparations.
38. Fixed dose combination of metoclopramide with systemically absorbed drugs except fixed dose combination of metoclopramide with aspirin/paracetamol.
39. Fixed dose combination or centrally acting antitussive with antihistaminics having atropine like activity in expectorants.
40. Preparations claiming to combat cough associated with asthma containing centrally acting antitussive and/or antihistaminics.
41. Liquid oral tonic preparations containing glycerophosphates and/or other phosphates and/or central nervous system stimulant and such preparations containing alchohol more than 20 proof.
42. Fixed dose combination containing pectin and/or kaolin with any drug which is systemically absorbed from GI tract except for combination of pectin and/or kaolin with drugs not systemically absorbed.
43. Chloral Hydrate as a drug
44. Dover's powder IP
45. Dover's powder tablets IP
46. Antidiarrhoeal formulations containing kaolin or pectin or attapulgite or activated charcoal.
47. Antidiarrhoeal formulations containing phthalyl sulfathiazole or sulfaguanidine or succinyl sulphathiazole.

Contd....

...Contd.

48. Antidiarrhoeal formulations containing neomycin or streptomycin or dihydrostreptomycin including their respective salts or esters.
49. Liquid oral antidiarrhoeals or any other dosage form for paediatric use containing diphenoxylate or atropine or belladonna including their salts and esters or metabolites, hyoscyamine or their extracts or their alkaloids.
50. Liquid oral antidiarrhoeals of any other dosage form for paediatric use containing halogenated hydroxyquinolines.
51. Fixed dose combination of anti-diarrhoeals with electrolytes.
52. Patent and proprietary oral rehydration salts other than those conforming to the specified parameters.
53. Fixed dose combination of oxphenbutazone or phenylbutazone with any other drug.
54. Fixed dose combination of analgin with any other drug.
55. Fixed dose combination of dextropropoxyphene with any other drug other than anti-spasmodics and/ or non-steroidal antiinflammatory drugs (NSAIDs).
56. Fixed dose combination of a drug, standards of which are prescribed in the Second Schedule to the said Act with an Ayurvedic, Siddha or Unani drug.
57. Mepacrine hydrochloride (Quinacrine and its salts) in any dosage form for female sterilization or contraception.
58. Fenfluramine and dexfenfluramine.
59. Fixed dose combination of diazepam and diphenhydramine hydrochloride.
60. Cosmetics licensed as toothpaste/tooth powder containing tobacco.
61. Parenteral preparations containing fixed dose combination of streptomycin with penicillin.
62. Fixed dose combination of vitamin B_1, vitamin B_6, and vitamin B_{12} for human use.
63. Fixed dose combination of haemoglobin in any form (natural or synthetic).
64. Fixed dose combination of pancreatin or pancrelipase containing amylase, protease and lipase with any other enzyme.
65. Fixed dose combination of nitrofurantoin and trimethoprim.
66. Fixed dose combination of phenobarbitone with any anti-asthamatic drugs.
67. Fixed dose combination of phenobarbitone with hyoscine and/or hyoscyamine.
68. Fixed dose combination of phenobarbitone with ergotamine and/or belladona.
69. Fixed dose combination of haloperidol with any anti-cholinergic agent including propantheline bromide.
70. Fixed dose combination of nalidixic acid with any anti-amoebics including metronidazole.
71. Fixed dose combination of loperamide hydrochloride with furazolidone.
72. Fixed dose combination of cyproheptadine with lysine or peptone.
73. Astemizole
74. Terfenadine
75. Phenformin
76. Rofecoxib.
77. Valdecoxib & its formulation.

List of drugs and fixed dose combination prohibited for manufacturing and sale through Govt. of India (Ministry of Health & Family Welfare) Gazette notification GSR 578 (E) Dated 23-7-83 Amended from time to time.

(Published in the Gazette of India, Extraordinary Part-II; Section 3 Subsection (i), Ministry or Health & Family Welfare, Govt. of India notification).

Index

A

B

C

D

E

F

G

H

I

J

K

L

M

N

O

P

T

❑❑❑